HUMAN AGEING AND LATER LIFE

MULTIDISCIPLINARY PERSPECTIVES

Edited by Anthony M. Warnes
Department of Geography and
Age Concern Institute of Gerontology
King's College
University of London

Edward Arn
A division of Hodder & Stoughton
LONDON MELBOURNE AUCKLAND

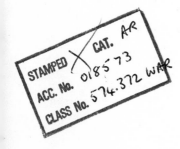
© 1989 Age Concern Institute of Gerontology

First published in Great Britain 1989

British Library Cataloguing in Publication Data

Human ageing and later life.
1. Man. Ageing
I. Warnes, A.M. (Anthony M)
II. Age Concern Institute of Gerontology
612'.67

ISBN 0–304–42953–4

Typeset in 10/11pt Melior by Wearside Tradespools, Fulwell,
Sunderland
Printed and bound in Great Britain for Edward Arnold, the
educational academic and medical publishing division of Hodder
and Stoughton Limited, 41 Bedford Square, London WC1B 3DQ
by St Edmundsbury Press Limited, Bury St Edmunds, Suffolk

CONTENTS

NOTES ON THE CONTRIBUTORS

Mark Abrams BSc, PhD, has had a pioneering and distinguished role in British social research. He was formerly Director of the Survey Research Unit of the Social Science Research Council and the founder Director of the Age Concern Research Unit. Among his many contributions to the study of elderly people in Britain, the two volumes of *Beyond Three Score and Ten* (Age Concern England, Mitcham, 1978 and 1980) have been particularly used. He has recently published *The Elderly Shopper* (Age Concern England, 1986) and is currently working on a social history of Britain's elderly population. He is a member of the Advisory Council of the Age Concern Institute of Gerontology.

Toni C. Antonucci PhD, is an Associate Research Scientist at the Institute for Social Research, Associate Professor of Psychology in the Department of Family Practice, and Adjunct Associate Professor in the Department of Psychology at The University of Michigan. A developmental psychologist by training, her research has focused on social relationships over the life span. Her published research includes mother–infant attachment relationships, three-generational intra-family relationships and adult interpersonal relationships. Dr Antonucci is currently the recipient of a Research Career Development Award from the US National Institute on Aging.

Janet Askham BA, PhD, is Assistant Director of the Age Concern Institute of Gerontology and responsible for its important service development projects and the associated evaluation research. Formerly a senior member of the Age Concern Research Unit, she has long experience of social research with elderly people. She is a research sociologist with particular interests in ageing and old age, the family and chronic illness, and her publications have included *Fertility and Deprivation* (Cambridge University Press), *Identity and Stability in Marriage* (Cambridge University Press), and *The Elderly Mentally Frail: Should We Prescribe Community Care* (King Edward's Hospital Fund).

Alan H. Bittles MA, PhD, FIBiol, is Senior Lecturer in the Department of Anatomy and Human Biology, King's College, University of London. His main interest in ageing relates to changes detectable at the cellular level, with human diploid fibroblast cultures as the research model. His publications have included studies of the free amino acid pool and peptidase profiles of fibroblasts *in vitro* and, most recently, the investigation of changing cellular energy requirements with ageing and their wider consequences. He has edited with Kenneth Collins *The Biology of Human Ageing* (Cambridge University Press, 1986).

Andrew Blaikie MA, PhD, is Lecturer in Gerontology at the Centre for Extra-Mural Studies, Birkbeck College, University of London. Recently added to his role as principal tutor for the Certificate and Diploma in Gerontology has been a major commitment to a new Diploma in Mid- and Later-Life Planning. He is currently researching with John Macnicol the social history of old age in the inter-war period, a project funded by the Economic and Social Research Council. He has published several articles on pressure groups, social policy and retirement in the earlier twentieth century. He is an Associate Lecturer at the Age Concern Institute of Gerontology.

Sally Greengross MA, has been with Age Concern England for ten years and became Director in June 1987. Among her many roles, she is Joint Coordinator of *Eurolink Age*, a European Community wide network of communication between politicians, administrators and elderly people's organisations, and Vice President of the *International Federation of Aging*, a Fellow of the Royal Society of Health. She writes, lectures and broadcasts frequently in Britain and other countries on a wide range of issues concerning policy and practice relating to older people. She is Joint Chairman of the Board of Management of the Age Concern Institute of Gerontology.

Brian H. Groombridge MA, is Professor of Adult Education and the recently-retired Director of the Department of Extra-Mural Studies in the University of London. Following early contact with various French universities of the third age, he was a co-founder and the first Chairman of the University of the Third Age in London. He has acted as a consultant in ageing to UNESCO and his publications include *Education and Retirement* (National Institute of Adult Education, London, 1960). With long experience of adult education and the role of broadcasting in education, his recent interests are reflected in his paper, 'Learning, education and later life', a declaration on behalf of the seminal Anglo-French seminar at Wye College. He is a member of the Advisory Council of the Age Concern Institute of Gerontology.

Emily M.D. Grundy MA, MSc, PhD, is a Lecturer in Social Gerontology at the Age Concern Institute of Gerontology, King's College London. Her interests include the migration of people in middle and later life, household composition and change, trends in morbidity and mortality and the demography of ageing. She has published a considerable number of articles on these topics, including articles in *Age and Ageing, Ageing and Society, The British Medical Journal, European Journal of Population, Journal of Biosocial Science* and the *Journal of the American Geriatrics Society*, and contributions to several recent books. She is the Course Tutor for the new Master in Science in Gerontology at King's College London.

Alan R. Hipkiss BSc (Tech), PhD, is Senior Lecturer in Biochemistry and a Joint-Chairman of the Special Interest Group in Ageing of the Faculty of Life Sciences at King's College, University of London. He also lectures in the biology of ageing at the University's Centre for Extra-Mural Studies, has been a Visiting Professor in the Department of Biology, University of Ottawa and a Visiting Research Professor at the Dartmouth College Medical School, Hanover, New Hampshire, USA and at the Université Claude-Bernard, Lyon, France. His research interests include the mechanisms of the selective breakdown of altered proteins in mammalian and bacterial cells. Among the most recent of his publications are articles on age-related changes in protein catabolism in the bovine lens.

James S. Jackson PhD, is a Professor in Psychology in the Department of Psychology and Research Scientist in the Research Center for Group Dynamics at The University of Michigan. A social psychologist, his research has focused on social reinforcement processes, attitude change, self-esteem and personal and group identity development. More recently his work has shifted to national surveys of the American black population including the National Survey of Black Americans, the National Three Generation Family Study and the National Black Election Study.

John S. Macnicol MA, PhD, is Lecturer in Social Policy at Royal Holloway and Bedford New College, University of London. He has published extensively in the history of social policy, and is currently working with Andrew Blaikie on a project funded by the Economic and Social Research Council on the social history of old age in the inter-war period. He is also researching the concept of an 'underclass' and general trends in the welfare state since 1945.

James McEwen MB, CHB, DIH, FFCM, MFOM, is Henry Mechån Professor of Public Health, University of Glasgow. Formerly he was Professor and Chairman of the Department of Community Medicine in the School of Medicine and Dentistry, King's College, University of London. He was also Director of Community Medicine for Camberwell Health Authority, London. His research interests include: measures of perceived health; inequalities and health; evaluation of health care; and health promotion in the workplace. He has published many scientific papers on measures of self-rated health, has been a consultant to the World Health Organization and worked in Sudan and other African countries. With S.M. Hunt and S.P. McKenna he has recently published *Measuring Health Status* (Croom Helm, 1986).

Sally J. Redfern BSc, PhD, SRN, is a Senior Lecturer in the Department of Nursing Studies at King's College London. She was a Ward Sister and a Research Nurse for a Regional Health Authority before moving to Chelsea College, now part of King's College. She has been a Visiting Professor at the Care Research Unit in the University of Lund, Sweden. Her current research interests include interpersonal communication between nurses and elderly people, and the quality of life and care of old people in various institutions. Her publications include *Issues in Nursing Research* (Macmillan, London, 1983) and *Nursing Elderly People* (Churchill Livingstone, 1986).

Cameron G. Swift PhD, FRCP, since 1986 has been Professor of Health Care of the Elderly at the School of Medicine and Dentistry of King's College, University of London. He has previously worked in the University Medical Schools at Cardiff and Dundee and has recently been appointed as Vice-Chairman of the Training Committee of the British Geriatrics Society. His research focuses on the efficacy and administration of drugs in treating elderly people and his most recent publication is a major edited collection on *Clinical Pharmacology in the Elderly* (Marcel Dekker, New York). He is a member of the Board of Management and the Advisory Council of the Age Concern Institute of Gerontology and has been closely involved in the development of health and medical options for the new Masters course in Gerontology at King's College.

Anthony M. Warnes BA, PhD, is Head of the Department of Geography at King's College London and has been closely involved from its inception with the Age Concern Institute of Gerontology. He has been a Visiting Professor at the Departments of Geography and Gerontology in the University of South Florida, Tampa, and has recently delivered invited lectures at the gerontology institutes at the Universities of Michigan, Florida at Gainesville, and at Brookdale (New York). He is Secretary of the British Society of Gerontology and the Review Editor of *Ageing and Society* (Cambridge University Press). His research interests include demography, housing, social networks and support systems, and the situation of elderly people in less developed countries. His books include *Geographical Perspectives on the Elderly* (Wiley, 1982) and *Elderly People and Ageing* (Université de Lille-Flandres-Artois, 1987).

Robert A. Weale BSc, MSc, MPhil, PhD, DSc, is an Honorary Senior Research Fellow at the Age Concern Institute of Gerontology, Emeritus Professor of Visual Science in the University of London and an Honorary Consultant at the Moorfields Eye Hospital, London. His publications include *The Ageing Eye* (H.K. Lewis, London, 1963) and *A Biography of the Eye: Development, Growth and Age* (H.K. Lewis, London, 1982). As a consultant of the World Health Organization he is concerned with gerontological matters in developing countries and he continues to pursue and publish experimental work on the crystalline lens and cataracts.

Sally Greengross

Director, Age Concern England
Joint Chairman, Board of Management
Age Concern Institute of Gerontology
King's College
University of London

FOREWORD

It is a great privilege for me to have been invited to introduce the first book in the newly created series of the Age Concern Institute of Gerontology (ACIOG) at King's College London. The Institute's birth in January 1986 was the result of a marriage of minds between many people at both Age Concern and King's; the first, an action-oriented agency which works with older people, the other, one of the most respected colleges of the University of London. Without the inspired leadership given by both my predecessor as Director of Age Concern England, David Hobman, and the Principal of King's College, Professor Stewart Sutherland, or the determined efforts of Jonathan Barker, Anthony Warnes and Janet Askham, the Institute would not have been born.

The philosophy underlying the Institute's combination of research, teaching, and the development and evaluation of practical action, derives largely from its multidisciplinary approach to the better understanding of ageing processes. The results of academic achievement must reach a wide audience else their benefit and influence remain restricted or are but slowly taken up and developed. All those concerned with this series are determined that the books will be based on well-conducted research, careful reflection, and good writing. Several of the later titles in the series will aim deliberately to bring specialised fields to a wide audience.

This book demonstrates the scope and challenge of gerontological inquiry and understanding. It has been prompted by the inaugural series of public lectures with which the ambitions and range of interests of ACIOG were announced. The lectures ranged from fundamental biological questions about ageing, through topics relating to the varied and changing circumstances of elderly people, to discussions of ethical, policy and practice issues. Many of the speakers were members of the staffs of Age Concern England and King's College, and we were delighted that friends and supporters from elsewhere in the University of London, from other of the young but vigorously growing centres of gerontological study in Britain, and from two long-established multidisciplinary institutes in the United States accepted our invitations to help form a coherent and stimulating programme.

The lectures were a solid basis for this book, but gerontologists are an unusually active group of people and not all could develop a chapter among their many other commitments. But the range of interest has been preserved with new recruits, many of whom reflect ACIOG's development within King's College and the links it has forged in London and elsewhere. Their contributions are remarkably diverse, and in this demonstrate the immense challenge facing the field's teachers, researchers, policy-makers and organisations such as Age Concern England. It is his long association with this voluntary body that permits a special welcome for the contribution from Mark Abrams, who has pioneered social research concerning elderly people and was the first Director of the Age Concern Research Unit.

All the authors have contributed to a book which has become more than its parts: it reflects the wide range of interests and questions that face those involved in the study of gerontology and which a multidisciplinary research and teaching institute will address. It is not a comprehensive survey or an introductory teaching text; it is comprised of research-based chapters that highlight some of the key scientific, scholarly, policy and practice issues of the late 1980s. The subjects range over basic biology, practical physiology, geriatric and community medicine, nursing studies, the history of social policy, social care practice, demography, the analysis of social statistics and educational theory. The last three chapters attempt to point to the way ahead and include discussions of a number of priority research and policy questions. Many readers will find some of the material unfamiliar and difficult: this is because few of us have yet benefited from the multidisciplinary training which the Institute and this series seeks to produce. We are only beginning to define the necessary syllabus and the most effective approaches.

Human Ageing and Later Life is being published at a significant time for the Age Concern Institute of Gerontology at King's College London. The appointment of its first Director, Professor Anthea Tinker, was made at the beginning of 1988 and the first students on the new MSc in Gerontology have been enrolled. The Institute, unique in its philosophy, its foundation and its purpose, should serve as a catalyst in pointing the way forward to some important gerontological developments in Britain. By raising the level of knowledge, of discussion and of innovative ideas in practice, older people in this country and elsewhere should benefit from its far-reaching potential to enhance academic excellence and the expansion and dissemination of knowledge.

1989   S.G.

Part One

AGEING PROCESSES

Alan Hipkiss

Department of Biochemistry
and

Alan Bittles

Department of Anatomy and Human Biology
King's College
University of London

1 BASIC BIOLOGICAL ASPECTS OF AGEING

INTRODUCTION

For most species on this planet, with the possible exception of micro-organisms, life inevitably leads to death. However, from a different perspective the existence of the vast variety of extant species testifies to the transmission from generation to generation of the genes which encode molecular information and thereby determine the structure and function of all living organisms. In other words, while the individual multicellular organism ages and dies, the information contained within that individual's germ cells (egg or sperm) normally 'lives' almost indefinitely and so escapes the fate of the somatic cells, i.e. those cells which are not germ cells. Manifestly the germ cells are not independently viable, since they cannot exist or unite with germ cells of opposite mating type in the absence of somatic cells (e.g. skin, blood, nerve, brain and heart) which support them. Does this mean that the advent of sex brought about the inevitability of mortality or immortality? Support for both viewpoints can be found. Many bacteria, though capable of genetic recombination (i.e. sexual reproduction), can divide indefinitely. Other micro-organisms can divide asexually for a limited number of times (around 60) before senescence and eventual death occurs – but if sexual reproduction takes place, the division clock is reset to zero. In the context of this book, ageing in the human is primarily concerned with the somatic cells of an individual. Nevertheless, it should be borne in mind that the individual germ line is not immune from age-related effects, as shown by the correlation between the incidence of certain human genetic abnormalities such as Down's syndrome and advancing maternal age.

THEORIES OF AGEING

Ageing is a multifaceted process. Consequently, the many attempts to explain ageing rather than simply to describe its progress are likely to fail to meet the requisite criteria originally suggested by Strehler (1977): universality, intrinsicality, progressiveness and deleteriousness. Perhaps the very use of the term 'ageing' is misleading, by its suggestion of a delineated set of changes which lead to senescence and finally death. A different perspective is provided if we use the phrase 'failure to survive'. As there are many ways of dying, are there many ways of ageing? All attempts first to understand the events which accompany or encompass ageing, and then to provide a theoretical basis for any explanation, should therefore be sufficiently unrestricted to allow as wide an interpretation as possible. It is accepted by most biologists that ageing ultimately has a molecular basis and that, whatever the changes in molecular structures or functions which accompany or cause ageing, these changes are manifested as deleterious alterations in cellular, organ and organismic behaviour. In other words, reductionist philosophy still has a useful application. However, the holistic caveat that cells, organs and organisms consist of interacting molecules is retained, i.e. the whole is indeed greater than the sum of its constituent parts.

Ageing of organisms

Theories which attempt to explain ageing at the level of the whole organism include:

(i) wear and tear theories which suggest that ageing is caused by the gradual wearing out of non-replaceable body constituents;

(ii) accumulation theories which argue that ageing results from the accumulation of toxic metabolites;

(iii) exhaustion theories which suggest that ageing follows the steady exhaustion of irreplaceable substances;

(iv) endocrine changes which hypothesise that ageing is a consequence of variations in the levels of certain hormones.

Ageing of cells

Many researchers in this field have assumed that at the cellular and molecular levels ageing brings about a loss of information which prevents either successful and complete cellular renewal or intracellular molecular replacement. The following examples provide a short and selective list of theories of ageing operating on this scale.

(i) *Somatic mutation theory.* This suggests that in both fixed and dividing cells, ageing is caused by a loss of information due to mutation or damage in the cell's information store, otherwise known as deoxyribonucleic acid or DNA. The DNA 'store' is located in the cell nucleus.

(ii) *Error theory.* This suggests that ageing is the result of an increase in erroneous gene replication and expression, that defective proteins subsequently accumulate, and that these in turn cause further decreases in the accuracy of protein synthesis and the eventual onset of an error catastrophe.

(iii) *Free radical theory.* This suggests that the toxic by-products of oxygen metabolism (oxygen free radicals) react with DNA, proteins and lipids, thereby causing defects in information storage, information retrieval and enzyme and membrane functions.

(iv) *Cross-linkage theory.* This suggests that excess cross-linking between protein molecules may evoke some age-related changes in protein properties. Causes of cross-linking can be both enzymic and non-enzymic. The latter are slow when mediated by glucose but occur more rapidly with other sugars; DNA also may be subjected to sugar-mediated cross-linking.

(v) *Programmed ageing theory.* This suggests that ageing is a pre-programmed process, like growth and differentiation, specified by one or more ageing genes.

AGE-RELATED CHANGES IN HUMAN PHYSIOLOGICAL FUNCTIONS

Many measurable physiological parameters decline in the elderly, although whether reported declines are as inevitable as once supposed is open to question. Tests or experiments performed at the cellular or subcellular levels should be free from conscious or subconscious expectations or environmental influences. Age-related changes in almost all aspects of cellular structure and function have been described.

The declining function with age of the reproductive system in the female is well characterised, but the fundamental causes of ovulatory failure and age-related infertility are not understood. In humans and other mammals the explanation is not simply a lack of oöcytes because they remain present when ovulation has ceased. It has been suggested that there is a minimum threshold number of follicle cells (which develop into oöcytes) to maintain ovulatory function; the system appears to cut out gradually as this number is approached. Explanations have been proposed in terms both of the deleterious effects of certain ovarian secretions and the effects of hormones from the hypothalamus and pituitary glands, especially oestradiol-mediated dysfunction of the hypothalamic-pituitary secretory system. The age-associated loss of fertility appears to be related to at least three failures: that of the ageing ovum or fertilisation; those intrinsic to the uterus; and that connected with hormonal support for pregnancy.

The secretion of hormones from the endocrine glands changes during ageing, in most cases showing a decline with advancing years. This is clearly seen in the case of hormones which regulate growth. Cellular growth is controlled essentially by a specific polypeptide called growth hormone which is released from the pituitary gland. Among elderly people, the pulsed release of this hormone, which normally occurs during the early stages of sleep, is significantly lowered or even absent. Interestingly, the drug L-dopa restores the pulsed release of growth hormone in elderly rats. This suggests that the hypothalamus could have an important role in regulating growth hormone release. Another important hormone is somatostatin, also produced by the hypothalamus as well as other tissues, the levels of which increase in later life, apparently inhibiting the release of growth hormone. The regulatory mechanisms of the production and release of somatostatin, however, are poorly understood.

In the laboratory rat, the release of insulin from the pancreas in response to elevated blood glucose levels is also impaired with age and the increased levels of somatostatin may provide part of the explanation. Longitudinal studies with healthy humans indicate no age-related decline in insulin release, although there is still a measure of age-related glucose intolerance. This partly illustrates the nature of the difficulties in extrapolating from animal model experiments to the human condition. However, a major function of insulin is to facilitate the entry of glucose into certain tissues and to inhibit the release of fatty acids into the bloodstream from others. In old animals and humans alike, changes in responsiveness to insulin have been reported which are due to either a decline in the number of insulin receptors on the cell surfaces of that tissue, or a decreased avidity of the receptors for insulin attachment. In summary, it is not obvious how or why endocrine functions alter with age, but it is clear that we are dealing with a complex set of interacting factors and that the balance between their functions is critical.

Changes in the nervous system certainly occur. The fact that in humans the neurones do not divide after formation implies that they must possess a very effective homeostatic mechanism to maintain both their integrity and function for many years. It is probably not the case that we are losing many millions of neurones from our brains throughout life as once was believed; recent studies have shown that while some losses do occur, these are confined to specific brain regions. Net losses of proteins and gangliosides (a major component of the nerve sheath) only occur to a significant extent in the caudate nucleus part of the brain. A careful study of brain tissues from aged humans without Alzheimer's disease has shown that there is loss of function of the cholinergic system, that is a decline in the neurotransmitter substance acetylcholine, probably due to decreased production by the enzyme acetylcholine synthetase. In contrast, there does not seem to be a decline with age in the cholinoreceptor cells, i.e. those cells which are stimulated by acetylcholine. In the case of a second neurotransmitter, serotonin, although the level does not decline with age, the number of serotonin receptors does. Other human transmitter substances – somatostatin, substance P and δ-amino butyric acid – may change to some extent, but only the acetylcholine and serotonin systems have been found consistently to show large declines with age.

There is considerable evidence that, even in 'normal' ageing, neuronal proteins may form aggregates, called tangles, paired helical filaments and amyloid plaque. In Alzheimer's disease, these structures are formed from the neuronal cells in large quantities, and appreciable brain atrophy occurs, especially in the hippocampus, as well as significant declines in the synthesis of the neurotransmitters acetylcholine and serotonin. Because the cholinergic neurones plus the serotonin- and noradrenalin-associated neurones constitute only 12 per cent of the total, the major loss of neurones in Alzheimer's disease must occur in some other unidentified class of neuronal cells. The enzymes involved in the oxidation of glucose to provide energy are also reduced by 50 per cent in Alzheimer's dementia. In the genetic disorder Down's syndrome an accumulation of amyloid, plaque and tangles occurs, as well as deficits in acetylcholine production. Recent studies have shown that the amyloid found in both Alzheimer's disease and Down's syndrome is composed of the same protein fragment, encoded by a gene on chromosome 21, of which there is an extra copy in Down's syndrome.

The immune system declines in efficiency with age, not only with respect to foreign organisms and molecules (by recognising surface proteins and polysaccharides), but also with respect to self-recognition as shown by the age-related increased incidence of autoimmune diseases in both humans and animals. Qualitative changes in the cells which mediate the immune response, the T and B lymphocytes, appear to be the cause, rather than a deficit in absolute cell numbers. Thus, when challenged by an antigen, the number of *effective* cells (either T or B cells) is fewer in old animals and humans. Furthermore, a decline in T cell function precedes the decline in soluble antibody production by the B cells, probably because helper T cells are required for the appropriate antibody protein production by B cells. The likely explanation of these events is partly that the thymus gland, in which T cells develop their immunocompetence, appears to regress and involute quite early in life, but it still retains immunological functions. Although there is inadequate insight into the mechanisms of thymus function, it is becoming clear that this organ profoundly affects the production of sufficient effective T cells from the pluripotent stem cells of the bone marrow. In addition, age-related changes in the ability of stem cells to divide has been observed, suggesting that the changes in this physiological system are complex. Further age-related defects in the immune system can be demonstrated, such as the failure to deliver soluble antibodies to their site of action, as shown by their low levels in nasal and respiratory secretions despite high levels in serum. The immune response occurs in that the antibody is produced, but it fails to be secreted at the site of infection. This may explain in part the high incidence of and mortality from pneumonia in the elderly.

The major age-related change in the skeletal system is the decrease in bone mass observed in post-menopausal females; a smaller and slower decline occurs in males. It is thought that this does not reflect a change in calcium metabolism, but instead is an aberration in the control of the turnover of the major bone protein, collagen. Normally bone collagen is replaced by processes of breakdown and resynthesis at a rate of between five and ten per cent each year with no net loss of material. The process involves two cell types with dissimilar functions, namely the osteoclast and the osteoblast. The osteoclasts excavate small canals in the bone by secreting specific enzymes which selectively degrade the collagen. Following the osteoclasts, the osteoblasts line the walls of the newly excavated canals and then secrete new bone protein collagen. An important feature of this process is the control of the osteoclasts by two opposed hormones, parathyroid hormone and calcitonin. Parathyroid hormone stimulates osteoclast activity; calcitonin inhibits it. Calcitonin is secreted by the thyroid gland under the stimulation of oestrogen and testosterone. At menopause the level of oestrogen falls dramatically, thus causing a sharp fall in calcitonin and reduced modulation of osteoclast activity. Osteoclastic collagen removal is accelerated without a corresponding increase in osteoblast function to replace the depleted protein. Consequently, it is possible to lose about 30 per cent of the bone mass in a decade. Hormone replacement therapy using oestrogen restores control of the osteoclasts. The attendant risks of endometrial cancer are reduced by the inclusion of progesterone, which prevents proliferation of the endometrium (the lining of the uterus). In men the decline in testosterone levels is much slower and only relatively small declines in bone mass occur.

Vision frequently changes during the middle and later years. There are two ways in which the function of eye lenses change with age. Firstly, the ability of the lens to change shape gradually decreases with age, due in part to increasingly tight packing of cells in the core which produces an inability to focus on near objects. Another change which affects most elderly people is decreased sensitivity to light. Less light reaches the light-sensitive surface, the retina, because more is scattered or absorbed. It seems that the proteins (the crystallins) contained within the cells of the lens core, which are usually in free solution, slowly form very small aggregates over the years. These tend to absorb or scatter the light rather than allow its uninterrupted transmission. A pathological version of this process occurs in the senile cataract: in this condition altered crystallins form very large aggregates which are highly insoluble and optically opaque. Further discussion of age-related changes in the human eye are developed in Chapter 4.

AGE-RELATED CHANGES AT THE CELLULAR AND MOLECULAR LEVELS

Proliferative ability and protein synthesis are frequently found to decline with age. Although numerous theories have been advanced, searches at the molecular level to explain these decrements have for the most part proved disappointing. Many questions in the biology of ageing are simply stated but difficult to answer. One conundrum opens by querying whether an old organism is composed of old cells which in turn are composed of old molecules. If so, it proceeds, can old cells made from old molecules be rejuvenated when placed in a young environment? Complementary questions are whether an old organism can be rejuvenated if young cells are introduced into it, and whether an old cell can be made young again upon the introduction of young molecules.

To attempt to answer these questions, it is necessary to outline some of the important cellular differences between the organs of the human body. Some body components comprise cells which divide almost continuously through-out life, for example, blood cell precursors in the bone marrow, skin and the lining of the alimentary tract. Others, such as liver, kidney, brain and muscle, have cells which though capable of division normally do so only rarely. Organs may also possess cells which never divide, for example, peripheral nerve cells, mature red blood cells and the eye lens core. In each of these arbitrary classes age-related effects can be demonstrated, which implies that 'ageing' occurs in cells which possess no genetic material (e.g. the red blood cell and lens core), as well as in the remainder which contain the full genetic complement. This is important because the genetic material DNA determines the structure and function of all intracellular and extracellular components, and without in-formation inside the cell no new macromolecules such as proteins can be synthesized. Thus, should protein molecules inside the cells of the lens core or the red blood cell become damaged, they cannot be replaced. DNA directly specifies the structure of all cellular proteins. There are many thousands of different types of proteins in most animal cells and they perform both structural and catalytic roles, the latter including the synthesis of more proteins. Cells which cannot make additional protein are severely handicapped since they depend for their survival only on pre-existing protein molecules.

Cells that cannot, or do not, divide but which possess a nucleus containing DNA can synthesize essential new proteins required either for the cell's specialised function or to replace damaged or malfunctioning molecules. Assuming that DNA, the protein synthetic machinery, and all other necessary functions remain unaltered with time, the cell theoretically should be able to function indefinitely. However, this does not seem to be the case. Many of the theories previously outlined address this dilemma. Cells which divide rapidly would simply be expected to replace malfunctional cells with effective ones, but again there is evidence that the replacement cells also may show symptoms of ageing.

Returning to the questions posed above: some cells in an old organism are as old (or almost as old) as the organism itself, for instance, lens core cells and neurones which do not divide. No evidence has been found for the possible rejuvenation of these old cells, and most biologists would consider it highly unlikely. Cell and organ transplant experiments from young to old hosts and vice versa have yielded equivocal results, although young cells remain young even in an old host while the host remains old. The transplantation of young nuclei into old cytoplasm and the reverse have suggested that there are roles for both the cytoplasm and the nucleus as determinants of ageing and that the effect of senescence is dominant. However, in most cases the conclusions are at best tentative and much work remains to be carried out.

Because age-related molecular changes have been described in all three of the above classes of cells, manifesting themselves at cellular, organ and organism levels, biologists have been searching for a molecular basis or bases of the ageing process. It is, however, naïve to expect that there is a single cause of ageing. In many studies of the biology of the ageing process, whether in animals or humans, one finds the question of causality either implied or stated directly in a form which reflects the experimenter's own research interests and which often excludes or inadequately recognises the possibility of other contributory factors.

The consideration of effects and causes leads us to another contentious area: whether we can clearly distinguish between the effects of ageing and its causes.

For example, an age-related decline in a physiological function might be a cause of death, but what was the fundamental cause of that decline? In the case of the immune system, is the decline in operational efficiency only a secondary consequence of some other primary process? Similarly, the precipitation of the lens protein crystallin as a senile cataract is certainly the cause of an age-associated loss of vision. However, there are several possible immediate causes of these changes in lens proteins which themselves could be primary or secondary manifestations of another (as yet unknown) age-associated event.

What cellular and subcellular changes could explain ageing or its symptoms?
So far the discussion has focused firstly at the cellular and then at the molecular level. While a full description of animal and human cell molecular biology is not appropriate here, to develop the argument for the non-biologist it will be helpful to outline further areas of cellular structure and metabolism.

Most cells in the body are specialised and perform a specific function. In order to maintain their function, cells must be supplied with a potential source of energy (normally glucose or fatty acids) which can be converted into usable energy. This energy is required for the synthesis of very large molecules (macromolecules) such as the proteins which are used as catalysts or in cellular structures, DNA which provides information storage, polysaccharides which provide energy storage, and lipids which serve both for energy storage and as structural elements in cell membranes. All of these processes take place within the cell and each step along the biochemical pathway requires a specific (separate) protein catalyst. Many different types of protein catalysts are known and in total over 200 million protein molecules co-exist inside each cell. Each individual protein molecule, whether catalyst or structural, is specified by DNA inherited from both parents. It is DNA which specifies from which amino acids the protein is made. Assembly of amino acids into protein requires the expenditure of energy.

Protein synthesis occurs in the cytoplasm of the cell while the information store (DNA) is located in the nucleus. This problem is overcome by the synthesis of smaller, mobile, blueprint molecules called messenger RNA on to which the instructions from DNA are copied. The messenger RNA is then transported from the nucleus to the cytoplasm where it is used directly as a template for protein production. All of these steps also require the presence of specific proteins, and the actual assembly of amino acids into protein occurs on protein/RNA complexes called ribosomes. So, in order for a cell to replicate itself, an information store (DNA) and a protein biosynthetic apparatus (ribosomes) are required. If either the functional DNA or the protein biosynthetic mechanism is absent the cell is incapable of self-replication and will sooner or later die. It will therefore be understood that some theories of ageing have been based on changes in the efficiency and accuracy of the processes of information retrieval and utilisation in protein biosynthesis.

SYSTEMS OF MOLECULAR REPAIR AND MAINTENANCE IN AGEING

The cells comprising our major organs have to function in a hostile environment. Both cells and organs are continuously under attack from physical, chemical and biological adversaries. Heat, cold, ultraviolet (UV) light and X-irradiation can alter, reversibly or irreversibly, the structure and hence function of DNA, RNA, protein or membrane lipids. Oxygen which is necessary for the efficient release of energy from food is also toxic, because highly reactive oxygen free radicals can be generated as by-products within the cells and damage DNA, RNA, protein and membrane lipids. Even the most common sugar, glucose, can react with proteins and so alter their properties and hence physiological function. Biological adversaries for humans range from macro-predators, whether 'lions and tigers' or next-door neighbours, to microscopic bacteria and viruses. Defence systems are therefore required at both the macro- and micro-levels to ensure survival from not only biological foes but also the chemical and physical onslaught to which our cells are continuously subjected.

Systems to combat the effects of environmentally-induced damage to our intracellular macromolecules have been identified. One such system involves a set of enzymes which carry out DNA repair; here the portion of DNA damaged by UV light, X-rays or free radicals is selectively eliminated and a com-plementary new segment synthesised and joined with the remainder of the macromolecule. Similarly, other enzymes selectively destroy protein mole-cules of abnormal structure which have resulted from errors in synthesis or environmental insults. Damage to membrane lipids principally brought about by oxygen free radicals is controlled by a battery of antioxidants, such as vitamin C, vitamin E, uric acid and the enzyme superoxide dismutase. Many of the processes for the maintenance of the status quo, called homoeostatic systems, are carried out by proteins which are themselves subject to environ-mentally-induced insults, and whose production requires accurate messenger RNA synthesis in the nucleus and protein synthesis on the ribosomes in the cytoplasm. Hence, if ageing is associated with a cellular malfunction, it may result from the inactivation of a specific function necessary for immediate survival and/or a failure to correct environmentally-induced damage. A de-ficiency in the intracellular release of energy will affect both immediate cellular function and the homoeostatic systems, many of which are energy dependent.

IS THERE AN AGEING GENE?

It is established that the maximum life span of an organism is genetically controlled. Mice rarely live for more than three years, whereas man can live for up to 120 years. Furthermore, there is evidence that human longevity does have a genetic component. Considerable effort has been applied to the search for mutant animals whose maximal life span is extended, however only reductions in survival have been detected. Two rare inherited disorders in humans, Werner's syndrome and progeria, appear to be a consequence of mutant genes and result in considerably reduced life expectancy, but again it is unlikely that these defective genes can be primary determinants of maximal life span.

A line of investigation which could reveal useful information is the study of transformed or tumour-forming cells. Transformation confers indefinite prolif-erative capacity and an escape from the prior cellular senescent and mortality properties. Research is therefore attempting to identify and characterise the bases of their indefinite survival. Studies of fusions between transformed and untransformed cells show that in some cases the resulting hybrids regain their mortality; in other words the senescence factor (whatever it is) dominates immortality. With the aid of DNA recombinant technology, the next few years may identify which genes are responsible.

COMMON FEATURES OF AGEING IN HUMAN CELLS AND POSSIBLE CAUSAL MECHANISMS

It is probable that the most common age-associated intracellular event is the accumulation of altered proteins. Examples are enzymes with altered heat stability, catalytic activity and immuno-reactivity; the age pigments, lipofuscin granules, often found in muscles and nerves, which are protein-lipid complexes resulting from incomplete breakdown of oxygen free radical-induced protein-lipid crosslinks; insoluble protein precipitates occurring as senile cataracts in the cells of eye lens core; and the amyloid bodies, neuritic plaque and neurofibrillar tangles in the aged brain which are especially prevalent in Alzheimer's dementia. The description of these symptoms does not identify the reasons for the production or accumulation of the altered proteins. Possible age-related causes include increasingly inaccurate protein biosynthesis (now considered to be unlikely by many researchers in the field); a change in the postsynthetic metabolism of the proteins; an alteration in gene expression resulting in unbalanced protein synthesis; and a decline in one or more of the homoeostatic systems, such as a reduction in antioxidant activities, in DNA repair, or in the elimination of erroneous proteins. Although any one or indeed a combination of these events could explain the observed symptoms, we still need to explain why they occur only in later life. This returns us to the question of whether ageing is genetically programmed or if it is a result of continuously occurring random deleterious events which eventually result in the inactivation of homoeostatic processes.

Another common observation is that the rate of protein biosynthesis declines in many aged tissues: this would result in a decrease in the rate of replacement of cellular proteins including those responsible for intracellular homoeostasis. But the environmentally derived insults to DNA, protein and lipid continue at a constant rate, thus we can envisage a point at which the homoeostatic systems cannot eliminate all damaged macromolecules. Some evidence exists for such a scenario; decreased superoxide dismutase activity has been detected in maturing red blood cells and in ageing liver; a decreased ability to degrade certain forms of abnormal proteins has been found in maturing erythroid cells, the liver of aged mice, in senescent human cells in culture and in cells of the lens core (possibly the oldest cells in the body which are formed *in utero* and have not since undergone replication). The possible importance of homoeostatic processes in ageing is also indicated by the finding that intracellular DNA repair capacity is highest in species which live longest. These ideas are dealt with in more detail in Chapters 2 and 3.

MODEL SYSTEMS FOR THE STUDY OF THE AGEING PROCESS

Although the investigation of ageing in human individuals is obviously desirable, it is equally clear that such studies are logistically and economically taxing and may be difficult to justify on ethical grounds. Nevertheless, the test battery approach, whereby individuals of different ages are subjected to multiple biochemical, physiological and psychological tests, has been modified and utilised in several centres (e.g. Boston and Gothenberg), and has produced useful information. This approach tells much about the ageing individual but generates little new knowledge of the ageing process *per se*. In addition, it may be difficult to differentiate between 'normal' ageing and early, pathological manifestations of disease. Alternative approaches have been employed to overcome these problems, namely either the use of an animal model, generally the mouse, or the culture of human cells in the laboratory. Studies on ageing mice have the intrinsic problem of interspecific extrapolation of findings; for instance, is a two year old mouse equivalent to a middle-aged human being, and is the mouse subject to the same range of age-related conditions as the human? It should be remembered that, although the life span of laboratory rodents can be increased by dietary restriction (specifically of calories), there is no published evidence that similar dietary regimes have a life-extending effect on humans. Given that calorie restriction is the *only* factor known to increase longevity in any animal model, and given its inapplicability to the human condition, one must question whether information appropriate to human ageing can be obtained from animal models. On the other hand, animal studies obviously have their place in comparative research programmes into ageing.

The demonstration that cells obtained from human tissue have finite, reproducible life spans when cultured in the laboratory and that they exhibit many of the age-related changes observed *in vivo*, has led to the widespread adoption of such cell cultures as appropriate investigatory tools for ageing studies. The fact that human cells derived from the skin or lung, such as fibroblasts, undergo senescence in culture shows that ageing has an intrinsic cellular basis and is not solely a consequence of defective intercellular communication. This does not preclude changes in secretory hormone levels having important effects at all stages of life including old age. But are these changes, i.e. altered hormone secretion, secondary to the primary age-related event which controls this cellular function? Perhaps the cultured fibroblast will provide a vital clue to the question, 'what causes cells (or at least fibroblasts) to age?'. However, as previously stated, it is probable that given the complexity of cells and their variety, there will be no single cause of ageing for all cells. The onset of senescence may even be induced by different factors in specific cell types.

Changes in fibroblast structure and function have been detected during *in vitro* senescence. Cell surface and membrane properties, and membrane protein composition, change during fibroblast ageing. By definition these changes would be anticipated to interfere substantially with intracellular organisation, especially energy and nutrient provision, and therefore could limit all cellular functions including nucleic acid and protein biosynthesis. Of special interest are the mitochondria, subcellular organelles which are widely distributed in most cells of the mammalian species. Mitochondria play a crucial role in the oxygen-dependent release of energy from food, and because of their intimate association with oxygen, they are major sites of oxygen free radical generation. As discussed in Chapter 3, a deterioration in mitochondrial structure has been detected with ageing which could affect energy provision. Alterations in the physical, chemical and biochemical properties of some but not all proteins have been reported also to accompany senescence, with changes in DNA replication enzymes being especially critical. Defective catabolism of some types of aberrant proteins has been shown which could result from reductions in the activities of appropriate homoeostatic enzymes or in the provision of energy for their selective function. Premature senescence has been reported to be induced by agents which cause increased erroneous protein synthesis. This has been interpreted by some as support for the error theory of ageing, however there is no firm evidence that protein synthetic error rates increase either during *in vitro* ageing or in any other ageing system.

IMMEDIATE, MEDIUM AND LONG-TERM DEVELOPMENTS

It used to be claimed that there were as many theories of ageing as there were investigators in the field. In recent years the number of investigators has increased and there has been no appreciable decline in the variety of ageing theories advanced. An exception is the error theory, perhaps because unlike many of the other theories it is amenable to experimental test. The topics attracting current investigation in cellular ageing include oxygen free radical involvement in DNA, protein and membrane damage, mitochondrial degeneration, defective protein breakdown, changes in postsynthetic protein modification, and non-enzymic protein and nucleic acid glycosylation (cross-linkage). Support for each of these and other proposed events has and will continue to be found, but it is unlikely that any one 'theory' of ageing will be sufficiently convincing to explain all age-dependent changes. It will continue to be difficult to distinguish between cause and effect. The idea of a specific gene which triggers ageing after a set time during development is open to debate. However, it is obvious that the organism has to be genetically programmed to survive up to and beyond the cessation of its own fertility or to the time when its offspring are themselves capable of independent life and reproduction. Can we regard the run-down of the maintenance systems necessary for cell duplication and sexual reproduction as directly programmed events? If we regard ageing as 'a failure to survive' and then think of what is required for survival, we see that continued effectiveness of the maintenance system required for successful cellular function and reproduction is a genetically determined process. On the other hand, its decline could occur randomly, because the maintenance system is itself affected by the end results of the very chemical and biological hazards it should eliminate. Changes in some homoeostatic processes with age provide support for this view.

The potential application of biology to human ageing may not be immediate. Major problems presently recognised in the ageing population are neurological disorders, particularly Alzheimer's dementia, with its attendant intra-neuronal protein aggregation products; osteoporosis, which involves a change in the relative rates of bone protein synthesis and breakdown such that the latter exceeds the former; senile cataracts, associated with an accumulation of altered and insoluble lens protein; kidney failure; the incidence of heart and circulatory diseases, both environmentally or self-induced; increased susceptibility to infection due to the decreased efficiency of immune surveillance and the associated increase in autoimmune disease; and the increased incidence of tumours. In many of these cases biology is able to identify the changes which occur and in a few even suggest possible causes and ameliorative measures. An example is the prevention and treatment of osteoporosis, where hormone replacement therapy appears to restore the balance of proteins and exercise is additionally beneficial. Perhaps we should place more emphasis on the study of those processes which prevent age-related changes from occurring, and also upon systems which ordinarily facilitate the removal of altered macromolecules. If a fully functional homoeostatic system is indeed important to combat ageing decrements, then one could ensure that the diet of elderly individuals contained sufficient antioxidants, the necessary co-factors and the full range of required amino acids so that synthesis of the homoeostatic enzymes was not limited.

AN INTRODUCTORY READING LIST

This chapter has been written with a non-biological audience in mind. Those wishing to pursue the subject in greater depth may find the following texts a useful next step.

Adelman, R.C. and Dekker, E.E. (Eds) (1986). *Modification of Proteins During Aging*. CRC Press, New York.

Adelman, R.C. and Roth, G.S. (Eds) (1983). *Testing the Theories of Aging*. CRC Press, New York.

Adelman, R.C. and Roth, G.S. (Eds) (1985). *Altered Proteins and Aging*. CRC Press, New York.

Bergener, M., Ermini, M. and Stahelin, H.B. (Eds) (1985). *Thresholds in Ageing*. Academic Press, London.

Bergener, M., Ermini, M. and Stahelin, H.B. (Eds) (1986). *Dimensions in Ageing*. Academic Press, London.

Bittles, A.H. and Collins, K.J. (Eds) (1986). *The Biology of Human Ageing*. Cambridge University Press, Cambridge.

Comfort, A. (1982). *Biology of Senescence*, 3rd edition. Churchill Livingstone, Edinburgh.

Coni, N. (1984). *Ageing: The Facts*. Oxford University Press, Oxford.

Evered, D. and Whelan, J. (Eds) (1988). *Research and the Ageing Population*. John Wiley & Sons, Chichester.

Rothstein, M. (Ed.) (1983, 1985, 1987). *Review of Biological Research on Aging*, Volumes 1, 2 and 3. Alan R. Liss, New York.

Roy, A.K. and Chatterjee, B. (Eds) (1984). *Molecular Basis of Ageing*. Academic Press, London.

Scarpelli, D.G. and Migaki, G. (Eds) (1984). *Comparative Pathobiology of Major Age-Related Diseases: Current Status and Research Frontiers*. Alan R. Liss, New York.

Strehler, B.L. (1977). *Time, Cells and Ageing*, 2nd edition. Academic Press, London.

Alan Hipkiss

Department of Biochemistry
King's College
University of London

2 THE PRODUCTION AND REMOVAL OF ABNORMAL PROTEINS: A KEY QUESTION IN THE BIOLOGY OF AGEING

INTRODUCTION

One of the most common observations made of ageing organisms, tissues and cells, is the occurrence of protein molecules whose structures, when compared to the equivalent molecules in nonsenescent material, have become altered in some important way. Among the many examples of such molecules and associated effects, the following have attracted particular interest.

1. Enzyme molecules with decreased catalytic activity (specific activity), altered heat-lability and ultraviolet spectral properties.
2. The altered forms of neuronal proteins which during normal ageing accumulate in aggregate forms down as tangles, plaque and amyloid. These occur in large amounts in Alzheimer's disease.
3. The crystallins of the lens which aggregate progressively with age thus decreasing light transmission and increasing scattering. This phenomenon is considerably amplified in the pathological condition of the senile cataract.
4. The aggregations of proteins with lipids which form lipofuscin granules characteristic of aged neuronal and muscle tissues.
5. The increase in autoimmune phenomena with age is an indication of altered immune function deriving either from alterations in antibody production and/or structure, as well as antigenic changes in 'self'.
6. The changes in connective tissue where collagen becomes increasingly cross-linked with age.

From this brief list of well-documented phenomena it is clear that to further our understanding of the role of molecular processes in human ageing, three issues need to be more thoroughly investigated. Firstly, improved understanding of the production and removal of altered or abnormal proteins is required. Secondly, it must be determined if either the formation or removal of altered proteins changes during ageing and, thirdly, molecular gerontology needs to develop sufficient understanding of the molecular bases of these age-related events to assess whether they can be regulated (Mann, 1985; Rogozinski, Blumenfield and Seifter, 1983).

As with all studies based upon phenomenological symptomology, the caveat applies that many or most of the changes are probably not causal to the ageing process and are more likely to be consequences of other unspecified, inadequately understood or unrecognised processes. This caution is particularly necessary when dealing with the biology of life forms whose somatic cells do not proliferate indefinitely, and therefore have a limited life span.

ALTERED AND ABNORMAL PROTEINS: DEFINITIONS, SOURCES AND FORMATION

The structure of an altered or an abnormal protein deviates significantly from that of the normal gene product. Typical examples are:

1. mutant proteins containing amino acid substitutions or which are prematurely terminated or truncated;
2. denatured or improperly folded proteins;
3. proteins with unregulated cross-linking;
4. protein fragments;
5. improperly processed polypeptides;
6. under- or over-modified proteins.

The accumulation of abnormal proteins can derive from an increase in their synthesis and/or a decrease in their removal. They can be produced by several processes, a selection of which will be briefly described, and any one of which could account for some of the age-related changes in altered polypeptides which have been detected in aged cells and tissues.

Errors in protein biosynthesis

The most error-prone step in protein biosynthesis is in translation, namely the binding of the cognate aminoacyl transfer ribonucleic acid (tRNA) to the correct codon in the messenger RNA on the ribosome. Despite the editing role of aminoacyl tRNA synthetase at the aminoacylation step and the additional editing role on the ribosome itself, misincorporation has been found to occur at a measurable frequency at least *in vitro*. The frequency of misincorporation varies from codon to codon. A mean of three errors in 10^4 codons is often quoted. It should be remembered, however, that this average takes no account of the amino acid content of the protein and the codon usage during its synthesis. Many workers have attempted to determine whether translational error rates increase with ageing, as predicted by the error-catastrophe theory of ageing. The detection of ribosomal ambiguity mutations (RAM) in bacteria, in which there is an increased level of translational inaccuracy from a mutation in a ribosomal protein, stimulated these enquiries because it provided another example of the possibility of error-feedback into the accuracy maintenance apparatus of the cell. However no consistent evidence has been produced to demonstrate an age-related increase in the protein biosynthetic error rate (Filion and Laughrea, 1985; Rothstein, 1987).

It is interesting to note that in some cases an increase in the error rate elicits responses similar to those found with senescence. For example, the addition of agents, such as paromomycin, which increase translational error rates in cultured human fibroblasts, does eventually promote the premature senescence and death of these cells. Even in the bacterium *Escherichia coli*, which normally does not age, continuous treatment with a low dose of the error-inducing antibiotic streptomycin after ten cell doublings causes the cessation of growth, a decreased ability to degrade abnormal proteins, and finally the death of the cells (Carrier, Kogut and Hipkiss, 1984). (The selective proteolysis of aberrant proteins will be considered below.) Cell-free extracts of untreated cells were able to degrade the abnormal proteins which had accumulated in the 'old' bacteria. These experiments demonstrate that it is possible to induce an error-feedback phenomenon by experimentally increasing the inaccuracy of the protein biosynthetic system, but the absence of convincing evidence for changes in the accuracy of protein biosynthesis during 'normal' ageing suggests that an error-feedback does not occur in the 'wild'. Altered proteins could arise from transcriptional errors. However ribonucleotide incorporation is far more accurate than translation and occurs at a frequency of around one in 10^6. Nonetheless, there is little evidence for an age-related increase in error frequency at the transcriptional step.

Deoxyribonucleic acid (DNA) replication is the most accurate step in macromolecule biosynthesis. The DNA error-detection and repair systems carried out by proteins are well characterised, and it is therefore theoretically possible for an error-feedback to occur in DNA replication (Tice and Setlow, 1985). There is, however, little direct evidence for age-related changes in the accuracy of DNA replication, but many cells show age-related increases in chromosomal damage and other abnormalities associated with the nucleus. Whether these changes in chromosome function and structure result from changes in the DNA or in protein is not known. The possibility of a correlation between ageing and the systems which eliminate damaged DNA is intriguing because of the relationship between the 'efficiency' of DNA repair and the maximal life span of mammalian species. The relationship between changes in DNA repair efficiency and the production of altered proteins remains to be clearly demonstrated.

Changes in the amino acid composition of mature proteins with age
Slow changes in amino acid composition can occur some considerable time after synthesis of the protein; the speed at which each change occurs depends upon the nature of the amino acid concerned and the polypeptide environment in which it is found. The spontaneous deamidation of asparagine and glutamine residues to aspartic and glutamic acid residues respectively, immediately increases the overall negative charge and places a carboxyl group (usually charged negative) in a position where evolution had 'placed' a neutral amide function (Beutler, 1986). Major changes in both protein structure and function may result.

Racemization of the normal *laevo* (L) stereochemical configuration of certain of the amino acid residues to the alternative *dextro* (D) form occurs at a slow but measurable rate. Aspartic acid and serine residues are most prone to racemization with rates between 0.1 and 0.3 per cent per annum. Its effects are seen most markedly in the crystallin protein of the eye's lens and in the enamel of teeth, because these proteins are replaced either very slowly or not at all – hence there is sufficient time for accumulation of the altered proteins. Indeed, the senile cataract found in the lens core has a higher incidence of D-amino acids, which may indicate that amino acid racemization has a role in the cataractogenesis of the major lens protein.

Proteins modified by oxygen free radicals and related species
Recent studies have revealed that oxygen free radicals, which are present to some degree in all oxygenated tissues, can modify proteins by oxidising certain amino acid residues, most commonly tyrosine, proline, histidine and methionine. They can also cleave peptide bonds to produce protein fragments. Both enzymic and non-enzymic routes of reactive radical generation have been described (Harman, 1987). The term 'mixed functional oxidase reaction' has been used to describe the former process. The degree to which the oxidation reactions occur is dependent upon several factors, including those involved in free radical generation and the antioxidant systems which should eliminate free radicals before they exert their detrimental effects. The position of the peptide bond cleavage can depend on metal ion availability (e.g. copper or iron) and the amino acid sequences with their different affinities for such ions.

Mixed functional oxidase-induced damage is thought to involve modification of specific histidine residues, but the surrounding amino acids are important. The presence of substrate or co-enzyme can also protect an enzyme from free radical attack. Not only can oxygen free radicals induce peptide bond cleavage but these highly reactive species can induce protein cross-linking to produce very high molecular weight aggregates of the altered protein and lipids. The senile cataract and lipofuscin granules both appear to contain cross-linked polypeptides. Reactive free radicals are also induced by ionising radiations such as ultraviolet and X-irradiation which may produce similar effects on cellular protein molecules. In cultured human fibroblasts, mixed functional oxidase-damaged protein accumulates with *in vitro* age; fibroblasts obtained from premature ageing syndromes (progeria and Werner's syndrome) show elevated amounts of mixed functional oxidase-modified protein sooner than age-matched controls.

Oxygen free radicals can also damage DNA which, if not repaired, could give rise to the production of altered, mutant, proteins (Saul, Gee and Ames, 1987). The degree to which free radical modification of DNA occurs will be dependent both on the efficacy of the cellular antioxidant system which eliminates the free radicals before they affect cellular macromolecules and the effectiveness of the DNA repair apparatus. Should altered proteins be produced from free radical modified DNA, the abnormal protein elimination system might be expected to facilitate their removal.

Cleavage by proteases

In most cells proteins are continuously turned over, the degradative components being carried out intracellularly, primarily by cytoplasmic and lysosomal proteases (Reznick *et al.*, 1985). The immediate products of the initial peptide bond cleavage are protein fragments (aberrant protein molecules by definition). Each protein species appears to be degraded at a specific rate: the molecular determinants of the catabolism of normal cellular proteins are being actively debated in a search for an understanding of this phenomenon. Changes in cellular physiology, such as starvation, can accelerate the breakdown of normal cellular proteins by activating lysosomal function. Hormones such as insulin and glucagon are both known to effect the regulation of lysosomal proteolytic function, although the mechanisms by which both the selective proteolysis and its control are brought about are not fully understood. If the intracellular calcium concentration increases, either because of an increased rate of calcium entry into the cell, or from environmentally-induced membrane damage which allows the intracellular calcium levels to rise, normal proteins can be cleaved by the intracellular proteolytic enzyme called calpain, a calcium-activated neutral protease. Oxygen free radicals may be involved, not only because they can damage cell membranes through the presence of protein, but principally because of the ability of the free radicals to induce the formation of lipid peroxides, which then cause chain reactions, so amplifying the original molecular trauma and allowing further calcium entry and calpain activation. Antioxidant activity is therefore important for the control of the calpain-induced peptide bond cleavage which produces the 'unscheduled' formation of protein fragments.

Protein denaturation and misfolding

Protein structure is determined by a large number of interacting forces; frequently only a limited number of structures are physiologically functional. The three-dimensional structure of a protein is influenced by its immediate environment, especially ionic strength, temperature, the concentration of hydrogen ions (pH) and the availability of (stabilising) ligands and cofactors. Alterations in protein structure often produce molecules without the correct conformation to carry out their proper physiological function. Although these denaturation events occur continuously, the denatured molecules do not normally accumulate in the cell because they are selectively degraded by the cytosolic proteolytic system, which also degrades erroneously synthesized proteins (see pp. 23–4). It has been suggested that a protein's spontaneous denaturation rate in fact determines its intracellular half-life. It is interesting to consider that in certain organisms, such as fruit flies, growth at a low temperature increases maximal life span. Whether the expected lower rate of protein denaturation at lower temperatures is involved in this response is unknown. As most events occur relatively slowly at low temperatures, it is likely that the life-extending effects result from decreased rates of insult from the numerous agents known to be involved, directly or indirectly, in the production of altered proteins.

Changes in postsynthetic modification

Many proteins are modified after synthesis, especially those destined to be exported from the cell. Many types of modification occur, each catalysed by specific enzymes of which many are located in the golgi apparatus with others present outside the cell. The attachment of polysaccharide to specific amino acid residues, sometimes amounting to one half of the molecular mass, is required for glycoprotein production. Collagen precursors are glycosylated to a variable extent depending on the type of collagen and the site of its usage.

Other intracellular modifications include hydroxylation, methylation, acetylation, carboxylation, phosphorylation and sulphation. Whether all those polypeptides which are either under- or over-modified are detected by the aberrant protein degradation system and thereby removed is not known. The attachment of non-protein ligands such as metal ions, cofactors and co-enzymes also occurs. This is exceptionally well demonstrated in the case of haemoglobin biosynthesis, during the later stages of which the haem group is attached to the globin. Globin chains which are misfolded and to which the haem group cannot be attached have been clearly shown to be selectively broken down by the aberrant protein degradative apparatus in erythroid cells (Daniels et al., 1983).

Protein processing is another form of postsynthetic modification where a large polypeptide is converted into the one or more smaller active gene product(s) by cleavage of specific peptide bonds. Failure to carry out the correct cleavages may generate abnormal polypeptides. Some evidence for age-associated improper polypeptide precursor processing has been found in the case of the hormone somatostatin: a high molecular weight form which is a possible precursor has been detected in aged rodents.

Non-enzymic, spontaneous protein modification also occurs. Most of the modifications involve the attachment of glucose to a protein's amino groups. Interestingly, glucose is the slowest sugar to carry out this non-enzymic glycosylation, whereas other sugars such as galactose and fructose spontaneously attach to the protein at much faster rates. In diabetics elevated serum glucose levels are reflected by the occurrence of glycosylated haemoglobin, which usefully provides a monitor of the effectiveness or otherwise of the patient's control of his or her glucose level. In long lived proteins, cross-linking between the glycosylated proteins can occur. This has not been detected in short-lived proteins, because they are removed before the slower cross-linking events take place. However the proteins of the lens core are made *in utero* where no protein replacement occurs, and among these non-enzymic glycosylation can be readily detected, especially in diabetics. It is thought that the coloured (brunescent) cataracts isolated from elderly people and from diabetics arise as a result of the non-enzymic glycosylation and subsequent cross-linking and precipitation of the modified crystallin molecules (Monnier and Cerami, 1983).

Glycosylation may also be involved in the alterations to proteins associated with age-related changes in immune response. It is conceivable that there are time-related changes, such as glycosylation and cross-linking, in those body proteins which turn over very slowly to produce 'new or different' proteins. These would be detected by the immune system as non-self, producing the auto-immune phenomena frequently detected with ageing.

FATES OF ABNORMAL PROTEINS

Aggregation
When cells are manipulated to produce proteins of altered amino-acid composition or chain length, the aberrant polypeptides which result often form multipeptide and high molecular weight aggregates. The formation of these aggregates occurs even more readily when the proteolytic system, which selectively degrades aberrant proteins, is saturated with substrate. The nature of the association between the chains appears essentially to be non-covalent. A similar aggregation and decrease in solubility is frequently seen during protein denaturation.

There are several situations in which protein aggregation is a required function. For example, during collagen and keratin synthesis the proteins are secreted from the cells in soluble form, then to be converted into less soluble aggregated forms which are initially held together by hydrophobic forces. Cross-linking between adjacent polypeptide chains through lysine or histidine residues then occurs which decreases further protein solubility and increases the strength of the interpeptide interaction. During the formation of the blood clot which follows the initial conversion of the soluble fibrinogen monomers to the insoluble fibrin multimeric aggregate or clot, further strengthening is brought about by calcium-dependent transglutaminase (factor 13). Its effect is to create cross-links between the glutamine and lysine residues. Such cross-links are refractory to attack by the enzymes which are usually responsible for the elimination of aggregated error proteins.

The α- and β-crystallins in the lens are very high molecular weight multimeric proteins which are held together by various forces including a limited number of disulphide bonds. During the formation of the cataract, however, the number of these bonds between the polypeptide chains increases as a result either of a decrease in the lens' glutathione concentration, which normally keeps most of the crystallin thiol groups in the reduced state, or of changes in the conformation of the crystallins. These permit disulphide bond formation between those parts of the protein molecules which are normally insufficiently close for the bonding to occur.

Non-enzymic glycosylation of proteins results eventually in the formation of interpeptide cross-links. While the nature of the chemistry is both complex and uncertain, it is clear that the rate at which these aggregates are formed is dependent on the nature of the sugar to which the protein is exposed. Glucose is the least reactive sugar, whereas trioses like dihydroxyacetone and glyceraldehyde react almost instantaneously, producing a coloured cross-linked protein complex. These and related trioses are common intermediates in the major pathway of intracellular glucose breakdown (glycolysis) which occurs almost universally. However, it is not known if any of the intracellular proteins become glycosylated by these very reactive sugar molecules, or, if this is the case, what the implications would be. It is theoretically possible that some of the altered proteins which accumulate with age are derived from such postsynthetic changes in their chemistry.

Intracellular proteolysis of abnormal proteins

It is clear that most cells which synthesize proteins possess the ability to degrade, selectively and rapidly, abnormal proteins, including the many mutants, those with shortened chain length and those which do not have the proper ligand or associated cofactor. During the past decade, the proteolytic system or systems responsible for this intracellular 'housekeeping' have been studied in both eukaryotic and procaryotic cells. Some surprising and apparently paradoxical features have emerged.

The degradation of aberrant proteins is frequently but not always energy-dependent (i.e. ATP-dependent). This is surprising because protein biosynthesis is energy-dependent and a superficial understanding of energetics would not suggest that energy is required to reverse an energy-consuming process. A partial explanation lies in the discovery of an ATP-dependent proteolytic enzyme in the 'simple' bacterium *Escherichia coli* and that this enzyme is often required for the initiation of the degradation of this micro-organism's aberrant proteins. At least one more ATP-dependent protease has recently been detected in *Escherichia coli.* When the synthesis of the aberrant proteins exceeds the degradation capacity of the bacterial proteolytic system, the altered polypeptides frequently aggregate, presumably because of the exposed hydrophobic polypeptide surfaces (Katayama-Fujimura, Gottesman and Maurizi, 1987; Kemshead and Hipkiss, 1974).

Research in mammalian cells has also demonstrated that aberrant proteins frequently aggregate before catabolism and that saturation or inhibition of the degradative apparatus causes the non-degraded polypeptides to accumulate as aggregates of increased size. There is, however, another factor which causes the molecular weight of the substrate protein to increase during degradation. All eukaryotic cells contain a small peptide ubiquitin, with an approximate molecular weight of 9000. Prior to a proteolytic attack upon an abnormal protein, a number of ubiquitin molecules become covalently linked to the aberrant protein amino groups to produce a polyubiquitinated protein. Then an ATP-dependent protease, which recognises the much modified polyubiquitinated protein as a substrate, selectively and rapidly degrades the protein. The system responsible for the attachment of ubiquitin, and the subsequent catabolism of the polyubiquitinated conjugates, is located in the non-lysosomal, cytosolic fraction. Once more ATP is required, this time for both the degradation of the conjugate and to attach the ubiquitin to the potential proteolytic substrate. However, the purified ubiquitin-dependent proteolytic system from the reticulocyte, although active against monomeric aberrant globin chains, appears not to function when presented with the very high molecular weight forms of aggregated aberrant protein which accumulate in those reticulocytes which are synthesizing abnormal gene products in large amounts. Because both whole cell and reticulocyte cell-free preparations could degrade the high molecular weight aggregate, another uncharacterised component of the aberrant protein degradation system is clearly required for the disaggregation stage of this surprising and intriguing process.

Of considerable interest is the very recent finding that the enzyme which attaches the ubiquitin to the protein destined for degradation is actually the same protein (RAD 6) which is also important in DNA repair. This evidence suggests that one polypeptide chain carries out separate roles in two very important intracellular homoeostatic functions: DNA repair and the elimination of erroneous proteins. The full significance of this observation to any ageing cell or organism has yet to be explored.

The degradation of some polypeptide fragments, particularly those with low molecular weight, does not require the participation of ATP or ubiquitin. The proteases responsible for the selective degradation of proteins which have been oxidised by oxygen free radicals have also been shown to be ATP-dependent but ubiquitin-independent. The mitochondria of eukaryotic cells have been reported to possess a protease similar to the ATP-dependent protease found in *E. coli*. In both bacteria and nucleated cells, the synthesis of aberrant proteins can induce the biosynthesis of the so-called heat-shock or stress proteins, some of which are proteases, and which in eukaryotes include ubiquitin. This implies that the cell can respond to the production of aberrant proteins by increasing its ability to degrade them (Findlay and Varshavsky, 1985).

It was stated on page 20 that aberrant proteins frequently form high molecular weight aggregates, however it is not certain if the ubiquitin system as presently understood is sufficient for the catabolism of the multimers. It is interesting that one stress protein called hsp 70, the DNA K gene product, is known to play a role in the dissociation of protein clathrate complexes (Chirico, Waters and Blobel, 1988). One speculates that this protein has an important role in the disaggregation of aberrant proteins prior to the proteolytic events. Saturation of the proteases with aberrant proteins or inhibition of proteolytic enzymes both increase the formation of high molecular weight complexes of abnormal proteins. Similarly, in the reticulocyte where cell maturation is accompanied by a decline in proteolytic activity, abnormal proteins accumulate almost exclusively in the form of high molecular weight aggregates. Mixing experiments have shown that cell-free preparations of less mature reticulocytes are able to degrade the accumulated aberrant protein complexes which more mature cells were unable to catabolise.

It is clear, therefore, that cells normally possess at least one system which can selectively remove aggregated and unaggregated abnormal proteins. It has also been shown that if the systems become overloaded or saturated, the cell can respond by producing more of the required enzymes. It should be noted that the stress response does not occur in reticulocytes or in the cells of the lens core because they have lost their nuclei at an earlier stage of their development.

THE ACCUMULATION OF ABNORMAL PROTEINS IN AGED CELLS

The reasons for the accumulation with time of abnormal proteins is a key question in biological gerontology. First principles lead us to alternative but not necessarily mutually exclusive answers: either the production of aberrant proteins increases or their removal decreases.

Increased production of abnormal proteins
Previous sections have outlined the various routes by which aberrant cellular polypeptides arise. In this section the evidence for age-related increases in

aberrant gene expression, protein oxidation, denaturation or modification will be briefly considered.

Increased aberrant gene expression
One of the predictions of the error-catastrophe theory of ageing was that with age there will be increases in erroneous gene duplication and hence gene expression which give rise to a catastrophic accumulation of erroneous polypeptides so that the cell ceases to be viable. While there are many examples of cells having an increased incidence of chromosomal abnormalites with age, it has proved difficult to determine the precise molecular basis for such changes (Hannawalt, 1987). There is little evidence for increased errors in DNA synthesis in aged cells, nor for the proposition that there are increases in erroneous RNA transcription or translation with age. However, it has been shown in cultured human fibroblasts that an increased synthesis of altered proteins, as brought about by treatment with a miscoding drug, does decrease the life span of these cells.

Increased rate of spontaneous changes in protein composition
Some of the spontaneous changes to which long-lived proteins are subject, for example, deamidation and racemisation, are expected to occur at a constant rate since they are not dependent on any biological function. However, it has been shown that more racemised protein is detected in old erythrocytes. It has been suggested that the activity of a system which re-racemises the D-amino acid residues through a methylation process itself declines during the life span of the erythrocyte. A similar observation has been reported of the lens core.

The rates of non-enzymic oxygen free radical production might not be expected to vary with cell age but, should the antioxidant levels alter or the superoxide dismutase activity fall, as has been detected, then the incidence of free radical damage to cellular protein might increase with cell age. Increases in the activity of mixed functional oxidases or the supply cofactors, such as NAD(P)H oxidase, cytochrome p450, xanthine oxidase, H_2O_2, quinones, ATP, ADP and non-haem iron-sulphur proteins, could also increase the rate of free radical generation.

Changes in sugar utilisation which results in increased intracellular mono-saccharide concentrations could increase the rate of spontaneous non-enzymic glycosylation. Some workers have produced evidence in cultured human fibroblasts which suggests that these cells switch from mitochondrial ATP generation to glycolytic production of ATP as a result of the degeneration of mitochondria (see Chapter 3). Increased flux through the glycolytic pathway might increase the steady-state levels of the more reactive sugars (especially trioses) and thereby increase the rate of non-enzymically modified proteins. Why the mitochondria seem to degenerate is not known; it has been suggested that these organelles themselves play an important role in the ageing process. It is interesting to note that mitochondria are the major source of oxygen free radical generation and that there may be only a finite ability to counteract any damaging effects on the organelle's macromolecules (protein, DNA and lipids).

Decreased removal of altered proteins
There is clear evidence that those cells (erythroid cells and lens core) which are predestined to lose their ability to synthesize proteins are also defective in their ability to degrade abnormal polypeptides. Furthermore, should abnormal proteins occur in these cells, the aberrant molecules accumulate as high molecular weight aggregates. The lens core is low in ubiquitin and the enzymes

required for ubiquitin conjugation and the subsequent metabolism of any altered, polyubiquitinated product. One must consider the possibility that in other cases where aberrant proteins accumulate with age, such as in the neuronally-associated amyloid, plaque and tangles, changes in the efficacy of the proteolytic apparatus could be partly responsible. There are reports that during the *in vitro* senescence of cultured human fibroblasts, there is a decline in the ability to degrade some protein fragments (Wharton and Hipkiss, 1985), and protein oxidation products, and an age-related decline in the degradation of puromycin-peptides (i.e. truncated proteins) in mouse liver has also been shown, but as yet few studies using neuronal tissue have been published.

Recent studies of Alzheimer's disease suggest a role for protein catabolism in this condition and possibly in ageing in general. One form of aberrant protein which accumulates in the brain during normal ageing and in very large amounts in Alzheimer's dementia is called amyloid, a multipeptide aggregate of a 43 amino acid residue protein fragment termed the A4 protein (Kitiguchi *et al.*, 1988). This, in turn, appears to be derived from a neuronal cell surface protein about 695, 751 or 770 amino acid residues long. The gene for the A4 protein precursor is located on chromosome 21 which is the extra chromosome in Down's syndrome. Down's syndrome patients also produce large amounts of amyloid in the brain. It is not known why so much of the A4 protein is produced in either the Alzheimer's or the Down's condition. Perhaps one or more of its precursors, the 695, 751 or 770 amino acid residue proteins, are produced in quantities which exceed the catabolic system's ability to cope with it; but why does only the A4 protein accumulate? Perhaps the A4 protein, being almost totally hydrophobic and forming β-sheet multimers, is more refractive to degradation than the remainder of the precursor molecule. It certainly does appear that the breakdown of the protein is incomplete. Tantalisingly it seems that the two larger A4 precursor molecules possess a protease inhibitory sequence which, one speculates, exerts some effect on the catabolism of either A4 or its precursors.

Another example of the incomplete breakdown of neuronal protein is seen in Alzheimer's dementia. This involves paired helical filaments, which are found in small amounts in the brain during normal ageing and in large amounts in Alzheimer's condition, and, as the name implies, are an aggregated form of neuronally-derived proteins. As ubiquitin is found conjugated to them, this appears to be another case of incomplete degradation of an altered protein (Mori, Kondo and Ihara, 1987). Clearly we have much to learn about the catabolism of neuronal proteins and its relationship to ageing. In fact little is known about protein breakdown in general in neuronal tissues. Can neuronal cells carry out the heat shock response and thereby increase the intracellular levels of at least some of the degradative enzymes? Is the A4 protein itself susceptible to degradation in other tissues? Is neuronal tissue low in certain proteases and do these activities remain constant during ageing? Does the high oxygen requirement of neuronal tissues predispose them to oxidative damage? Do the antioxidative systems of the brain decline with age? The homoeostatic systems may slowly decline in efficacy to the point at which there is insufficient activity to remove the altered proteins as they are produced. This allows the accumulation of altered protein and protein fragments. It is particularly likely that protein fragments interact indiscriminately with other cellular macromolecules and interfere with cellular functions. *Nature* does not usually allow the intracellular accumulation of protein fragments because the large battery of enzymes, many with overlapping specificities, facilitates the rapid removal of proteolytic degradative intermediates. However, it has not been demonstrated that the altered proteins which accumulate are themselves pathogenic; it is conceivable that they represent a non-pathological symptom of the absence of another process which is necessary for effective cellular function.

Even less is known about the catabolism of non-enzymically modified proteins. It has been reported that extracellular cross-linked proteins are recognised by scavenging macrophages and mast cells and thus removed, but why do these altered proteins accumulate with age? Does the efficiency of the scavenging cells change with age (Cerami, 1986)? Very little work has been carried out on intracellular cross-linked proteins and whether they are selectively degraded by the homoeostatic proteolytic systems. Interestingly, both ubiquitin conjugation and some ATP-independent proteolytic activities require the availability of the substrate amino groups, but the non-enzymic protein glycosylation and the subsequent cross-linking which occurs at such amino groups would have the effect of permanently eliminating them from recognition by the degradative apparatus. Such modified proteins might therefore show a decreased susceptibility towards the degradative enzymes.

AGE-RELATED DECLINE IN THE REMOVAL OF ABERRANT PROTEINS

The homoeostatic protein degradative system which is responsible for the elimination of altered proteins is itself composed of protein molecules subject to all the postsynthetic modifications and damage which have been described. It is therefore likely that these proteins are also subjected to the same catalogue of insults as the substrates they are supposed to remove, and one envisages that with time there would be a slow decline in degradative activity, especially if the protease replacement rate, i.e. its turnover, is at its highest in young cells and at its lowest in the oldest. At some point the rate of removal of aberrant proteins could become slower than their rate of formation. Thus, one might speculate that in long-lived species there would have to be a high initial level of protease activity: the number of insults to the protein molecules of the homoeostatic system required to lower its functional activity below that necessary for the immediate removal of altered gene products will be greater than in cells of short-lived species. Such measurements have not yet been made, although a similar correlation has been observed for some aspects of DNA repair.

Most nucleated cells are capable of the heat-shock response which involves synthesis of extra proteases and other proteins; altered proteins can also induce the heat-shock response. It is unclear whether this occurs properly in old cells in response to the accumulation of the altered proteins. Perhaps the conformation of the accumulated proteins is insufficiently altered to provoke the response; perhaps the type of altered proteins are not susceptible to proteolysis; or perhaps old cells have a restricted ability to carry out the heat-shock response.

Many proteases are controlled by endogenous inhibitors (mostly polypeptides) and it is possible that the age-related changes outlined above result from changes in protease inhibitor activity or concentration. Unfortunately, because the degradative apparatuses have not been sufficiently characterised, not enough is known about the subtle control and modulation of the critical proteases during cell growth and development. However, the intriguing detection of a protease inhibitor sequence in some of the A4 precursor molecules suggests that this might be an informative line of investigation.

Finally, it is possible that the protein biosynthetic rate could itself determine the proteolytic capacity of the cell towards altered gene products, (e.g. protein fragments). Because mRNA translation is the most error-prone step in gene expression, it follows that to facilitate the rapid removal of error protein, cells which contain more of the ribosomes involved in protein synthesis might possess high levels of the relevant proteases. Support for a relationship between protein synthesis rates and maximal degradative activity towards aberrant proteins has been found in two strains of bacteria, *Escherichia coli* and *Arthro bacter* sp. 55 (Potier *et al.*, 1987). In *E. coli* the maximal rate of error protein catabolism increased logarithmically with the growth rate. It will be important to determine if such a correlation holds for eukaryotic cells, for another common observation of ageing cells is that the rates of protein biosynthesis are lowered. This may be related to the fact that most Metazoa have a finite size limit and it is necessary for these organisms to decrease their protein biosynthetic rate when maximal size (maturity) is reached. Interestingly, transformed cells capable of unlimited duplication synthesize protein at rapid rates and do not show senescence. However, their maximal rates of error protein elimination have not been determined.

CONCLUSION

Many of the problems associated with the production and removal of altered proteins now attract considerable attention, and it is likely that at least some of the factors which promote their production or inhibit their removal will be identified. The conditions can already be envisaged in which abnormal proteins accumulate faster or sooner, as when lower amounts than normal of important proteolytic enzymes or oxygen free radical scavengers are present. If it should prove possible to identify such individuals by assay of accessible tissue such as blood, then the avoidance of situations which provoke the formation of altered proteins or which ensure sufficient antioxidant intake could be beneficial. In the long term it might be possible to activate or reactivate the relevant protease or antioxidant gene or protein, which would increase selectively homoeostatic enzymes to normal levels. Whether the prevention of the accumulation of altered proteins will itself prolong life span is entirely unknown, because it has not been clearly demonstrated that the altered proteins which accumulate are pathogenic in themselves and detrimental to cellular function. These molecules could be non-pathogenic, benign material, and symptomatic of other unidentified homoeostatic defects that prevent cellular proliferation.

The evidence to suggest that the processes which eliminate altered proteins decrease with age is accumulating. Explanations for this decline must lie partly in the intrinsic instability of protein molecules of the cellular homoeostatic proteolytic apparatus and partly in the possible modulation of the enzymes involved. Ageing may be inevitable in complex organisms; indeed it is surprising that we live so long given the multiplicity of insults to which our cells are continuously subjected. Only the homoeostatic systems enable our survival. Maybe if we wish either to live longer or to resist the ravages of time, we should design further homoeostatic systems to repair the repair systems. Whether this is biologically feasible is uncertain, due to the energetic and informational demands upon the cell. The moral and ethical acceptability of such a proposal is another debate.

REFERENCES

A fully documented version of the paper, citing over 80 research papers, is available from the author. The following list concentrates on the principal and most recent papers. Readers new to the biology of ageing should read Chapter 1 before this paper. Students of the biology of ageing will find the collection of papers in H.R. Warner *et al.* (Eds) a particularly useful collection for further reading.

Beutler, E. (1986). Planned obsolescence in human and in other biosystems. *Perspectives in Biology and Medicine*, **29**, 175–9.

Carrier, M.J., Kogut, M. and Hipkiss, A.R. (1984). Changes in intracellular proteolysis in *Escherichia coli* during prolonged growth with a low concentration of dihydrostreptomycin. *FEMS: Microbiology Letters*, **22**, 223–7.

Cerami, A. (1986). Aging of proteins and nucleic acids: what is the role for glucose? *Trends in Biochemical Sciences*, **11**, 311–14.

Chirico, W., Waters, M.G. and Blobel, G. (1988). 70K heat shock protein stimulates protein translocation into microsomes. *Nature*, **332**, 805–10.

Daniels, R.S., McKay, M.J., Atkinson, E.M., Worthington, V.C. and Hipkiss, A.R. (1983). Subcellular distribution of abnormal proteins in rabbit reticulocytes: effects of cellular maturation, phenylhydrazine and inhibitors of ATP synthesis. *FEBS Letters*, **156**, 145–50.

Filion, A.M. and Laughrea, M. (1985). Translational fidelity in the aging mammal: studies with an accurate *in vitro* system on aged rats. *Mechanisms of Aging and Development*, **29**, 125–42.

Findlay, D. and Varshavsky, A. (1985). The ubiquitin system: functions and mechanisms. *Trends in Biochemical Sciences*, **10**, 343–6.

Hannawalt, P.C. (1987). On the role of DNA damage and repair processes in aging: evidence for and against. In H.R. Warner *et al.* (Eds), op. cit., pp. 183–98.

Harman, D. (1987). The free radical theory of aging. In H.R. Warner *et al.* (Eds), op. cit., pp. 81–7.

Katayama-Fujimura, Y., Gottesman, S. and Maurizi, R.M. (1987). A multiple component, ATP-dependent protease from *Escherichia coli*. *Journal of Biological Chemistry*, **262**, 4477–85.

Kemshead, J.T. and Hipkiss, A.R. (1974). Degradation of abnormal proteins in *Escherichia coli*: relative susceptibility of canavanyl proteins and puromycin-peptides to *in vitro* proteolysis. *European Journal of Biochemistry*, **45**, 535–40.

Kitiguchi, N., Takahashi, Y., Tokushima, Y., Shiojiri, S. and Ito, H. (1988). Novel precursor of Alzheimer's disease amyloid protein shows protease inhibitory activity. *Nature*, **331**, 530–2.

Mann, D.M.A. (1985). The neuropathology of Alzheimer's disease: a review with pathogenic, etiological and therapeutic considerations. *Mechanisms of Aging and Development*, **31**, 213–55.

Monnier, V.M. and Cerami, A. (1983). Detection of nonenzymic browning products in the human lens. *Biochimica et Biophysica Acta*, **760**, 97–101.

Mori, H., Kondo, J. and Ihara, Y. (1987). Ubiquitin is a component of paired helical filaments. *Science*, **235**, 1641–4.

Potier, P., Drevet, P., Gounot, A-M. and Hipkiss, A.R. (1987). Protein turnover in a psychrotrophic bacterium: proteolysis in extracts of cells grown at different temperatures. *FEMS Letters*, **44**, 267–71.

Reznick, A., Dovrat, A., Rosenfelder, L., Shpund, S. and Gershon, D. (1985). Defective enzyme molecules in cells of aging animals are partly denatured, totally inactive normal degradation products. In *Modifications of Proteins During Aging*, R.C. Adelman and E.E. Dekker (Eds), pp. 69–82. Alan R. Liss, New York.

Rogozinski, S., Blumenfield, O.O. and Seifter, S. (1983). The non-enzymic glycosylation of collagen. *Archives of Biochemistry and Biophysics*, **221**, 428–36.

Rothstein, M. (1987). Evidence for and against the error catastrophe theory. In H.R. Warner *et al.* (Eds), op. cit., pp. 139–56.

Saul, R.L., Gee, P. and Ames, B.N. (1987). Free radicals, DNA damage and aging. In H.R. Warner *et al.* (Eds), op. cit., pp. 113–29.

Tice, R. and Setlow, R. (1985). DNA repair and replication in aging organisms and cells. In *Handbook of the Biology of Aging*, C.E. Finch and E.L. Schneider (Eds), pp. 173–224. Raven Press, New York.

Warner, H.R., Butler, R.N., Sprott, R.L. and Schneider, E.L. (Eds) (1987). *Modern Biological Theories of Aging*, Aging Series vol. 31. Raven Press, New York.

Wharton, S.A. and Hipkiss, A.R. (1985). The degradation of proteins and peptides of different sizes by homogenates of human MRC 5 lung fibroblasts. *FEBS Letters*, **184**, 249–53.

Alan Bittles

Department of Anatomy and Human Biology
King's College
University of London

3 THE ROLE OF MITOCHONDRIA IN CELLULAR AGEING

INTRODUCTION

During the study of change through time in any biological system, it is frequently difficult to differentiate between causal factors and secondary effects. This is certainly the case in human ageing where the number and complexity of the changes involved may be inextricably bound up with underlying disease symptoms. To be preoccupied with the identification of primary age changes may appear to be of limited immediate consequence, especially to clinicians working in specialties in which the elderly are over-represented. Does it really matter whether the condition under investigation, and possibly requiring treatment, is a primary or a secondary manifestation of ageing? However, in order to successfully unravel the natural histories of many disease entities common in, or even unique to, elderly people, a deeper understanding of the basic cellular mechanism(s) associated with ageing must be a logical starting point.

Throughout the animal and insect world ageing is accompanied by a generalised loss of function. A recent evolutionary explanation advanced for this loss of function, the disposable soma theory, is based on the premise that a balance must be struck between the requirements of the various energy-utilising functions to be met during the life span of an individual (Kirkwood, 1977; Kirkwood and Holliday, 1986). In this respect the allocation of energy resources between reproduction and for the maintenance and repair of non-reproductive body tissue would be of particular importance. The theory therefore proposes that by opting for the strategy of an acceptably rapid rate of reproduction, thus ensuring the future of the species, individual members of that species age because a less than optimal supply of energy is available to facilitate essential cellular maintenance tasks. In somatic cells these can vary from the prevention and removal of damage to deoxyribonucleic acid (DNA), the basic cellular information store, through the surveillance of overall accuracy in macromolecular synthesis and degradation of defective proteins, to the preservation of the functional competence of the immune system.

If the predictions of the disposable soma theory are correct, there should be evidence of an impairment in the energy supply to somatic cells with ageing, and, further, any factor or factors which impede the supply of energy to such cells may precipitate, or at least exacerbate, ageing. It follows that study of the pathways by which individuals produce energy at the cellular level should represent a fruitful area of primary research into ageing. In humans, as in other mammals and insects, energy production is principally the role of the mitochondria, organelles which are found in virtually all cells. The intention of this chapter is to review briefly the means by which mitochondria fulfil their energy-producing role and to examine the experimental evidence for and

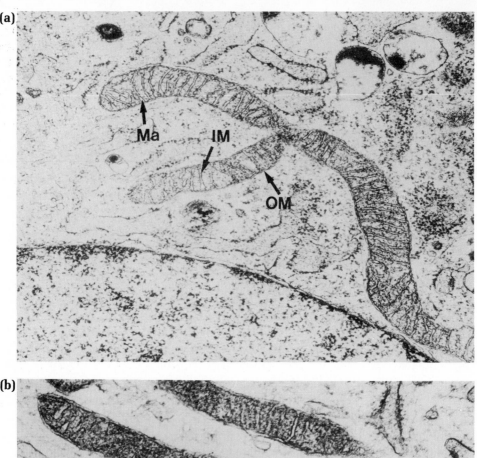

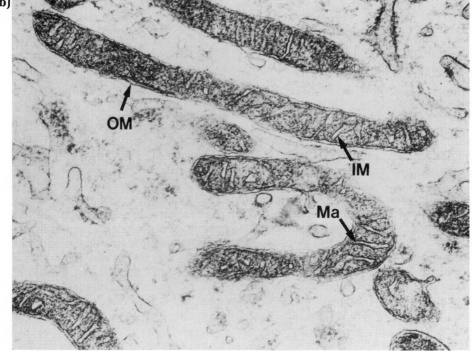

Fig. 3.1 Transmission electron micrographs of human diploid fibroblasts at cell population doubling (CPD): **(a)** CPD 23 and **(b)** CPD 59. The maximum life span of this cell strain is 60 ± 3 CPD. In the cells at CPD 23 **(a)**, the mitochondrial outer membrane (OM), inner membrane (IM) and matrix (Ma) are clearly distinguishable and appear functionally intact. At CPD 59 **(b)**, there is marked degeneration of both the OM and IM. Magnification $\times 35\,000$. Reproduced by kind permission of Dr Yula Sambuy.

against current hypotheses which seek to link ageing to loss of mitochondrial function.

ENERGY PRODUCTION BY THE MITOCHONDRIA

In mammalian systems energy can be obtained from a variety of dietary sources, principally carbohydrates, fats and amino acids derived from protein catabolism. The immediate form of energy used by cells for chemical and mechanical work is adenosine triphosphate (ATP), which is synthesised from the original dietary components either anaerobically (without oxygen) or by the more efficient aerobic pathway. An indication of the relative efficiencies of the two systems is that while one mole of glucose gives two moles of ATP via anaerobic glycolysis, the equivalent yield in the aerobic pathway is 36 moles. In aerobic organisms such as man, energy production is dependent on the tricarboxylic acid (TCA) cycle and the electron transport chain, along which high-energy hydrogen atoms are passed in a series of oxidation-reduction reactions. At the end of the chain the atoms are trapped (or coupled) by the attachment of inorganic phosphate to adenosine diphosphate (ADP) giving ATP, in the process known as oxidative phosphorylation.

The enzymes of the TCA cycle are present in the mitochondrial matrix while the respiratory complexes responsible for electron transport and the enzyme catalysing ATP synthesis, oligomycin-sensitive ATPase, are located in the inner mitochondrial membrane (Tzagoloff, 1983). This means that for optimal efficiency of aerobic ATP synthesis, the maintenance of mitochondrial inner membrane integrity is essential. Most studies aimed at measuring the integrity of the inner membrane have tended to concentrate either on age-related compositional changes or on a search for altered specific activities of the enzymes located therein. However, a more comprehensive assessment of overall mitochondrial competence is provided by two indices (Hansford, 1981): phosphorylation efficiency (P/O) measured in terms of phosphate esterified per unit of oxygen consumed, and the respiratory control (RC) ratio which compares maximal potential activity of the aerobic pathway (state 3 respiration) with respiration in the resting mode (state 4).

MITOCHONDRIAL NUMBERS, SIZE AND STRUCTURE IN AGEING

The currently favoured rationale linking a decline in mitochondrial function with ageing is based on the free radical theory (Harman, 1956). This suggests that changes generally considered as characteristic of ageing can most convincingly be attributed to the destructive action of highly reactive intermediates (free radicals), such as the superoxide radical, and hydrogen peroxide generated in mitochondria as by-products of cellular respiration. Since respiration takes place in the inner mitochondrial membrane, which is rich in polyunsaturated lipids, logically the greatest degree of damage inflicted by free radicals would be expected at this site with peroxidation of membrane lipids and consequent loss of function. A further prediction implicit in the free radical theory is that the rate of mitochondrial ageing/decline should be approximately proportional to the level of oxygen consumption, which effectively raises mitochondria to the status of biological clocks determining cellular life span (Harman, 1983). Some proponents of the free radical theory believe that cellular ageing is the end result of a fundamental imbalance between the

Table 3.1 Age-related changes in mitochondrial number, size and structure.

	Insects	Rodents	Man
Decrease in number	Housefly (Rockstein and Bhatnagar, 1965)	Rat liver (Shamoto, 1968) Mouse liver Mouse heart (Herbener, 1976)	Hepatic cells (Tauchi and Sato, 1968; 1985)
Increase in size	Blowfly, fruitfly, housefly, honeybee, mosquito (Chesky, 1978; Sohal, 1978)	Rat liver (Wilson and Franks, 1975) Rat testis (Johnson, 1984)	Hepatic cells (Tauchi and Sato 1968; 1985)
Structural changes	Blowfly (Sacktor and Shimada, 1972)	Rat pineal (Johnson, 1980)	Lymphocytes (Beregi and Regius, 1983; Beregi, 1986)

disorganising effects of oxygen radicals and mitochondrial DNA (mtDNA) repair (Miquel and Fleming, 1984). Criticism of this hypothesis has centred on the fact that an mtDNA repair system has yet to be demonstrated and the potentially beneficial effect of mitochondrial replication in diluting out defective genomes may have been underestimated (Hart and Turturro, 1987). Significantly, studies on mtDNA during the life span of human cells *in vitro* failed to detect age-related changes in the integrity of the mitochondrial genome or in numbers of mtDNA genomes per cell (Shmookler Reis and Goldstein, 1983).

As is clearly seen in Fig. 3.1, major structural alterations can be observed if mitochondria from young and very old cells are compared. A number of the basic age-related changes in mitochondria, common to many species, are listed in Table 3.1. While it is tempting to accept pan-specific data of this nature as convincing evidence for a central, evolution-driven mitochondrial role in ageing, it is important to stress that the case for suggesting observed alterations in mitochondrial morphology were responsible for the onset and gradual progression of ageing, rather than merely being part of the general expression of senescence, is difficult to sustain. In virtually all cases the insects and rodents studied were old, often close to the end of their expected life span. This also applies to the human examples. The changes reported in lymphocyte and liver cell mitochondria were detected in people between 60 and 80 years of age. Is it reasonable to accept these data as evidence for a causative mitochondrial role in ageing, when they appear to imply that in man ageing does not commence, or at least changes associated with ageing are not expressed, until the seventh decade?

MITOCHONDRIAL ENERGY SUPPLY AND AGEING

For ethical as well as logistical reasons more detailed investigations into mitochondrial function have not and cannot be directly conducted on human subjects. As a result, studies which have been carried out (for example, on the maintenance of the energy supply with ageing) have concentrated on experimental models, principally using insect species and tissue from rodents, or on normal human cells grown in the laboratory from small biopsy samples. The basic problems involved in extrapolating experimental findings from one species to another have been briefly discussed in Chapter 1, and a detailed summary on the use of cultured human cells in ageing research, with ageing defined in terms of the cumulative cell population doubling level (CPD), is set out in Bittles and Sambuy (1986).

In general, the age-related findings obtained from insect and rodent based models have been essentially complementary with respect to mitochondrial energy production. An uncoupling of oxidative phosphorylation was observed in blowflies (Tribe and Ashhurst, 1972) and isolated rat liver (Weinbach and Garbus, 1956), with depressed maximal (state 3) respiration (Weindruch *et al.*, 1980) and reduced ATP synthesis (Clandinnin and Innis, 1983). As declines in mitochondrial protein synthesis (Bailey and Webster, 1984), especially of the inner membrane-matrix proteins (Marcus *et al.*, 1982), and changes in lipids of the inner membrane-matrix compartments have been reported (Clandinnin and Innis, 1983; Lewin and Timiras, 1984), the reduction in ATP production with ageing has been ascribed both to altered mitochondrial membrane protein and membrane lipid composition. However, since lipid changes were claimed in rats at only four months of age, that is, in animals which had just attained sexual maturity (Clandinnin and Innis, 1983), their relationship to ageing could be considered speculative. Investigators have also attempted to test the free radical theory as applied to mitochondrial function. There was no change with ageing in activity of the free radical scavenging enzyme superoxide dismutase (Nohl *et al.*, 1979) and a range of antioxidants, including vitamin E, failed to show any beneficial effect on mitochondrial structural or functional changes in old animals (Johnson *et al.*, 1975; Horrum *et al.*, 1987).

Data from ageing human cells *in vitro* have been less supportive of a role for mitochondrial decline as a cause of ageing. The lower numbers and the greater proportion of abnormal mitochondria reported in the cells of elderly individuals (Table 3.1) were confirmed in some studies of human fibroblasts aged in the laboratory (Lipetz and Cristofalo, 1972; Johnson, 1979) but not in others (Goldstein and Korczak, 1981; Goldstein *et al.*, 1984). Age-related reductions in mitochondrial proton-motive force (Goldstein and Korczak, 1981) and membrane potential (Rugolo and Lenarz, 1987) have been observed, but no change in the activity of oligomycin-sensitive ATPase was detected, even in old cells (Harper *et al.*, 1987). A study of mitochondrial membrane antigens, using antimitochondrial antibodies present in the sera of patients with primary biliary cirrhosis (Ghadiminejad *et al.*, 1987), revealed the presence of antigenic changes in the outer but not the inner membranes of old human fibroblasts, with loss of specific antigens. This would suggest that if there were indeed energy changes with ageing, they may primarily be caused by defects in the outer membrane transport of essential cell nutrients rather than a reduction in oxidative phosphorylation.

The apparent discrepancies between the insect and rodent findings and those obtained with cultured human cells is somewhat puzzling and currently beyond resolution. Two possible explanations can be advanced. There may be a genuine difference between humans and other species in mitochondrial susceptibility to ageing and free radical attack but, given the pan-specific similarities in mitochondrial changes with ageing shown in Table 3.1, this appears improbable. Alternatively, since it is known that anaerobic glycolysis provides a large component of the energy needs of cultured human cells (Sumbilla *et al.*, 1981), it could be that free radical production during cellular life span *in vitro* does not match the levels attained in insects and rodents. Hence the mitochondrial inner membrane of cultured human cells would be less exposed to the resultant effects of free radical attack.

THE STUDY OF AGEING AS AN ENERGY CRISIS

All available evidence, whether from insects, small mammals or human cell cultures, indicates major perturbations in the cellular energy supply with ageing. As indicated above, experimental evidence for a causative role in ageing for mitochondrial decline is currently somewhat equivocal. This may be due not only to variation according to the experimental system and approach adopted, but also because significant age-dependent differences in phosphorylation efficiency (P/O) or in the respiratory control (RC) ratio remain to be proven. A major increase in the utilisation of glucose via anaerobic glycolysis is known to occur in cultured human cells (Bittles and Harper, 1984), with a critical point in mid life span that coincides with altered cellular nucleoprotein organisation (Puvion-Dutilleul *et al.*, 1982). Yet recent studies (Bittles *et al.*, 1988) appear to show that increased glycolysis commences independently of a reduction in the efficiency of oxidative phosphorylation (Fig. 3.2). If mitochondria remain functional with increasing life span *in vitro*, as appears to be indicated by the antimycin A inhibition data, is the concomitant increase in anaerobic glycolysis evidence of a greater cellular energy requirement with ageing? For which specific reactions would such additional energy be required?

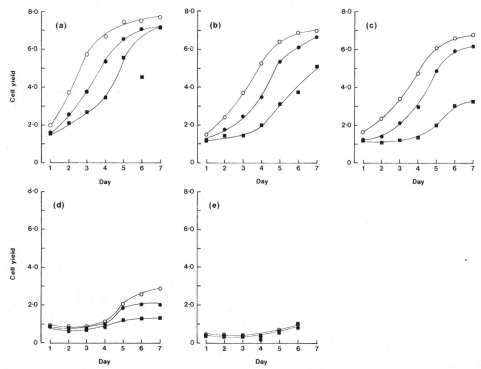

Fig. 3.2 Cell growth and inhibition studies conducted on human diploid fibroblasts at **(a)** CPD 23, **(b)** CPD 33, **(c)** CPD 43, **(d)** CPD 53 and **(e)** CPD 61. The maximum life span of this cell strain is 60 ± 3 CPD. As the cells age their proliferative capacity diminishes becoming particularly marked in the control cells (o—o) after CPD 43. Addition to the growth medium of 3 mM 2-deoxyglucose (■—■), an inhibitor of glucose transport and therefore of glycolysis has a progressively greater effect as the cells age, indicating greater reliance on glycolysis as an energy source. By comparison, the inhibitory effect of 100 nM antimycin A (●—●), which blocks operation of the electron transport chain and thus inhibits aerobic ATP production by the cells, appears not to alter with increasing cell age *in vitro*.

Furthermore, what repercussions, if any, can be predicted to stem from the shift to glycolysis in ageing cells?

Although much less efficient than the aerobic energy-producing pathway, anaerobic glycolysis has the distinct benefit of greater rapidity in ATP synthesis. Therefore, it could have considerable benefits as a means of satisfying short-term cellular energy requirements. However, in many areas of cellular metabolism, a major shift to increased utilisation of one pathway typically may be compensated by a reduction in the activity of one or more others. In young cells a small proportion of the available glucose is degraded via the hexose monophosphate shunt (HMS), where it is a substrate for the synthesis of RNA, DNA and nucleotide enzymes, and the production of nicotinamide adenine dinucleotide phosphate (NADPH), which serves as a hydrogen and electron donor in reductive biosynthesis (Condon et al., 1971). As the proportion of glucose used in anaerobic glycolysis increases, so the probability rises that a limitation will be placed on glucose entering the HMS, which ultimately could restrict nucleic acid synthesis. If, at the same time, NADPH production was adversely affected, there would be a decline in the availability of reduced glutathione, thus tending to negate the ability of cells to mop up hydrogen peroxide and organic peroxides and placing membrane lipids at risk.

A recent report indicated that although the enzymes responsible for catalysing the HMS remain functional in old cells, there is indeed a reduction of more than 50 per cent in glucose flux through the pathway and a significant reduction in the NADPH/NADP ratio (Jongkind et al., 1987). Therefore a logical explanation can be provided for the decline with ageing in the growth of cultured human cells, culminating in senescence and cessation of growth. The next investigative steps must be to identify how and why the switch to anaerobic glycolysis starts in cultured cells, then to determine whether similar changes also occur in animals and/or insects, and, finally, to see if this major change in the pattern of energy supply can be confirmed in human subjects. Only at that point can its real significance in terms of human ageing be assessed.

REFERENCES

Bailey, P.J. and Webster, G.C. (1984). Lowered rates of protein synthesis by mitochondria isolated from organisms of increasing age. *Mechanisms of Ageing and Development*, **24**, 233–41.

Beregi, E. (1986). Relationship between ageing of the immune system and ageing of the whole organism. In *Dimensions in Ageing*, M. Bergener, M. Ermini and H.B. Stahelin (Eds), pp. 35–50. Academic Press, London.

Beregi, E. and Regius, O. (1983). Relationship of mitochondrial damage in human lymphocytes and age. *Aktuelle Gerontologie*, **13**, 226–8.

Bittles, A.H. and Harper, N. (1984). Increased glycolysis in ageing cultured human diploid fibroblasts. *Bioscience Reports*, **4**, 751–6.

Bittles, A.H., Monks, N. and Baum, H. (1988). Differential growth inhibition of human diploid fibroblasts by 2-deoxyglucose and antimycin A with ageing *in vitro*. *Gerontology*, **34**, 236–41.

Bittles, A.H. and Sambuy, Y. (1986). Human cell culture systems in the study of ageing. In *The Biology of Human Ageing*, A.H. Bittles and K.J. Collins (Eds), pp. 49–66. Cambridge University Press, Cambridge.

Chesky, J.A. (1978). Comparative aspects of declining muscle function. In *Aging in Muscle*, G. Kaldor and W.J. Di Battista (Eds), pp. 179–210. Raven Press, New York.

Clandinnin, M.T. and Innis, S.M. (1983). Does mitochondrial ATP synthesis decline as a function of change in the membrane environment with ageing? *Mechanisms of Ageing and Development*, **22**, 205–8.

Condon, M.A.A., Oski, F.A., Di Mauro, S. and Mellman, W.J. (1971). Glycolytic difference between foetal and non-foetal human fibroblast lines. *Nature, New Biology*, **229**, 214–15.

Ghadiminejad, I., Harper, N., Bittles, A.H. and Baum, H. (1987). Age-dependent loss of a mitochondrial antigen in cultured human diploid fibroblasts. *Biochemical Society Transactions*, **15**, 1177–8.

Goldstein, S. and Korczak, L.B. (1981). Status of mitochondria in living human fibroblasts during growth and senescence *in vitro*: use of the laser dye Rhodamine 123. *Journal of Cell Biology*, **91**, 392–8.

Goldstein, S., Moerman, E.J. and Porter, K. (1984). High-voltage electron microscopy of human diploid fibroblasts during ageing *in vitro*: morphometric analysis of mitochondria. *Experimental Cell Research*, **154**, 101–11.

Hansford, R.G. (1981). Energy metabolism. In *Handbook of Biochemistry in Aging*, J.R. Florini (Ed.), pp. 137–62. CRC Press, Boca Raton, Florida.

Harman, D. (1956). Aging: a theory based on free radical and radiation chemistry. *Journal of Gerontology*, **11**, 298–300.

Harman, D. (1983). Free radical theory of aging: consequences of mitochondrial aging. *Age*, **6**, 86–94.

Harper, N., Ghadiminejad, I., Baum, H. and Bittles, A.H. (1987). Mitochondrial enzyme activity during *in vitro* ageing of human diploid fibroblasts. *Biochemical Society Transactions*, **15**, 1176–7.

Hart, R.W. and Turturro, A. (1987). Review of recent biological research in the theories of aging. In *Review of Biological Research in Aging*, Vol. 3, M. Rothstein (Ed.), pp. 15–21. Alan R. Liss, New York.

Herbener, G.H. (1976). A morphometric study of age-dependent changes in mitochondrial populations in mouse liver and heart. *Journal of Gerontology*, **31**, 8–12.

Horrum, M.A., Harman, D. and Tobin, R.B. (1987). Free radical theory of aging: effects of antioxidants on mitochondrial function. *Age*, **10**, 58–61.

Johnson, J.E. (1979). Fine structure of IMR-90 cells in culture as examined by scanning and transmission electron microscopy. *Mechanisms of Ageing and Development*, **10**, 405–43.

Johnson, J.E. (1980). Fine structural alterations in the aging rat pineal gland. *Experimental Aging Research*, **6**, 189–211.

Johnson, J.E. (1984). *In vivo* and *in vitro* comparisons of age-related fine structural changes in cell components. In *Aging and Cell Structure*, Vol. 2, J.E. Johnson (Ed.), pp. 37–88. Plenum Press, New York.

Johnson, J.E., Mehler, W.R. and Miquel, J. (1975). A fine structural study of degenerative changes in the dorsal column nuclei of aging mice. Lack of protection by vitamin E. *Journal of Gerontology*, **30**, 395–411.

Jongkind, J.F., Verkerk, A. and Poot, M. (1987). Glucose flux through the hexose monophosphate shunt and NADP(H) levels during *in vitro* ageing of human skin fibroblasts. *Gerontology*, **33**, 281–6.

Kirkwood, T.B.L. (1977). Evolution of ageing. *Nature*, **270**, 301–4.

Kirkwood, T.B.L. and Holliday, R. (1986). Ageing as a consequence of natural selection. In *The Biology of Human Ageing*, A.H. Bittles and K.J. Collins (Eds), pp. 1–16. Cambridge University Press, Cambridge.

Lewin, M.B. and Timiras, P.S. (1984). Lipid changes with ageing in cardiac mitochondrial membranes. *Mechanisms of Ageing and Development*, **24**, 343–52.

Lipetz, J. and Cristofalo, V.J. (1972). Ultrastructural changes accompanying the ageing of human diploid cells in culture. *Journal of Ultrastructure Research*, **39**, 43–56.

Marcus, D.L., Ibrahim, N.G. and Freeman, M.L. (1982). Age-related decline in the biosynthesis of mitochondrial inner membrane proteins. *Experimental Gerontology*, **17**, 333–41.

Miquel, J. and Fleming, J.E. (1984). A two-step hypothesis on the mechanisms of *in vitro* cell aging: cell differentiation followed by intrinsic mutagenesis. *Experimental Gerontology*, **19**, 31–6.

Nohl, H., Hegner, D. and Summer, K.H. (1979). Responses of mitochondrial superoxide dismutase, catalase and glutathione peroxidase activities to aging. *Mechanisms of Ageing and Development*, **11**, 145–51.

Puvion-Dutilleul, F., Azzarone, B. and Macieira-Coelho, A. (1982). Comparison between proliferative changes and nuclear events during ageing of human fibroblasts *in vitro*. *Mechanisms of Ageing and Development*, **20**, 75–92.

Rockstein, M. and Bhatnagar, P. (1965). Age changes in size and number of the giant mitochondria in the common house fly (*Musca domestica L.*). *Journal of Insect Physiology*, **11**, 481–91.

Rugolo, M. and Lenarz, G. (1987). Monitoring of the mitochondrial and plasma membrane potentials in human fibroblasts by tetraphenylphosphonium ion distribution. *Journal of Bioenergetics and Biomembranes*, **19**, 705–18.

Sacktor, B. and Shimada, Y. (1972). Degenerative changes in the mitochondria of flight muscle from ageing blowflies. *Journal of Cell Biology*, **512**, 465–77.

Shamoto, M. (1968). Age differences in the ultrastructure of hepatic cells of thyroxine-treated rats. *Journal of Gerontology*, **23**, 1–8.

Shmookler Reis, R.J. and Goldstein, S. (1983). Mitochondrial DNA in mortal and immortal human cells: genome number, integrity and methylation. *Journal of Biological Chemistry*, **258**, 9078–85.

Sohal, R.S. (1978). Aging changes in the structure and function of the insect heart. In *Aging in Muscle*, G. Kaldor and W.J. Di Battista (Eds), pp. 211–26. Raven Press, New York.

Sumbilla, C.M., Zielke, C.L., Reed, W.D., Ozand, P.T. and Zielke, H.R. (1981). Comparison of the oxidation of glutamine, glucose, ketone bodies and fatty acids by human diploid fibroblasts. *Biochimica et Biophysica Acta*, **675**, 301–4.

Tauchi, H. and Sato, T. (1968). Age changes in size and number of mitochondria of human hepatic cells. *Journal of Gerontology*, **23**, 454–61.

Tauchi, H. and Sato, T. (1985). Cellular change in senescence: possible factors influencing the process of cellular ageing. In *Thresholds in Ageing*, M. Bergener, M. Ermini and H.B. Stahelin, (Eds), pp. 91–113. Academic Press, London.

Tribe, M.A. and Ashhurst, D.E. (1972). Biochemical and structural variation in the flight muscle mitochondria of aging blowflies, *Calliphora erythrocephala*. *Journal of Cell Science*, **10**, 443–69.

Tzagoloff, A. (1983). *Mitochondria*. Plenum Press, New York and London.

Weinbach, E.C. and Garbus, J. (1956). Age and oxidative phosphorylation in rat liver and brain. *Nature*, **178**, 1225–6.

Weindruch, R.H., Cheung, M.K., Verity, M.A. and Walford, R.L. (1980). Modification of mitochondrial respiration by ageing and dietary restriction. *Mechanisms of Ageing and Development*, **12**, 375–92.

Wilson, P.D. and Franks, L.M. (1975). The effect of age on mitochondrial ultrastructure. *Gerontologia*, **21**, 81–94.

Robert Weale

Age Concern Institute of Gerontology
King's College
University of London

4 EYES AND AGE: VIEWS ON VISUAL HEALTH PROMOTION

Eyesight represents a crossroad between the body and the mind in several respects. If we do not see well we may draw wrong conclusions about the outside world: at best we may misread a word or two; at worst we may miss seeing an obstacle which may be a physical danger. However, poor co-ordination may in some cases produce effects similar to those due to faulty vision. The conclusion to be drawn from this is that we should never make our own diagnosis when there is something wrong. Eye complaints do not go away; they should always receive professional attention, and sooner rather than later: delay can magnify problems.

WHAT DOES THE EYE LOOK LIKE?

The eye is frequently compared with a camera, as Fig. 4.1 illustrates. When we look at an object, light rays pass from it to the glassy surface of the eye, known, because of its hardness, as the cornea. These rays then traverse the pupil which

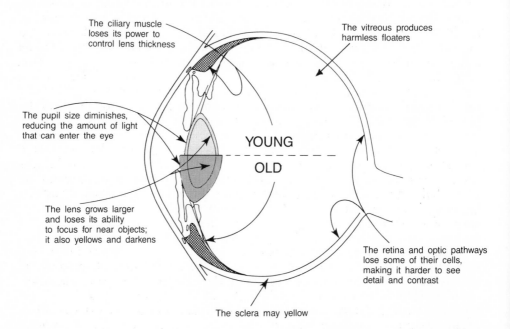

The ciliary muscle loses its power to control lens thickness

The vitreous produces harmless floaters

The pupil size diminishes, reducing the amount of light that can enter the eye

YOUNG

OLD

The lens grows larger and loses its ability to focus for near objects; it also yellows and darkens

The retina and optic pathways lose some of their cells, making it harder to see detail and contrast

The sclera may yellow

Fig. 4.1 Principal differences between the young and the old eye.

is an aperture in the coloured iris. Just behind this black hole, and invisible unless diseased, there is the crystalline lens. The rest of the ocular volume is filled with a jelly, called the vitreous humour. This serves to maintain the spherical shape of the eye, without which smooth eye movements would be impossible. The cornea and the crystalline lens together fulfil the role in photography of the camera lens, forming a minute upside-down image of the outside world on the retina lining most of the inside of the eye.

The retina is an extremely fine and complicated tissue which plays the part of the photographic film: when light rays impinge on it a sequence of chemical changes are initiated. These are converted into electrical impulses, passed by the optic nerve to the brain. Sometimes we 'see the light' i.e. we see phosphenes, shapeless, luminous indications of retinal strain which could lead to detachment. This may happen particularly to short-sighted people. This is an important alarm signal: an eye specialist should be consulted without delay. Although such a symptom is not unknown in young people, it is more likely to occur at a later age – in about one person in three hundred.

SOME ASPECTS OF OCULAR AGEING

While it is impossible to discuss in this chapter the many changes that occur in the eye with advancing years (Weale, 1982), some can be usefully noted because they enable us to think of ways of overcoming certain attendant difficulties. It also needs stating that, because we value our eyes and because the way they work is not straightforward, they may cause concern for no good reason. It is indisputable that the long-term prospects for the eyesight of the elderly are, at best, circumscribed. We live longer and longer, and, as in other parts of medicine, this tends to lead to the manifestation of changes in the body unencountered in the relative brevity of earlier lives. It is no exaggeration to say that prolonging life implicitly tends to promote blindness. The extension of our years of health has, on the whole, been more successful than that of our useful sight. But progress is being made in ophthalmology as in other biomedical fields. Whereas glaucoma, to give one example, was once dreaded because the increased intra-ocular pressure causing this disease could lead to blindness, its effects can now be controlled given a timely diagnosis.

We can easily distinguish old eyes from young ones by the folds and 'crow's feet' in the skin around them. Ageing of the skin is not, of course, confined to the tissue surrounding the eyes: what happens here is merely a result of the general loosening, softening and loss of elasticity of the dermis. These changes rarely affect eyesight. In some cases the lower eyelid may become very loose and tears which are constantly produced fail to flow through the punctum, a small aperture in the inner corner, into the nose. Excessive watering of the eyes needs careful wiping sideways, not downwards, otherwise the problem is likely to worsen. It is also a good idea to wipe each eye with a separate part of a handkerchief or tissue especially if one has a cold. When the eyes tend to be dry expert advice should be sought: a reduction of tear flow as we get older is normal but dryness is not.

Another normal change affects the iris and the pupil of the eye. In general, elderly people have much smaller pupils than the young, and more of the coloured irides can be seen. There is a tendency for the latter to become paler, especially amongst blue-eyed people. This is partly due to the loss of the black pigment, melanin, which underlies the coloured portion. In extreme cases pigmentary particles may clog the channels through which the aqueous humour leaves the eye. This flows through the anterior chamber between the iris and the inner surface of the cornea, and helps to keep the eye spherical. A rise in the intra-ocular pressure, which can be caused by clogging, may lead to glaucoma. Its symptoms can be either ocular pain or the appearance of rainbow-coloured fringes of peripheral vision. About one person in fifty is at some risk, especially those with a family history of this disorder. This is another problem which does not go away, and irreversible damage may ensue if expert advice is not sought at an early stage.

Diminution of the pupils has normal and potentially harmful effects. The pupil admits light to the retina, and the smaller it becomes the less light is available for sight. This is of little consequence by day when there is usually a surfeit of light. But, once it is dark, a reduced pupil can be awkward or a handicap. The situation is aggravated by the fact that our light-sensitive retinae become less responsive as we get older. Age therefore leads to a double handicap: retinae receive less light than they used to, and they also become less efficient in utilising that which they do receive. An increase in illumination provides a remedy, but this must not be done in an indiscriminate way.

READING GLASSES

The need for reading glasses is the most widespread manifestation of ocular ageing. It happens so commonly that gerontologists do not consider it so much a defect as part of normal life. The nub of the problem can be explained by returning to the photographic analogy. When we are young our eyes behave like a camera with an automatic focusing system. Such a camera needs no range adjustment by the photographer: it is directed at the object to be photographed, and the micro-system does the rest. The crystalline lens fulfils this role in the youthful eye (see Fig. 4.1).

When one looks at a nearby object, three events occur by reflex of the appropriate nerves. Firstly, our eyes turn inwards toward the common point of gaze; this ensures that the object in sight is imaged on that retinal part in each eye which is specially developed to detect fine detail, namely the fovea. Secondly, the pupillary diameter constricts, particularly if the object is very close. Photographers will understand that this is equivalent to reducing the aperture of the camera, i.e. it is a way of bringing into focus objects not only in the plane of fixation but also those a few centimetres in front of, and behind, the point of gaze. If this did not occur location in space might prove difficult. Thirdly, the crystalline lens becomes thicker, and moves effectively slightly forward within the eye, thereby increasing the optical power of the eye. Note that a camera can achieve this only by movement of the lens.

These reflexes change with age, but it ought to be stressed that ageing begins in childhood. The reflexes are best developed in infants and progressively lose their efficiency. It is when we become aware of something being amiss that we start to fumble for reading glasses.

We have already noted that age causes a progressive diminution of the pupillary size, which is actually at its largest in early teenage. This reduction is paralleled by the decreasing ability of the lens to change shape to accommodate the imaging of nearby objects: we say that the power of accommodation is diminished, and finally lost, giving rise to presbyopia – literally eyesight of the elderly.

The causes of presbyopia are only now beginning to be understood. Although it has been argued that the process can be defied, experience does not bear this out. However, there are important variations in its incidence. In the United Kingdom the average onset of presbyopia is near the age of 45, while in warmer countries it occurs much earlier: near the equator the onset is estimated at around 30 years of age. Moreover, even in temperate zones significant variations occur. For example, if someone is short-sighted, and thus cannot see objects in the distance without glasses, there may not be any need for reading glasses for close work: such people frequently manage by simply removing the glasses they need out of doors.

THE AGEING CRYSTALLINE LENS

The loss of ability to accommodate is not the only problem associated with the crystalline lens. We noted earlier that the pupil controls the amount of light that reaches the retina, on occasion necessitating the provision of additional illumination to satisfy visual requirements. The lens also influences retinal illumination but in a different way. As well as providing an aid to focusing, it acts as a light filter.

The young lens is faintly yellow. With advancing years the colour becomes more intense and darker. Although this change is progressive, it accelerates after the age of about 40 years. The young lens characteristically transmits 30 per cent of the blue light of the sky, but at the age of 80 years it passes only one tenth of this amount (two to three per cent). Since the change is relatively slow, individuals are not normally aware of it happening: the sky does not appear dark in bright sunshine. But what does happen, and can be revealed by suitable tests, is that the balance of colours perceived differs between young and old. Those who prided themselves when young on their aesthetic sense should, in later years, be guided by younger eyes when choosing daring ties or textiles.

The reduction of the pupillary diameter and the yellowing and darkening of the crystalline lens together reduce the amount of light reaching the retina by a factor of three or more. This becomes important when light is scarce. Homes for, and of, the elderly should not minimise lighting in toilets, corridors and staircases: it is not sound economics to save a few pounds on lighting only to spend a great deal more on repairing broken legs or hips. The economics of lighting raise another problem in connection with the ageing lens, which has only lately received attention. It has been found that when blue light of the intensity of a clear sky strikes a crystalline lens the radiation is transformed within the lens into greenish light. This phenomenon, known as fluorescence, is widespread and associated particularly with ultraviolet light. If, for example, ultraviolet light is directed at teeth, real ones are easily distinguished from false, because the natural material fluoresces. In the lens, such fluorescence is harmless but irritating as it presents the retina with a 'haze' superimposed on the outside world. This makes for fuzzy vision. The remedy seems simple: the eyes ought to be screened from blue light if we are at all worried by the haze accompanying bright sunlight. They should either be shielded with the brim of a hat or a peak, or yellowish sunglasses should be worn. It remains to be investigated whether domestic fluorescent tubes, which radiate considerable amounts of ultraviolet light, cause some slight handicap to elderly people as a result of fluorescence. It is unlikely, both as regards natural daylight and artificial light, that all elderly people will be equally affected. Those suffering from a certain type of cataract are more likely to feel a little uncomfortable as a result of fluorescence.

A cataract is a disease of the lens which interferes with the normal passage of light. In a small number of people the haze associated with cataracts vanishes some time after it has first appeared. However, in most cases it either stays or intensifies. There are about a dozen different types of cataract associated with a variety of causes such as excessive heat from a steel furnace, radio-active material, certain poisons and old age. In the latter instance, one refers to senile cataract. It is not an inevitable effect in old age, even though it is the greatest cause of blindness in the world. It is thought that up to 40 million people, equivalent to almost two-thirds of the population of this country, are blind as a result of cataract. By far the greatest number of sufferers live in tropical or sub-tropical countries. This type of blindness is, however, preventable as the necessary surgery is now relatively simple, safe, and successful. It is primarily economic and cultural obstacles which prevent the speed and ubiquity of medical intervention needed to control this avoidable scourge.

In this country it has been estimated that about one person in a thousand is likely to develop a cataract soon after the age of 60. The prevalence rate doubles with age every six or seven years until, at the age of about 100 years, it has risen to something like one in ten. For reasons not yet clear, women are thought to be at a greater risk than men, although it is fair to say that not all studies have reached this conclusion (Halevi and Landau, 1962; Weale, 1981). Even amongst the elderly, some people are comparatively protected while others are more at risk. For example, many experts believe that those who are short-sighted (myopic) are more likely to develop a cataract than those whose eyesight is normal or long-sighted.

Even among those with medium-severe myopia, the chance of a cataract has been estimated to rise tenfold. Diabetes is also a well-established risk factor, although the associated cataract has to be distinguished from a strictly senile cataract. Diabetic cataracts happen to develop sometimes in later life, but their cause is known, unlike senile cataracts. Some experts believe that at least one of the sub-groups of senile cataract is due to the prolonged exposure of the eyes to sunlight (Zigman, 1980). This does not mean half an hour's stroll outdoors in northern Europe or even a fortnight's over-exposure in Florida. It is the result of spending decades of one's life in the sunniest climate zones, such as those of India, Arabia, or most parts of Africa, without any ocular protection. The link between strong sunlight and cataracts in inter-tropical regions is, however, in dispute, for these areas of the world may exert other possible causal influences which are rare, if not altogether absent, in temperate zones. One of them is the intensity and frequency of diarrhoea. It has recently been found in a study in India that, if a person has suffered from at least one really serious bout in his or her childhood, then there is a considerable likelihood of a cataract developing later in life: with two such bouts one is dealing almost with a certainty (Minassian et al., 1984).

While we are clearly unsure about the multifarious causes of this condition, as we have seen it is remediable by surgery. The precise details of the requisite operation do not concern us here. Suffice it to say that, under general anaesthesia, the specialist makes a small incision in the cornea of the eye (see Fig. 4.1), and removes part or all of the opacified lenticular tissue. In western countries in the past, and at present in the majority of the less industrialised and maximally affected countries, the cornea is then stitched so that the wound may be closed, and the healing processes can begin. Since the patient has lost the crystalline lens, vision is very out-of-focus: an external substitute is provided with rather thick and none too fetching glasses, or perhaps contact lenses. However, the technique of implanting a substitute lens into the eye is now so advanced that it is widely used in industrialised countries, including the UK. The lens is made of light plastic and its optical power is made to suit the patient's visual requirement. It is attached with two springs to the iris.

Sometimes a slight film is formed over the implant after the operation. This is no cause for alarm as it is easily removed by harmless laser treatment.

SENILE MACULAR DEGENERATION (SMD)

This condition is one of the prime causes of registrable blindness in the UK. It was noted earlier that the retinal region which subserves the perception of fine detail is called the fovea. Relatively good vision extends, however, a little beyond this area: clinically the larger region is called the macula, because earlier clinicians thought the fovea to be co-existensive with the yellow spot, or macula lutea, visible round the fovea when the inside of the eye is examined with an ophthalmoscope. The loss of acute vision is an early symptom of SMD. One distinguishes broadly at least two types of the disease, but what matters to the individual is its time course. In some cases it is arrested at a comparatively mild stage, in others it tends to be progressive. SMD is thought to be a degenerative disease, and no definite cause has so far been identified. However, this has not prevented speculation and a diverse range of aetiological studies from being pursued.

Both in glaucoma and perhaps in cataract, genetic factors have been implicated. As regards senile macular degeneration, they seem to be less obvious, but cannot be ruled out. The reason is that one of the so-called risk factors associated with SMD is the colour of the iris which is genetically determined. This does not mean that having a certain iris colour is the cause of the disease, but only that in a large population a significant correlation has been found between blue irides and the presence of the disease. However, since iris colour is a heritable characteristic, it is possible that this is also true of the predisposition for SMD. In point of fact, the situation is more complicated and more interesting than this brief sketch would indicate. Several studies have shown that there is an inverse relationship in the occurrence of certain types of cataract on the one hand to SMD on the other. Both in India and in southern Africa there is a large prevalence of cataract but comparatively little SMD. Even in Scotland, a country noted neither for its tropical conditions nor for alimentary epidemics, a statistically significant inverse relationship has been noted between the two ophthalmic conditions.

For this and other reasons, over-exposure to light has again been advanced as a possible cause of SMD (Mainster, 1987). That some types of cataract cut down the amount of light reaching the retina and therefore protect it from the rays allegedly generating SMD is a possible explanation. But what about the blue iris? Some 25 years ago it was found that blue irides, or more strictly non-brown ones, tend to be perforated and therefore to transmit a great deal of light through their tissues. Pupils normally constrict when strong light reaches the retina: the constriction is achieved by the extension of the tissues of the iris which unfold in the process. However, if the iris is perforated then the unfolding will reveal its perforations. Whereas it may be difficult for light to pass through the folded tissue, its passage will be facilitated once the iris is stretched flat. This means that throughout life non-brown irises will transmit more light than heavily pigmented ones. Among elderly people these associations may be strengthened because, as previously noted, their pupils tend to be permanently more constricted. While light has not therefore been demonstrated to be a principal cause of SMD, it is a prime candidate. The good news is that if this hypothesis were shown to be correct, an obvious cure would be at hand.

PROBLEMS OF PREVENTION

There are three broad areas of practical concern in relation to elderly people's sight. *(i)* What can be done to make things easier for those who have normal but senescent eyesight? *(ii)* What relief can be afforded to those affected by diseases prevalent amongst the elderly? *(iii)* How can we minimise, or altogether prevent, the occurrence of adverse eye conditions?

Adapting to senescent sight

Coping with normal losses of visual ability calls for common sense rather than research. Enough is known for us to be able to say confidently that, within limits, many elderly people benefit from better lighting of the right sort. The reason is that their perception of contrast, notably of smaller objects, is reduced, and improved illumination tends to compensate for this deficit.

Occasionally the lighting requirements of elderly people are antagonistic to those of the majority. But in the design of domestic environments there are many instances where minor alterations would be important improvements without causing any difficulty elsewhere. For example, modern light sockets would be more visible on white walls if the mobile switch stood out against the plastic mount. Any digital display of information about exits, time, toilets, first aid, and telephones should maximise visibility and legibility. In many cases adequate visibility of information may be achieved only by the introduction of self-luminous keyboards or alphanumerics. The cost is likely to be far out-weighed by the attendant advantages: sometimes, the problem is a lack of awareness, sometimes it is merely the absence of a mechanism for off-setting the costs borne by one party with the benefits reaped by another.

The operational solution to the widespread social problem of insensitivity is for young designers to provide themselves with glasses and filters which physically mimic the broad data of senescent eyesight. This would promote the modification of artefacts so as to make them more visible. An additional decremental factor ought to be allowed for, as the deficits due to senescence are not just optical: in other words, the enhancement of contrast should often be accompanied by one in size. But any improvement would be a step in the right direction.

The provision of relief from ocular disease

Not all curative procedures for diseases of the eye need involve surgery. For example, the effects of hypertension and some types of glaucoma can be dealt with by medication. There are reports that drugs are also effective in the treatment of certain types of cataract. But the verification of some claims takes a long time to complete, and doctors have also to satisfy themselves that any new drug, even if effective in its prime objective, is certain to be safe as regards possible side-effects.

One impediment to the timely diagnosis of disorders of the inner eye is the patient's tardy realisation that something may be wrong when there is neither pain nor visual handicap. There are at least two reasons for this sensory ignorance. We have two eyes that tend to cover for each other. Many people, not just the elderly, lead normal lives without being aware that one eye is defective; their good eye sees what the other overlooks. The other reason for not noticing a disorder is that it is normal for one eye to be dominant. That is to say, messages sent to the brain from one eye preponderate over those sent by the fellow eye, as has been demonstrated by electrical recordings from certain areas of the visual cortex at the rear of the brain.

A solution to these difficulties might be provided by basic health training for young and old, but mainly the latter, as they are more at risk. Any self-testing should be done on each eye in turn, while the other is covered. In this way one can do simple tests for fuzzy vision. Vision should normally be sharp, and, if a person has had acute and well-defined vision when young, then reduced acuity is not hard to detect.

A slightly more complicated but clinically more valuable test is to scan one's visual fields. This can be done by fixing a small object like a dark postage stamp to a light background at a distance of about one metre. One eye being covered, the other looks at the stamp, mere detection being what is wanted. Then the person proceeds to look away from the target in all possible directions in gradually increasing steps up to two or three metres distant. In some directions the nose will form an obstacle making the target invisible. In others, it will be the upper brow. But within easily learnt limits, the stamp should be visible except when the left eye looks roughly one-third of a metre to the right of the target, and, similarly, the right one to the left of it. In those two cases the target is imaged on the blind spot of each eye, and failure to see small targets at those points in the two separate visual fields is normal. If the stamp is consistently missed elsewhere then this may be clinically significant and needs attention.

Given the necessary understanding on the elderly person's part, such self-screening can only be useful. No competition with professional experts is at stake, no misdiagnosis can occur, and, at worst, we may have to deal with some false positive responses. The advantages of this type of health training are too obvious to need pleading.

The prevention of eye disorders

Applied gerontology can be divided into palliative and preventive branches, and these two approaches apply when the effects of ocular senescence are tackled. In large measure, the recommendations made above are palliative. When it comes to the prevention of deleterious effects, one finds oneself in a very different field, where research is at a premium, and where one more often needs to deal with the young than the old.

This paradox is easy to illustrate by a reference to the effects of smoking. The consequences of continued heavy smoking may not appear till in late years. Even then they may remain latent, and only be revealed if another systemic insult is experienced. Genetic disposition, environmental effects and accidents are difficult to disentangle, but, in so far as they may contribute cumulatively to any one condition, preventing them early on may play a role in later life.

As regards the eye, diabetes, a systemic disease, may cause retinal problems and also cataract. If the chance of diabetes occurring can be reduced, for example, by appropriate dietary means, the statistics of the concomitant ocular conditions will probably change. It is equally likely that hypertensive diseases of the eye may be altogether modified by a control of those diets known to lead to obesity. Where diet is involved one is moving from strictly clinical to cultural spheres, and nowhere is the problem of possible prevention illustrated in this context more clearly than when it comes to myopia. We have mentioned the correlation between myopia and cataract, and there may even exist a physiological link between the two conditions. This would not be an isolated example. The size of the crystalline lens and the incidence of some types of glaucoma are connected: the continual, lifelong growth of the lens is normal, but takes place differently in various ethnic groups. At present we do not know whether lenticular growth can be controlled: to do this would be useful because one could modify a predisposition for glaucoma in some people. It may be possible to control the incidence of myopia, because it has been found that the predisposition for this condition is increased significantly if one does at least two hours of close work every day when young.

CONCLUSION

It is fitting that one should return to the view which stresses that old age is merely the continuation of lifelong development. Its onset is indefinable, for senescence varies from person to person, from organ to organ, from tissue to tissue, and also from one part of the world to another. It is useful to repeat the distinction between the palliative and the explorer's approach to the problems that arise. As was indicated, some visual difficulties can be solved with a little thought and consideration for others. But the very consideration shown toward elderly people which the mores of earlier ages taught us, may now have to be extended to the young. For if there is a link between myopia and cataract, we may reduce the prevalence in old age of the latter by minimising the former amongst the young. However, reducing myopia may well involve an interference with the established pattern of schooling and further education.

The armed forces of the USA already suffer from a shortage of pilots with normal vision: too many of otherwise suitable candidates are myopic, presumably because they have been studious types. Would you entrust your personal safety or that of your country to semi-literate personnel in order that myopia may be less frequent and the incidence of senile cataracts reduced?

REFERENCES

Halevi, H.S. and Landau, J. (1962). Hospitalized senile cataract in different Jewish communities in Israel. *British Journal of Ophthalmology*, **46**, 285–90.

Mainster, M.A. (1987). Light and macular degeneration: a biophysical and clinical perspective. *Eye*, **1/2**, 304–10.

Minassian, D.C., Mehra, V. and Jones, B.R. (1984). Dehydrational crises from severe diarrhoea or heatstroke and risk of cataract. *The Lancet*, **1** (8380), 751–3.

Weale, R.A. (1981). Physical changes due to age and cataract. In *Mechanisms of Cataract Formation in the Human Lens*, G. Duncan (Ed.), pp. 47–70. Academic Press, London.

Weale, R.A. (1982). *A Biography of the Eye: Development – Growth – Age*. H.K. Lewis, London.

Zigman, S. (1981). Photochemical mechanisms in cataract formation. In *Mechanisms of Cataract Formation in the Human Lens*, G. Duncan (Ed.), pp. 117–49. Academic Press, London.

Anthony Warnes

Age Concern Institute of Gerontology
and Department of Geography
King's College
University of London

5 THE AGEING OF POPULATIONS

The uniformity of (the ageing) process is one of the earliest unpleasant discoveries that every individual has to make, and although we have many psychological expedients to blunt its impact, the fact of this effective fixity of the life span, and of the decline in activity and health that often determine it, is always in the background of the human mind.

(Comfort, 1979)

Viewed as a whole the 'problem of aging' is no problem at all. It is only the pessimistic way of looking at a great triumph of civilisation . . . with a peversity that is strictly human, we insist on considering the aggregate result of our individual success (at achieving our goal of individual survival) as a 'problem'.

(Notestein, 1954)

Inquisitiveness about the processes of individual and population ageing extends well beyond academic concerns in biology, medicine or the social sciences. Consciousness of and introspection upon ageing and mortality is surely universal among human beings; it evinces human intelligence and awareness. We are conscious of the ageing of ourselves and our children, parents and most intimate confidants, although it is also true that sometimes during periods of stability in our lives the passage of time appears to have been arrested. The accommodations that are made to the existence of ageing are not only personal and familial: since the emergence of literate cultures, they have been an important stimulus for among the most profound imaginative and philosophical treatises and a foundation for the most sophisticated and widely adopted religious doctrines.

This chapter has several themes and begins with an examination of the nature and connections between the ageing of individuals and the changing age structures of populations. The imprecise term, *'demographic ageing'*, refers to populations with an increasing share in the older age groups: the recent progress and projections of this phenomenon in various parts of the world and in some special populations will be reviewed. The final sections will examine the relationships between the most advanced stages of demographic ageing and the prevalence and age-distribution of certain measures of ill-health (morbidity) and social dependency, with emphasis upon the implications for social policies about retirement incomes, health and social service funding, and the support of frail elderly people and their carers.

Grateful acknowledgement is made to The Simon Population Trust for their support for some of the research reported in this chapter. Ashley Horsey, the research assistant on the project, prepared some of the projections and tabulations. My thanks also to Philip Rees of the University of Leeds for his contributions to our collaborative research.

DEFINITIONS AND USAGES OF AGEING

Senescence

Ageing as senescence is a 'general title for a group of effects that, in various phyla, lead to a decreasing expectation of life with increasing age' (Comfort, 1979). It is not intrinsic to all organisms; for example, bacteria can divide indefinitely and many plants are capable of unlimited vegetative propagation (Kirkwood and Holliday, 1986). While a maximum potential life span appears to be a characteristic of mammals and warm-blooded vertebrates, it is not established which species experience senescence, partly because in wild populations mortality due to environmental causes is so high that few members of a species attain long life. It is necessary to distinguish, as far as it is possible, the intrinsic age-related rise in susceptibility to death from the mortality associated with the duration of exposure to environmental insults. Glass beakers rarely have a long life, but not because an intrinsic chemical or structural characteristic increases the likelihood of breakage with time.

Age-distributions, mortality rates and survival curves

All biological populations are composed of individuals with variable character-istics and environmental exposures. The age of death of an individual is therefore a poor guide to the average expectation of life which must be determined by the probabilities of death at different ages in a large population. The survival curves for many mammals and for human populations until this

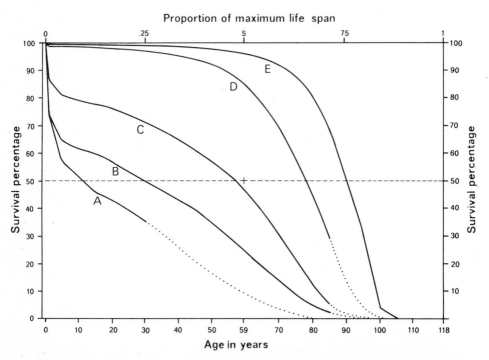

Fig. 5.1 Survival curves for various human populations: **A** Manchester, England, early 1840s (Playfair, 1845); **B** United States, non-white males, 1900–02 (NCHS, 1985); **C** United States, white males, 1900–02 (NCHS, 1985); **D** United States, total population, 1982 (NCHS, 1983); **E** Hypothetical western population with minimum disorders (Benjamin, 1986).

century reveal two major sources of mortality: that from the malign effects of predators, pestilence and privation; and that associated with the rising intrinsic susceptibility with age.

The range of mortality conditions among both contemporary and national populations in Britain during the last 150 years is quite remarkable. Mortality statistics for the insanitary and congested industrial towns of Lancashire during the early 1840s showed that a quarter of those born in Manchester died before one year of age: nearly half died before they attained 5 years of age (Fig. 5.1). So few people lived beyond the age of 60 years that it is impossible to assess the ageing effect on mortality schedules for these towns. Mortality which is more clearly associated with senescence is however evident among contemporary western populations, as exemplified by the life table for the United States in 1982 (curve D of Fig. 5.1). The survival curves from earlier dates show that infant and child mortality have been enormously reduced in recent decades. Death rates now remain very low until individuals reach their early fifties: thereafter the exponential increase in the probability of death is clearly apparent.

The forms of the mortality and survival curves in privileged human (or domesticated mammal) populations have been one starting point for an impressive range of theoretical ideas and empirical investigations concerning ageing. (For substantial reviews see Comfort, 1979; Warner et al., 1987.) One of the earliest formal descriptions of the relationship between age and mortality by Gompertz (1825) suggested that it approximated to a simple exponential, i.e. the rate of mortality starts at a relatively low level, the basal vulnerability, and

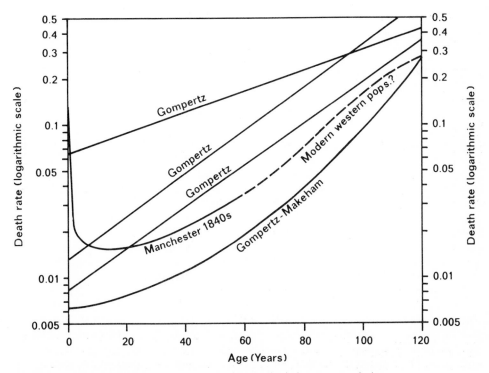

Fig. 5.2 The relationship between age and mortality in human populations.

with time increases at an increasing rate. The equation has been represented variously but the fundamentals can be set down as:

$$D_x = D_0 e^{ax}$$

or,

$$\ln(D_x) = \ln(D_0) + ax$$

where D_x is age specific mortality at age x; D_0 is the basal vulnerability (mortality rate at birth); a is the 'rate of actuarial ageing'; ln is lognormal or natural logarithm; and e is the base of natural logarithms.

The concept of basal vulnerability has been useful in fitting different populations to the function, for changes in D_0 have a more significant effect on initial mortality rates than on those in later life. As D_0 falls, the survival curve becomes more rectangularised, or has a longer initial period of low mortality, as with the contrast between curves A and D of Fig. 5.1 (Hart and Turturro, 1987). For privileged human and domestic animal populations, the fit is poor without the addition of another constant, known as the Makeham term, b, which increases further the rectangular form of the survival curve and allows a longer plateau of low mortality at younger ages:

$$D_x = (D_0 e^{ax}) + b$$

A Gompertz-Makeham and several Gompertz mortality functions are shown on Fig. 5.2. One feature of the mortality schedules of human populations which is not well represented by the Gompertz-Makeham function is the decline in mortality rates during the first days and months of life. This is a feature of the age–mortality relationships in 1840s Manchester, among the United States populations at the beginning of this century (curves B and C of Fig. 5.1), and in many Third World populations today. The substantial departure of these conditions from the Gompertz function is clearly shown on Fig. 5.2: they are better fitted by a second degree exponential of the form:

$$D_x = D_0 e^{-bx + ax^2}$$

or,

$$\ln(D_x) = \ln(D_0) - bx + ax^2$$

where b is the initial rate of worsening mortality.

Information is scarce about the form of the age–mortality relationship in extreme old age, say, over 85 years, but whether there is a moderation of the rate of increase of mortality among centenarians if not earlier is disputed (Barrett, 1985; Kannisto, 1988). Demographers and actuaries have not, until recently, been greatly concerned with the mortality of the few people that survive to these ages, but now an intensive interest exists in the changing lethality of the most common diseases of old age and the prevalence of different states of health. The mortality curve in extreme old age is tentatively represented by a third term in the Gompertz equation (Fig. 5.2).

Temporal change in the age distribution of populations

Populations are intriguingly dynamic and in biological examples it is as common for the average age to be declining as increasing. This has occurred more rarely in human populations, but if the birth rate rises, or if mortality in the first minutes or months of life declines, the average age falls. These dynamics apply to both special human populations and to the universes of human artefacts: the principles have been applied to phenomena as diverse as automobiles, lightbulbs and nuclear reactors. Gerontology is interested in these processes as they apply both to several special human populations, such as grandchildren, general practitioners or nurses, and to inanimate objects such as dwellings and residential institutions.

Public concern about the ageing of western populations has recently spread but sometimes the understanding is naïve and often 'ageing' is used loosely. A straightforward measure of ageing is the average age, but this abstract quantity conveys little meaning and is rarely employed. A more common usage is for 'ageing' to refer to an increase in either the absolute size of the elderly population or its relative share. This shifts the problem to the delineation of old age, a matter which is often seen as tedious and trivial but which requires consideration of far from facile questions of the way a society structures and characterises this period of life.

In contemporary western societies the elderly population is practically synonymous with those who have reached the ages during which the status of full-time employee is proscribed. Different ages are employed by nations in legislation or regulations about the age of entitlement to state pensions or old age benefits, or for privileged access to and charges for medical services. There is also considerable variation among nations in the directions of change of these eligibility ages. During much of the twentieth century, there has been a consensus among the representatives of labour, employers and social reformers for incremental reductions of the age of retirement. Extensions of the period of retirement have allowed the older population of a country to share in the rising material standard of life of western countries and permitted the labour force to be reduced during periods of economic recession. A contrary view; that early, mandatory retirement serves neither the interests of individuals nor of national economies; has also been evident, particularly in periods of labour shortage and among those who argue that at least for a minority of people work is a source of identity, self-esteem, satisfaction and social opportunity as well as income.

These questions are debated thoroughly elsewhere: demographic analysis must adopt a working definition of ageing and therefore a lower age boundary of being old. It is unhelpful if different national statistical organisations tabulate their age structures using different definitions. The most common recommendation is to use the age of 60 years as the cut off.

PROCESSES OF DEMOGRAPHIC AGEING

The age structure of a human population is a complex record of the demographic conditions which it has experienced over the previous century. It is influenced by the year-by-year histories of births or additions to the population, by the survival or life expectancy of successive cohorts, and by gains and losses through migration. For many large national populations, although not for countries as diverse as the USA, Israel, Kampuchea or the Republic of Ireland, external migrations during the last half century have been relatively unimportant. The principal task is therefore to understand the influence of the levels, age distributions and trends of mortality and fertility on population age structure.

In many biological populations only a minority of individuals attain even half of their potential life span. A very high rate of mortality, associated very often with a hostile environment, bears on individuals from the moment of birth. The resulting age structure is heavily weighted towards young individuals. We have seen that such conditions adequately describe extremely disadvantaged human populations. The effect can be sufficient to prevent a high proportion of individuals reaching an age at which they reproduce, which therefore interacts with fertility. But normally in these populations high fertility complements high mortality and the population pyramid is broad based and approaches a triangular form. The average age and the age distribution is a function of mortality and fertility in the recent past.

There is no better demonstration of the achievement of modern human societies than that their survival curves have been improved to the point at which a majority of lives attain half the potential life span. (Maximum human longevity, and whether it is changeable, is still in dispute: here it is assumed to be 118 years (Hayflick, 1987).) This remarkable and unprecedented change is associated with innumerable social, economic and technological changes – in particular the relative contributions of medical practice and of public hygiene have been vigorously debated (McKeown, 1976). The success in combating mortality, and in achieving such a marked change in the survival curve, has increased the importance of fertility fluctuations on age structure. If the annual total of births has been increasing over the last 80 years, the population pyramid will still have a broad base and sloping sides. If, however, the annual total of births has been falling, the pyramid may appear as a steepled church tower and may even have overhangs and will always be steep-sided. The age distribution will feature low percentages of the young and higher proportions of people aged more than half the life span.

These relationships have been described using long-term projections of populations with unchanging or stable age-specific fertility and mortality schedules. After many decades the population approaches a stationary age and sex structure, whether it is increasing or decreasing in size. These theoretical exercises demonstrate that at the levels of mortality which prevail in the world today, it is indisputably the level of fertility which has most influence on the average age and the elderly share of the population (Clark and Spengler, 1980). What is not yet fully understood, however, is the impact of substantial further improvements in late age mortality.

THE AGEING OF NATIONAL POPULATIONS IN THE TWENTIETH CENTURY

National populations have only recently departed from a relatively youthful age structure. As late as 1880, only France, Belgium, Sweden and Norway had more than one in twenty of their populations aged at least 65 years. But from that date, there has been a progressive diffusion of demographic ageing through the world's nations. Few countries in Africa, Latin America or southern Asia have yet been substantially affected, but we are at an interesting turning point. As fertility declines have recently spread to almost all countries of the world, the next few decades will see a rapid dissemination of demographic ageing. Little more than half of the world's present elderly population live in its less developed regions, but as soon as the end of the century, that share will have increased to 61 per cent (Warnes, 1987b).

Demographic ageing became established in north western Europe during the last two decades of the nineteenth century; it spread to southern Europe and the United States early in this century, and to Japan, Australasia and temperate South America after the Second World War. Very recently its first steps have become evident in several newly industrialising countries, such as Brazil, Korea and Thailand (Fig. 5.3). In each case, the onset of demographic ageing can be associated with a prior fall in fertility. The more recent the entry of a nation into the ageing transition, the more rapid has been the nation's rate of mortality decline, and consequently the greater has been the contribution from this cause to the increasing average age of the population.

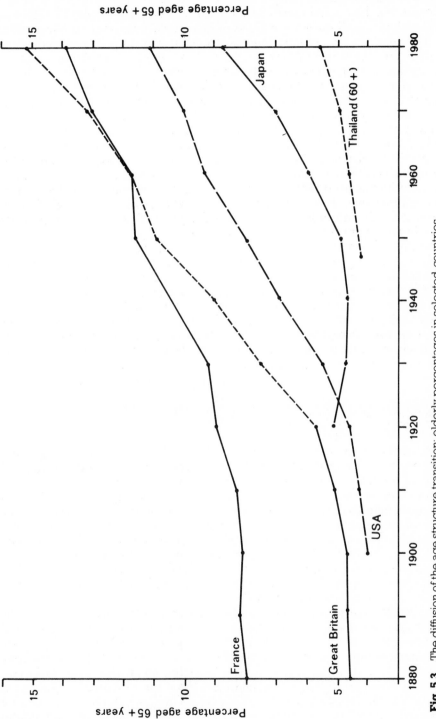

Fig. 5.3 The diffusion of the age structure transition: elderly percentages in selected countries.

Following the 1982 World Assembly on Aging, several United Nations Organization (UNO) publications have focused on the social and economic situation of elderly people throughout the world. *The World Aging Situation* is a digest of policy debates and demographic evidence based on the UNO 1982 medium growth variant population projections (UNO, 1985a); and a companion issue of the organisation's *Periodical on Aging* provides fuller statistical tables (UNO, 1985b). Together with the detailed census tabulations from the most developed nations, they enable an increasingly detailed global review of the presence of elderly people and the ageing of national populations.

Great Britain

The north-west European history of fertility and mortality since the late eighteenth century can be generalised into a sequence of changes known as the demographic transition. Substantial falls in death rates during the middle decades of the nineteenth century were followed in its last quarter by a substantial decline in fertility, and it was the latter which rapidly reduced the relative presence of children and initiated growth in the relative share of elderly people. Throughout the late nineteenth century the pensionable age population of Great Britain remained around 6.1 per cent although it increased each decade by 11 to 14 per cent (Warnes, 1987a). After 1911, the growth of the pensionable population rose to annual rates of over 2.2 per cent during 1921 to 1951. The total increased by 2.4 million during 1931 to 1951, to form more than one in eight (13.6 per cent) of the population. Since 1951, the growth in the relative share has slowed, although until the 1970s the absolute annual increase remained substantial. Not until the first decade of the next century, when the high post-1945 birth cohorts reach retirement, will there again be a substantial increase in the elderly population in Britain, and only if there are further substantial falls in fertility and late age mortality will the elderly share of the population increase substantially. Indeed, it can be said that the demographic ageing of the British population extended from around 1900 until around 1970.

Europe

During the later nineteenth century, France, Belgium and the Scandinavian countries had slightly higher elderly population percentages than Great Britain, but subsequently all nations of north western Europe have experienced a rapid rise in their relative and absolute elderly populations. By 1980, seventeen per cent of Sweden's population was aged 65 or more years, and 7.2 per cent were 75+ years. The Netherlands, the Republic of Ireland, Spain and Portugal lag behind as a consequence of their higher fertility (Table 5.1). In the early 1980s two-thirds of the 50 million people aged 65+ years in the nations of the Council of Europe were in West Germany, the United Kingdom, Italy and France. Apart from Turkey, where average female life expectancy was 65.5 years, the variation in mortality conditions was very low, with this index ranging from 79.6 years in Sweden to 75.0 in Ireland and 73.8 in Malta (Council of Europe, 1985).

The demographic experience of eastern European countries since 1939 has varied. High population losses during the Second World War, post-war emigration, low fertility in many countries after the mid-1950s, and rising mortality in the 1980s in some nations have produced more complex and variable age distributions. Albania's fertility is very high and in 1985 the average age of its population was around 22 years, compared to 36 years in Hungary and East Germany (Kostrubiec, 1987). Only the latter two countries

Table 5.1 The representation of elderly people in selected west European countries: 1950, 1970 and early 1980s. Data from Clarke (1987) and Council of Europe (1985).

| | Percentage 65+ years | | | Percentage 75+ years | | |
	c. 1950	*c.* 1970	early 1980s	*c.* 1950	*c.* 1970	early 1980s
Austria	10.6	14.2	14.2	3.2	4.7	6.5
Belgium	11.1	13.4	14.4	3.6	4.6	5.8
Denmark	9.1	12.4	14.9	2.9	4.5	6.3
France	11.8	13.4	12.8	4.1	5.0	6.3
Federal Republic of Germany	9.3	13.2	14.6	2.7	4.2	6.5
Greece	6.7	11.2	13.3	2.2	3.8	5.4
Ireland	10.7	11.3	10.7	3.7	4.2	3.9
Italy	8.2	10.6	13.3	2.6	3.8	4.8
Netherlands	7.7	10.2	11.8	2.4	3.7	4.9
Norway	9.7	12.9	15.5	3.6	4.7	6.4
Portugal	7.2	9.7	11.7	2.3	3.1	4.3
Spain	7.2	9.7	12.0	2.2	3.3	4.9
Sweden	10.2	13.8	17.0	3.4	5.0	7.2
Switzerland	9.6	11.4	14.0	3.0	3.9	6.2
Turkey	3.3	4.3	4.2	1.0	1.1	1.5
United Kingdom	10.7	12.8	14.9	3.5	4.6	6.3

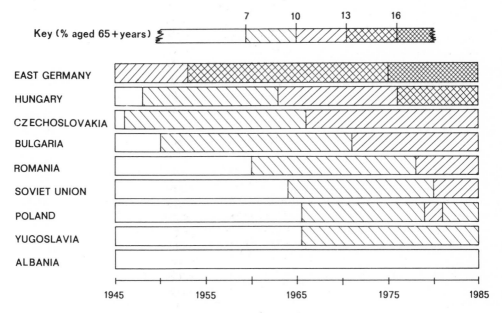

Fig. 5.4 The progress of ageing in east European countries.

have progressed to the high average ages found in western Europe. In the case of Poland, a rise in mortality from 1979/80 has reversed the process of demographic ageing (Fig. 5.4).

The United States and other developed nations

Non-European economically developed nations generally have higher fertility and a lower average age, partly as a result of the immigration of young adults. Being at an earlier stage of demographic ageing, they have higher rates of growth of their absolute and relative elderly populations. In the United States, for example, immigration and high fertility early this century are the cause of today's elderly population increases of around 1.8 per cent each year. The rate is likely to fall to around 0.4 per cent per annum during the 1990s.

> From an annual increase of approximately 600,000 (65+ years) persons currently, the number will reach a nadir of about 150,000 in 1999. This will be followed by a steady gain in the net additions after the year 2000.... For a seven year period in the 2020s, over 1.4 million persons will be added each year to the aged population. Thereafter, declining net additions are expected until net deficits are reached in the last years of the 2030s. (Myers, 1985)

The quality and detail of analyses of demographic ageing in the United States and of the fiscal and health-financing implications are unsurpassed (Rosenwaike, 1985; Siegel, 1980). They have not, however, prevented irrational, ideologically expedient and even alarmist interpreations of the trends, despite the nation's exceptional economic capacity to adjust to an ageing population, not least from the anticipated increases in its working population. The contribution of demographers to the debate has for the most part been constructive, but interpretations which take a narrow view of the ratio of the elderly to the working age groups, or which pose the economic interests of different age groups as antagonistic, do fuel fashionable concerns: some deserve the elicited critical response (Binney and Estes, 1988).

In Australia too, high rates of immigration and fertility during the 1950s and 1960s, and subsequent decreases, lie behind the rapid rates of absolute and relative elderly population growth during the late 1980s. 'Between 1971 and 1981 the number of Australians aged 65 years or more increased by one-third to 1.46 million and from 8.3 to 9.8 per cent of the population. Moreover, even more rapid growth of the older population is in store' (Hugo, 1986). The elderly population will reach around 3.5 million people by 2021 when it will form 14.6 per cent of the population. Even though Australia is at a relatively early stage of demographic ageing, it will soon pass the maximum rate of change. During the 1980s the 65+ years population will increase by another third, but during both the 1990s and in the first decade of the next century, the increase will be less than one-fifth. As elsewhere, however, there will be significant ageing within the 65+ years population, for example, a peak growth, by 57 per cent, of the 85+ years population is expected during the 1990s.

The situation in Japan has important differences in recent demographic history and in projections. As late as 1940, Japan had a young population with less than one in twenty aged 65 years or more. At the conclusion of the Second World War, the country faced economic chaos, national demoralisation and American occupation: it had to absorb seven million Japanese from its lost empire and cope with a population boom brought about by the rapid response of the death rate to medical and public health programmes. In a single decade the crude birth rate was halved, initially by the widespread practice of abortion. One consequence has been an unprecedently rapid rate of demographic ageing. By 1980, 9.1 per cent of its population was aged at least 65 years and it is projected that by 2015 the elderly share will increase to 21 per cent, among the highest in the world (Parant, 1987).

The less developed world

The fastest growth of elderly populations and the most challenging problems of service provision in the next decade will occur however in the less developed countries which since 1960 have experienced marked fertility declines. In 1980 the population aged 60 years or more ranged from 4.9 per cent in Africa to 16.9 per cent in Europe. Among individual countries the range was from 3.0 in Kenya (and less than 4 per cent in Malawi, Tanzania, Botswana and Nicaragua) to 21.9 in Sweden (and over 19 in Norway, East Germany, Denmark, the UK, Austria and Switzerland). Nearly a quarter (22 per cent) of the world's elderly population lived in Europe. The global distribution shows a latitudinal arrangement with, in general, inter-tropical regions having the least elderly age structures.

United Nations' population projections suggest that from 1980 until 2000 the world's elderly population will increase by 66 per cent, with a range from 95 per cent in Central America to 2.7 per cent in northern Europe. For individual countries the probable range is from less than one per cent in Sweden and Norway to over 125 per cent in Guatemala and Nicaragua. The global distribution is suggestive of an inverse correlation with the level of economic and social development. The largest absolute increase was projected to occur in China, with an expectation that 62 million will be added to the elderly population between 1975 and 2000. Among the other countries faced with a combination of high absolute and proportionate increases are the Soviet Union, India, Brazil, Indonesia, Mexico and Bangladesh. Projections for 2025 suggest that 14 per cent of the world's population will be aged 60+, that 71 per cent of these 1135 million people will be living in the less developed regions and fewer than 12 per cent in Europe.

In Latin America, all nations except Panama, the Dominican Republic and Haiti in the Caribbean and central America, and all the large republics except Brazil (6.1 per cent) in tropical latitudes had less than 6 per cent of their population aged 60 or more years in 1980. On the other hand, the elderly formed more than one in ten of the population of Barbados (12.5 per cent), Cuba (10.4 per cent), Argentina (12.7 per cent), and Uruguay (14.8 per cent). In many of the poorer countries of the continent, the elderly population is expected to continue to increase for some decades at between 2.5 and 3.5 per cent per year (Table 5.2).

A detailed investigation of the likely growth of the elderly population in Thailand and its capital city, Bangkok, has been undertaken (Warnes and Horsey, 1988). Thailand's population has grown fivefold since the 1920s to 53 million and that of Bangkok has grown even more rapidly, to reach 10.4 per cent of the national total in 1986. The elderly population (60+ years) of Thailand has only recently exceeded five per cent of the national total, but its present annual growth rate (3.8 per cent) is nearly fifty per cent higher than that for all age groups. Not only is it expected that there will be a slowing of population growth in Thailand as fertility falls, but rapid increases in demographic ageing are already predicted, especially in Bangkok, where presently there is an over-representation of the middle aged as a result of the substantial flows of rural migrants since the 1950s. It is quite possible that in no more than 30 years from now, Bangkok will have an elderly population share comparable to that of European nations today: the adjustments that individual families and the society will have to make in this short period puts into perspective our own concerns with demographic ageing, and the experience will be repeated in many parts of the Third World.

Table 5.2 Estimated and projected 60+ years population and annual rates of change: Latin America 1980, 2000 and 2025. Data from UN (1985a).

Nation	Estimated or projected population (thousands)						Average annual growth rate	
	1980 000s	%	2000 000s	%	2025 000s	%	80–00 %	00–25 %
Caribbean	2391	7.8	3701	8.5	8092	13.1	2.2	3.2
Barbados	33	12.5	34	10.6	82	21.5	0.1	3.6
Cuba	1016	10.4	1520	13.0	2752	20.3	2.0	2.4
Dominican Rep.	260	4.4	526	5.6	1515	10.4	3.6	4.3
Guadeloupe	31	9.4	46	13.0	87	21.1	2.0	2.6
Haiti	323	5.6	478	4.8	1025	5.6	2.0	3.1
Jamaica	192	8.8	247	8.6	551	14.6	1.3	3.3
Martinique	32	9.8	46	12.7	82	19.1	1.8	2.3
Puerto Rico	326	8.9	537	10.1	1321	20.4	2.5	3.7
Trinidad and Tobago	88	7.5	146	9.8	358	20.0	2.6	3.7
Windward Islands[1]	30	7.3	28	5.3	96	12.9	−0.3	5.0
Other Caribbean[2]	61	7.6	93	8.1	224	14.7	2.1	3.6
Central America[3]	4684	5.1	8866	5.7	23431	9.6	3.2	4.0
Costa Rica	124	5.6	251	7.4	683	14.0	3.6	4.1
El Salvador	245	5.1	485	5.6	1276	8.5	3.4	3.9
Guatemala	326	4.5	734	5.8	1899	8.7	4.1	3.9
Honduras	163	4.4	347	5.0	906	6.8	3.9	3.9
Mexico	3590	5.1	6615	5.7	17512	10.1	3.1	4.0
Nicaragua	106	3.9	194	3.8	595	6.1	3.1	4.6
Panama	122	6.4	224	7.9	530	13.5	3.1	3.5
Temperate South America[4]	4768	11.6	6886	13.3	10542	17.0	1.9	1.7
Argentina	3437	12.7	4857	14.6	6818	17.4	1.7	1.4
Chile	899	8.1	1471	9.9	3038	16.2	2.5	2.9
Uruguay	432	14.8	557	16.1	685	16.7	1.3	0.8
Tropical South America[5]	11484	5.8	21537	6.8	51253	10.3	3.2	3.5
Bolivia	290	5.2	489	5.0	1077	5.5	2.6	3.2
Brazil	7464	6.1	13995	7.5	31816	10.9	3.2	3.3
Colombia	1433	5.6	2589	6.8	6606	12.8	3.0	3.9
Ecuador	424	5.3	779	5.3	1935	7.5	3.1	3.7
Guyana	52	5.9	87	7.0	256	15.8	2.6	4.4
Paraguay	171	5.4	303	5.6	810	9.5	2.9	4.0
Peru	925	5.2	1693	5.5	4167	7.4	3.1	4.6
Surinam	22	5.7	34	4.9	81	7.4	2.2	3.5
Venezuela	698	4.5	1564	5.7	4494	10.5	4.1	4.3
Latin America	23328	6.4	40990	7.2	93317	10.8	2.9	3.3

1 Including Dominica, Grenada, Saint Lucia, Saint Vincent and the Grenadines.
2 Including Anguilla, Antigua and Barbuda, Bahamas, British Virgin Islands, Cayman Islands, Montserrat, Netherlands Antilles, Saint Christopher and Nevis, Turks and Caicos Islands, and United States Virgin Islands.
3 Including Belize.
4 Including Falkland Islands.
5 Including French Guiana.

AGE STRUCTURE AND LATE-AGE MORTALITY

As old people form a larger share of national populations, demographers' and politicians' attention shifts to the structure of the elderly population. A few elderly people are 40 years older than those reaching the years of retirement: the life histories of people born so far apart are likely to have been markedly different and their present circumstances will be quite variable. In 1981 the majority of people in Great Britain aged 60–64 years were married, whereas the majority of those aged at least 75 years were widowed and living alone (Warnes, 1987a). Some alarm has arisen about the circumstances of the 'oldest old' and the projections for increasing numbers of people aged 85 years or more (Rosenwaike, 1985; Suzman and Riley, 1985; Zones *et al.*, 1987). In Britain and other European countries, the numbers of people in the oldest age groups will vary in response to fluctuations in births earlier in this century. In the United States and Australia, the growth of the 'oldest old' population will be faster as a result of the higher rates of population growth throughout this century. In both the old and the new developed nations, a further important influence will be the future course of late-age mortality. Life expectancy at age 60 years has been improving erratically but strongly in many affluent nations. The key questions that arise are: What factors have brought about these improvements? How much further improvement can be expected and at what pace?

Until there is an understanding of the molecular and genetic mechanisms of human ageing, it is premature to contemplate significant alterations in the maximum human life span. Were this century's enormous improvements in living conditions for the most privileged sections of our populations spread to all, and if there were no counteracting influences from AIDS, drug abuse or declining standards of nutrition or physical fitness, then we might be surprised at the numbers of people living to be nonagenarians. There are several issues concerning future survival curves which can be discussed without assuming radical departures from present ageing effects upon individuals. One starting point is the recent improvement in late age mortality in Britain.

Mortality rates have been falling in Britain throughout this century, those specific to later ages more erratically than all-age mortality. Nothing comparable to the apparent irregular progress of mortality declines in the United States is evident in Britain (Brody, 1985). From 1961 until 1984 late-age mortality fell in Great Britain by about 20 per cent. Between 1970 and 1980 life expectancy at birth increased for males from 68.6 to 70.4 years and for females from 74.9 to 76.5 years, and life expectancy at age 60 years increased from 15.1 to 16.1 years

Table 5.3 Age-specific death rates per 1000, England and Wales 1961–1984. Data from OPCS (1985b).

Year	Males				Females			
	55–64	65–74	75–84	85+	55–64	65–74	75–84	85+
1961	21.9	54.7	124.4	256.9	10.8	30.9	87.8	214.1
1966	21.3	53.5	119.2	259.2	10.2	28.5	80.0	203.3
1971	20.1	50.5	113.0	231.8	10.0	26.1	73.6	185.7
1976	19.6	50.3	116.4	243.5	10.1	26.0	74.6	196.6
1981	17.7	45.6	105.2	226.5	9.5	24.1	66.2	178.2
1984	17.2	44.4	99.7	211.3	9.5	23.9	61.7	169.0
Ratios of change								
1984 : 1961	0.79	0.81	0.80	0.82	0.88	0.77	0.70	0.79
1984 : 1976	0.88	0.88	0.86	0.87	0.94	0.92	0.83	0.86

for males and from 19.7 to 20.6 years for females (Rees and Warnes, 1986). There have been only minor differences in the recent mortality improvement at different ages among the older population (see Table 5.3). On the other hand, recent mortality trends have shown interesting sex differentials, with the improvements among young elderly males (aged 55–64 years) tending to reduce their differential disadvantage in comparison to females. Mortality among those ten years older has improved faster for females and slower for males, resulting in an increasing sex differential until 1971. Since then there have been signs of a reversal. For the succeeding decennial age group (75–84 years), female mortality has been improving more rapidly than male mortality since at least 1931.

ELDERLY POPULATION PROJECTIONS

Population growth during the late nineteenth century in Great Britain was sufficiently high to have produced until the 1970s an increasing elderly population. The annual increase has, however, been unsteady during the last 30 years, and this will continue, largely as a consequence of the fluctuating annual totals of births during this century. Apart from the distortions from the two major European wars, economic growth during 1953–65 was associated with high birth rates, and the periods of recession during the inter-war years and since the early 1970s have been associated with low fertility.

Official projections of the size, age and sex structure of the population of Great Britain are produced every two years by the Government Actuary in association with the Office of Population Censuses and Surveys (OPCS). These employ cohort-survival projection methods based on extrapolations of recent trends in mortality, fertility and net international migration (Daykin, 1986). Unlike United States' or United Nations' projections, which provide alternative high and low growth projections, only one series is published in Britain. Recent OPCS projections indicate that the pensionable age population in England and Wales will increase from around 9.0 million in 1981 to 10.8 million in 2021. There will be large increases of the smaller cohorts in extreme old age and a fall of approximately 11 per cent in the population aged 65–74 years (OPCS, 1985). The 85+ years population has been growing during the 1980s at the exceptional annual rate of 3.8 per cent but this will moderate to 2.2 per cent during the 1990s and stabilise by the 2010s.

It should be emphasised that the increases in the very old population are largely a function of the projection's mortality assumptions. Alternative projections using constant mortality by Rees (1987) highlight the effect. The anticipated increase by 2006 in the population aged 85 years or more is reduced, for example, from 91 per cent in the OPCS projections to 19 per cent in the Rees projections. As the best informed commentators admit that we have only tentative understandings of the reasons for recent reductions in mortality, and of their periods of stasis and of descent, then there is little basis in understanding for the official assumptions of the course of mortality, and the largely mechanistic character of trend extrapolations must not be forgotten. Epidemiologists and demographers are, however, giving much attention to the improvement of our forecasts.

One approach to future late age mortality is to examine recent trends in the death rates attributable to specific causes, with emphasis upon the most common. If an understanding is reached of the reasons for recent changes in the rates, then in some cases it is possible to project the antecedent causal factor. For example, if we specify the relationship between the prevalence of smoking among those aged 20–29 years at one date and the rate of smoking-related mortality from lung cancer among the same cohort when aged 60–69 years, then estimates of the deaths from this cause could be projected 40 years ahead. Anderson and Ashwood (1985) have recently provided a summary of current British practice. For the ten leading causes of death they concluded that: (a) ischaemic heart disease should be considered separately for there were no grounds for expecting a deviation from recent trends; (b) a specific model relating past and present smoking to future lung cancer is feasible and could be a valuable indicator; (c) it may be possible to relate bronchitis, asthma and emphysema to past and anticipated levels of environmental pollutants; (d) there is inadequate evidence for any departure from the steady recent rates of mortality from malignant diseases apart from lung cancer; and (e) all other diseases should be aggregated and past trends extrapolated.

They predict substantial decreases in the male cause-specific mortality rate from lung cancers, but increases in the rates for females aged 75 years or more. Past trends in bronchitis, emphysema and asthma late-age mortality are quite different from those for lung cancer, there being no clear evidence of a cohort change as with smoking. The different trends for males and females are difficult to explain, but the authors point to an interaction between the contrasted levels and trends of smoking and exposure to atmospheric pollution. Their projections for males extrapolate the substantial declines in mortality since 1951 to suggest an approximate halving by the 2020s; but for females they suggest that no change will occur in the 1980s age-specific rates. Benjamin (1986) has undertaken a comparable but more speculative exercise, with assumptions that a number of the leading but avoidable present causes of death are radically reduced. His hypothetical schedule of age specific mortality rates may be close to the most benign that can reasonably be conceived. Its form, and the considerable room for further improvements that we may take as a goal, are illustrated as curve E on Fig. 5.1 (p. 48).

Similar exercises have become numerous in the United States. The country's Bureau of the Census projects age-specific mortality by using: extrapolations of recent trends; the assumption of an ultimate mortality level at a specified future date, towards which levels for intermediate years progress; and adjustments for recent trends in significant specific causes of death (Myers, 1981). In recent years, however, these procedures have repeatedly underestimated the improvement in late-age mortality. In both 1976 and 1980, the Bureau revised downward its forward projections of mortality. The reasons were primarily associated with declines in deaths from heart and vascular diseases, particularly among those aged 60–69 and 80 or more years. Until recently future mortality assumptions appeared to be serviceable and there was little interest in the variations between projected and actual numbers among the relatively small numbers of people surviving into their seventies. The situation has now radically changed, and there is considerable support for research into trends in cause-specific mortality by age and sex, the complications arising from the declining lethality of specific causes and the complementary growth of multiple causes of death.

A second approach to the description of future survival curves is less grounded in recent improvements in cause-specific mortalities and employs mathematical functions such as the Gompertz-Makeham equation to specify the age mortality relationships that will produce a given, higher, average life expectancy. An unusually ambitious theoretical exercise of this kind has been applied to evaluate the possible age structures of Europe's population from 1970 to 2150 (Bourgeois-Pichat, 1981). The projection methodology has three phases: in the first, detailed mortality projections for the period 1970/4–2000 produced by the United Nations for four regions of Europe are employed. These suggested a convergence among the regions' mortalities towards a life expectancy at birth of 72.3 years for men and 77.5 years for females. For the second phase, during the first half of the next century, Bourgeois-Pichat assumes that biomedical advances will enable the survival curve to progress steadily towards a level at which average life expectancy at birth is 100 years. In 2050 the crude death rate will reach a historic low, but thereafter, although he assumes that the survival curve is unchanging, the progressively greater average age of Europe's population will lead to increases in the crude death rate. Bourgeois-Pichat also assumes that a substantial fall after 2050 in the populations of European nations will be prevented by a recovery in fertility. This will rejuvenate the population, reducing the 65+ years from 43 per cent of the total in 2050 to 33 per cent in 2150.

A third approach is concerned with the quality and health of survivors as well as their number. It is attracting great interest from government spending and health service planners, because it is extending the methodology of population forecasting to the populations with different degrees of health, sickness and disability. A starting point is that the lethality of strokes, heart disease and other disorders is decreasing and, therefore, the average age of death is increasing. Some argue that the upward limit of survival potential is being approached and that in the future there will be less variation in the age of death. In other words, it is argued that the length of life of the longest lived will increase more slowly than the length of life of the majority, and that the survival curve will become more rectangular. Others, however, believe that there is considerable room for further 'rightward-shifts' in the survival curve (Fries and Crapo, 1981; Manton, 1982). The 'rectangularists' see the prevalence and the duration of chronic illnesses being reduced; the 'life extension' school forecasts the opposite. The outcome will have a profound effect on not only the quality of old age lives but also the requirement for acute and long-stay health and social care facilities. Governmental health and social security administrations are therefore keen to encourage the resolution of this debate, and in 1987 many substantial grants were awarded by the USA National Institute on Aging to pursue this research. The principal impediment is the scarcity of long-run, nationally representative and time series data on the health of the population, but important theoretical and model-refinement work has been published (Koizumi, 1982; Manton and Soldo, 1985).

The speculative nature of projections is clear in Bourgeois-Pichat's long-term exercise but is also true of short-term, extrapolative forecasts. Strictly, all projections have instructional rather than predictive value. Demographers stress this repeatedly but it is often forgotten by politicians and macroeconomists. All projections are founded on the present and the recent past and we tend to resist scenarios which indicate radical change. However, as the recent diffusion of the autoimmune deficiency virus and the recent declines in later life expectancy in some east European countries have reminded us, future mortality may worsen and is unpredictable.

AGEING IN SPECIAL POPULATIONS

Demography's first contribution to gerontology was to offer forecasts of the numbers of men and women at specified advanced ages. Now apparent is its potential to offer much more, both through a disaggregation of its projections by health status, and by the application of its sharp and proven tools to local rather than national territories, to household formation, and to categories of old people by income, housing tenure, marital status and dependency (Grundy, 1987; Rees, 1987).

Some recent work has examined projections of the age structure of two hypothetical settlements of elderly people, a retirement community of 1000 dwellings initially populated exclusively by married couples with the men aged 65 years and the women 62 years (Warnes, 1987c). The second is a 'sheltered housing' community of 1000 units initially populated by 700 widows aged 72 years, 100 widowers aged 68 years, and 200 married couples with husbands aged 70 years and their wives three years younger. Common to the retirement community and the sheltered housing populations is an initial asymmetrical wave of adjustment: the average age rises for a time and then falls. The form, amplitude and period of this wave varies according to the annual rate of turnover, the age at which people enter the settlement, life expectancy at entry, and the heterogeneity of the population.

In the sheltered housing population the initial phase lasts about 15 years, during which the average age increases from 70.5 to 77.1 years. For the retirement community, the first period lasts 19 years and the average age increases from 63.5 to 73.8 years, the population falls to 78.6 per cent of its starting value and the number of married couples decreases by 43 per cent. The second period of recovery is less marked in the sheltered housing population than in the retirement community but in both cases it extends over 11 years. Many other characteristics of these special populations may be studied using projection methodology, including the relationship between these quantitative demographic and household indicators and the functional and dependency status of the residents.

CONCLUSIONS

Demographic ageing, the progressive rise in the mean age, is only one of the forms of change in the age distributions of human populations that concern the gerontologist. It is widely discussed but there is much confusion about its progress, causes and implications. Most western European countries have, since the beginning of this century, experienced major changes in their age structures as a result of substantial falls in mortality and fertility. The United States, Australia and Japan are not far behind. Western countries have already accommodated most of the predicted increase in the elderly population: it is in the less developed countries that new and radical demographic ageing changes will occur during the next fifty years.

Western countries, including Britain, will experience fluctuations in the relative and absolute size of the elderly population, largely as a result of periods of low and high fertility. Further improvements in late age mortality are expected, however, and this will, for several decades, lead to a progressively higher mean age among people of retirement age. Demographic methods and findings have been of considerable value in forecasting the future numbers and age distribution of elderly people. But they have also been much misused, and more care and gerontological insight must be encouraged. There is considerable scope for projections of the characteristics of the elderly population and not just their number. It is important that we learn much more about the prevalence of disorders and different degrees of healthiness among the elderly population. The living arrangements and the psychological state of future elderly populations deserve more attention. Diverse quantitative and qualitative characteristics will be more critical for the welfare of the elderly population than its size.

While demographic researchers are turning to these topics with enthusiasm and imagination, and their contributions to gerontology are diversifying rapidly, there needs to be a greater appreciation of the cohort effects which can alter the age-specific prevalence of diseases and ill-health. Interpretations of population projections must be increasingly informed by an understanding of the changing sociology of later life. This is the lesson of careful study of the demography of ageing, and it should dispel false identifications of unprecedented increases in the size of the elderly population or simplistic alarms about the implications.

REFERENCES

Anderson, M. and Ashwood, F. (1985). Projection of mortality rates for the elderly. *Population Trends*, **42**, 22–9.

Barrett, J.C. (1985). The mortality of centenarians in England and Wales. *Archives of Gerontology and Geriatrics*, **4**, 211–18.

Benjamin, B. (1986). The prospects for mortality decline and consequent changes in age structure of population. In *The Biology of Human Ageing*, A.H. Bittles and K.J. Collins (Eds), pp. 133–54. Cambridge University Press, Cambridge.

Binney, E.A. and Estes, C.L. (1988). The retreat of the state and its transfer of responsibility: the intergenerational war. *International Journal of Health Services*, **18**(1), 83–96.

Bourgeois-Pichat, J. (1981). Le dilemme de le révolution démographique: croître ou vieillir. In *Aging: A Challenge to Science and Society*, A.J.J. Gilmore, A. Svanborg and M. Marois (Eds), pp. 260–78. Oxford University Press, Oxford.

Brody, J.A. (1985). Prospects for an aging population. *Nature*, **315**, 463–6.

Clark, R.L. and Spengler, J.J. (1980). *The Economics of Individual and Population Ageing*, Cambridge University Press, Cambridge.

Clarke, J.I. (1987). Ageing in Europe: introductory remarks. *Espaces, Populations, Sociétés*, 1987/1, 23–8.

Comfort, A. (1979). *The Biology of Senescence*, 3rd edition. Churchill Livingstone, Edinburgh.

Council of Europe (1985). *Recent Demographic Developments in the Member States of the Council of Europe.* Council of Europe, Strasbourg.

Daykin, C. (1986). Projecting the population of the United Kingdom. *Population Trends*, **44**, 28–33.

Fries, J.F. and Crapo, L.M. (1981). *Vitality and Aging: Implications of the Rectangular Curve.* Freeman, San Francisco.

Gompertz, B. (1825). On the nature of the function expressive of the law of human mortality and on a new mode of determining life contingencies. *Philosophical Transactions of the Royal Society*, **2**, 513–85.

Grundy, E. (1987). Migration and household change among the elderly in England and Wales. *Espaces, Population, Sociétés*, 1987/1, 109–23.

Hart, R.W. and Turturro, A. (1987). Evolution of life span in placental mammals. In *Modern Biological Theories of Aging*, H.R. Warner et al. (Eds), pp. 21–34. Raven Press, New York.

Hayflick, L. (1987). Origins of longevity. In *Modern Biological Theories of Aging*, H.R. Warner et al. (Eds), pp. 21–34. Raven Press, New York.

Hugo, G. (1986). *Population Aging in Australia: Implications for Social and Economic Policy.* Papers of the East-West Population Institute No. 98. Honolulu, Hawaii.

Kannisto, V. (1988). On the survival of centenarians and the span of life. *Population Studies*, **42**, 389–406.

Kirkwood, T.B.L. and Holliday, R. (1986). Ageing as a consequence of natural selection. In *The Biology of Human Ageing*, A.H. Bittles and K.J. Collins (Eds), pp. 1–16. Cambridge University Press, Cambridge.

Koizumi, A. (1982). Towards a healthy life in the twentieth century. In *Population Aging In Japan: Problems and Policy Issues in the Twenty-First Century*, T. Kuroda (Ed.). Population Research Institute, Nihon University, Tokyo.

Kostrubiec, B. (1987). Aperçu général du vieillissement des populations de la communauté des pays de l'Est. *Espaces, Populations, Sociétés*, 1987/2, 343–56.

Manton, K.G. (1982). Changing concepts of morbidity and mortality in the elderly population. *Milbank Memorial Fund Quarterly*, **60**(2), 183–244.

Manton, K.G. and Soldo, B.J. (1985). Dynamics of health changes in the oldest old: new perspectives and evidence. *Milbank Memorial Fund Quarterly*, **63**(2), 206–85.

McKeown, T. (1976). *The Modern Rise of Population*. Edward Arnold, London.

Myers, G.C. (1981). Future age projections and society. In *Aging: A Challenge to Science and Society*, A.J.J. Gilmore, A. Svanborg and M. Marois (Eds), pp. 248–59. Oxford University Press, Oxford.

Myers, G.C. (1985). Aging and worldwide population change. In *Handbook of Aging and the Social Sciences*, R.H. Binstock and E. Shanas (Eds), pp. 173–98. Van Nostrand Reinhold, New York.

Notestein, F. (1954). Some demographic aspects of aging. *Proceedings of the American Philosophical Society*, **98**, 38–47.

Office of Population Censuses and Surveys (OPCS) (1985). *Population Projections, 1983–2023*, Series PP2, No. 13. HMSO, London.

OPCS (1987). *Mortality Statistics: England and Wales, 1985*. HMSO, London.

Parant, A. (1987). Le vieillissement démographique: un nouveau défi pour le Japon. *Espaces, Populations, Sociétés*, 1987/2, 357–64.

Playfair, L. (1845). *Report on the State of the Large Towns in Lancashire*. Health of Towns Commission, HMSO, London.

Rees, P.H. (1987). How many old people will there be in the United Kingdom and where will they live? *Espaces, Populations, Sociétés*, 1987/1, 57–72.

Rees, P.H. and Warnes, A.M. (1986). 'Migration of the elderly in Great Britain', Working Paper 573, School of Geography, University of Leeds. In *Migration of the Elderly: An International Comparative Study*, A. Rogers and W. Serow (Eds), Institute of Behavioral Science, University of Colorado, Boulder, Colorado.

Rosenwaike, I. (1985). *The Extreme Aged in America*. Greenwood, Westport, Connecticut.

Siegel, J.S. (1980). Recent and prospective trends for the elderly population and implications for health care. In *Second Conference on the Epidemiology of Aging*, National Institute of Health Publication 80–969, S.G. Haynes and G. Feinleib (Eds), pp. 289–315. National Institute on Aging, Bethesda, Maryland.

Suzman, R. and Riley, M.W. (Eds) (1985). 'The Oldest Old', special issue. *Milbank Memorial Fund Quarterly*, **63**(2), 177–451.

United Nations Organization (UNO) (1985a). *The World Aging Situation*. UNO, New York.

UNO (1985b). *Periodical on Aging*, Vol. 1, No. 1, 1984. UNO, New York.

Warner, H.R., Butler, R.N., Sprott, R.L. and Schneider, E.L. (Eds) (1987).

Modern Biological Theories of Aging. Raven Press, New York.

Warnes, A.M. (1987a). The ageing of Britain's population: geographical dimensions. *Espaces, Populations, Sociétés*, 1987/2, 317–27.

Warnes, A.M. (1987b). Geographical locations and social relationships in developed and developing nations. In *Social Geography: Progress and Prospects*, M. Pacione (Ed.), Croom Helm, Beckenham, Kent.

Warnes, A.M. (1987c). *The ageing of residents in elderly housing schemes*, Working Paper 3. Age Concern Institute of Gerontology, King's College, London.

Warnes, A.M. and Horsey, A. (1988). *The elderly population of third world cities: projections for selected metropolitan areas.* King's College, London.

Zones, J.S., Estes, C. and Binney, E.A. (1987). Gender, public policy and the oldest old. *Ageing and Society*, **7**(3), 275–302.

Part Two

AGEING AND ELDERLY PEOPLE IN SOCIETY

Andrew Blaikie

Centre for Extra-Mural Studies
Birkbeck College
University of London
and

John Macnicol

Royal Holloway and Bedford New College
University of London

6 AGEING AND SOCIAL POLICY: A TWENTIETH CENTURY DILEMMA

INTRODUCTION

The unfolding of the twentieth century has seen old age emerge as a major social issue in advanced industrial societies. The lower birth rates that have existed since the late 1870s as part of the 'demographic transition' process, supplemented by improvements in longevity, have produced a profound effect on the age structures of such societies. In Britain there were 700 000 persons aged 65 and over in 1841, amounting to 4.5 per cent of the population. By 1901, they had risen to 1.5 million, but there was little change in the elderly's proportionate relationship to the rest of the population, since they still constituted only 5 per cent. By 1978, however, these figures had risen to 7.9 million and 14.5 per cent. Since the United Nations defines an 'aged population' as one with more than seven per cent of its members aged over 65 (Midwinter, 1985), then clearly Britain boasts a large, if passive, gerontocracy.

Whilst there can be little disputing the demographic evidence, historians are much less certain of how the experience of old age has altered qualitatively over time. Havighurst (1978) has declared that 'the twentieth century has transformed the elderly from an almost invisible group sheltered by the extended family to a highly visible group with a life of its own, with moral and legal claims on society, and with a certain amount of social and political power'. Yet many would argue that the change has been both more complex and less dramatic.

The ageing of the British population has been marked by two interconnected features. Firstly, there has been an increasing withdrawal of the elderly from the labour market: in the 1880s, nearly three-quarters of men aged 65 and over still worked; by the early 1950s this had fallen to one-third; and by 1982 only three per cent were working full-time and four per cent part-time (Hannah, 1986; Abrams, 1983). Whilst it is clear that rising unemployment has recently accelerated this shift, historians disagree on the precise causal sequence of long-term trends. It has come about partly because of the shift to an advanced industrial economy, with an increasingly specialised division of labour and the shake-out of elderly workers; partly it has been a product of greater prosperity and higher living standard expectations, giving rise to a desire for retirement; and it has partly been induced by both private and state pension schemes (notably with the imposition of the retirement condition for receipt of the state

We wish to acknowledge the support of the Economic and Social Research Council, under whose grant (G01 250016) some of the research for this paper was conducted.

pension in 1946) (Hannah, 1986). Thus the relationship between age-related government policy and the development of retirement is far from straightforward. Changing rates of retirement fail to coincide with the spread of state pensions (Johnson, 1985). Between the 1930s and the 1960s, despite clear booms and slumps in the economy, the withdrawal of men over 65 from paid labour appears to have been continuous rather than fluctuating. It is doubtful whether state pensions policies can themselves be made to account for this process, although profound changes in production techniques and industrial infrastructure have certainly influenced those policies.

Secondly, the twentieth century has witnessed an increasing reliance by elderly people on welfare provided by a paternalist state. Myles (1984) has argued that the modern welfare state is principally a welfare state for elderly people: in 1985–86 there were 9.4 million retirement pensioners, 1.7 million of whom claimed supplementary pensions (with an additional 600 000 eligible but not claiming). At £16 677 000, retirement pensions were by far the largest single item in the social security budget, costing nearly as much as the National Health Service and four times as much as child benefit (Central Statistical Office, 1987).

Radical analysts of old age tend to see this reliance on state welfare as part of a wider condition of *structured dependence* of the elderly which 'is being manufactured socially' with 'unnecessary' severity (Townsend, 1981). Age, class, race and gender make up four interconnected components of structured disadvantage. Older women, for example, often continue to shoulder a burden of domestic support well into their old age. Thus, while it is true that in advanced capitalist societies there is 'a general devaluation of skills, ability, knowledge and output of older workers' (Walker, 1985), and that the dependence of the elderly is structured in the sense that it bears a structural relationship to their prior labour market status, it must also follow that the status of an elderly person will vary greatly according to other factors (Taylor and Ford, 1983). There is, in short, an enormous variety of 'old age experiences' and a world of difference exists between, on the one hand, the retired male bank manager on a final-salary occupational pension, owning his own home and enjoying the fruits of accumulated lifetime savings and, on the other, the elderly widow of a manual labourer, solely reliant on the state pension and living in private rented accommodation.

THE EMERGENCE OF RETIREMENT

A good deal of the discussion surrounding the marginalisation of older people has emphasised the emergence of retirement as an institution and the structured dependence that follows in its wake – a dependence which is distinguished less by virtue of its inherent characteristics than through its sheer magnitude. Far from being a once-and-for-all recipe, it is the malleability and ambiguity of the notion of retirement that have permitted its deployment, with varying degrees of success, over recent decades. Phillipson (1983) argues, for example, that both policy and ideology in twentieth-century Britain have varied directly with one another as a function of the economy's manpower requirements. Thus, during the inter-war depression years older workers were considered to be less efficient than younger, less adaptable to changing processes of production and rapid technological change and the most dispensable in times of slump. Conversely, in the 'never had it so good' phase of the 1950s, their reliability, commitment and experience were emphasised as labour shortages became evident. The more recent, and escalating pattern of withdrawal from full-time work, together with the near collapse of part-time employment for the over-65s, again indicates the relative ease with which this 'reserve of labour' can be manipulated as part of an industrial management strategy (Phillipson, 1982).

Increased state intervention began with the filtering of society and social issues into categories based upon age differences during the later Victorian era. Notions of formal removal from the work-force and a lowering of pensionable age gained ascendancy in the 1920s and a piecemeal programme, sustained by the growth of such exclusionist thinking, eventually culminated in the introduction of the retirement condition in 1946. Today, as the postwar consensus crumbles, the spread of early retirement euphemistically betokens new levels of mass redundancy (Thane, 1978; Townsend, 1981). Even a cursory inspection of publications from each period will reveal many apt illustrations of the sometimes unwitting, sometimes conspiratorial, translation of ideology into implementation. It needs to be said, for instance, that before the Second World War the notion of retirement was more widespread than the practice, or, again, that the creation of today's retirees represents the effect, not the cause, of the welfare state (Guillemard, 1983). Ironically, it was Beveridge's 'full employment welfare state' that sanctioned the elimination of older operatives from the work-force at a time when they were most needed.

However, despite its functionalist, though radical underpinnings, the model of retirement as a means of social control does have some heuristic value. Biological and sociological definitions of old age have diverged over the course of the past century and such separation owes much to the gradual emergence of retirement as a fixed rite of passage, determined by chronological age, where once it was determined more flexibly according to the physiological and mental capacity of the individual (Thane, 1978). Secondly, we can state with some confidence that whenever competition exists from younger members of the labour force – times which generally correspond with periods of high unemployment – older workers will be marginalised.

The nature of such displacement, though in clear need of empirical investigation at the level of the region, type of industry or single firm (Riddle, 1984), is perhaps less significant than the standard of living to be enjoyed or suffered thereafter by its recipients. Structured dependence can imply a powerlessness on the part of older people, but retirement clearly has a differential impact according to income levels maintained while in work. Early retirement does not always entail a reduction in personal wealth and the spread of home ownership and both private and occupational pension schemes has occasioned greater economic security for some. Among 'elderly only' households, fewer people are owner occupiers than is the case generally: in 1981, 48 per cent, as against 56 per cent for the population at large. Nevertheless, the census found 'wide disparities in tenure between areas; thus owner occupiers comprised 64 per cent of 'elderly only' households in East Sussex but only 31 per cent of such households in Tyne and Wear' (Office of Population Censuses and Surveys, 1984). Increased choice and continued ability to consume have to be offset against the persistent and constraining poverty faced by generations of state retirement pensioners.

This variety of old age experiences creates problems for any historian wishing to treat the issue with sympathy and sensitivity. Two definitional puzzles immediately present themselves. Firstly, there is the tautology that old age is a 'problem' for welfare systems in advanced industrial societies, yet old age has usually been defined in terms of eligibility for those very same welfare systems. The age of 70 years was used in the 1908 pension scheme, 65 years was adopted from 1925, and 60 (women) and 65 (men) from 1940. While there is a similarity of retirement ages in all advanced industrial societies, the criteria for selecting these ages were often somewhat arbitrary, owing more to fiscal caution than an agreement about the onset of senescence (Thane, 1978; Graebner, 1980).

Secondly, the artificiality of these crude pensions-eligibility definitions of old age is further emphasised by anthropological evidence that pre-industrial societies have operated an enormous variety of cultural definitions of old age such as the menopause, toothlessness, grey hair, wrinkled skin and grand-parenthood. In some cultures, such as the Sambaru pastoral nomads of northern Kenya, powerful gerontocracies have existed, through which the old have conspired to oppress the young (for example, by denying them land); in others, explicit sanctions against the elderly (including parricide) have operated (Foner, 1984). In modern industrial societies the status of the elderly will be affected by cultural factors, particularly the existence of close kin contacts; hence Francis (1984) found that family support for a group of Jewish elderly was stronger in Leeds, England (despite a more comprehensive welfare state), than that enjoyed by a comparable group in Cleveland, Ohio, because the former had longer-established kinship networks.

A sympathetic position, therefore, would be one which maintained that crude age-related definitions of old age are arbitrary, unfair and hence ageist: it would follow Sheldon's famous statement in 1948 that old age is, 'a quality of mind and body whose time of onset varies from individual to individual, rather than a mere quantity expressed by a term of duration applicable to all' (Sheldon, 1948). Yet, on the other hand, many who campaign for the elderly have felt the need to deploy age-related definitions in order to present them as an identifiable, vulnerable client group, united in their dependence on a state welfare system that needs to be improved. For similar reasons, lobbyists for the elderly in the USA tend still to propagate, as part of their campaigning rationale, the 'veneration-to-degradation' thesis of the history of old age that is now largely discredited among British social historians. Thus, while it is undeniable that being old is likely to exacerbate the lack of access to resources that accompanies poverty, at the same time social and economic changes have complex effects on the status of the elderly, and much will depend on the prevailing political context in which the issue of old age is placed. This can be illustrated by some recent examples, which demonstrate that there have been striking thematic continuities in twentieth-century debates on the political economy of old age.

AN AGEING POPULATION

Since the late 1970s, there has been an increasing wave of concern over the growth of the proportion of elderly (particularly the very old) that is likely to take place over the next fifty years, and the social and economic consequences of the ageing population. In 1981 Shegog claimed, in the publication significantly entitled *The Impending Crisis of Old Age*, that one problem above all others was 'already casting an unmistakable shadow. This is the marked increase in the numbers of very elderly and frail people which will occur in Britain in the next twenty years, and the consequent profound effects on society and its social and health services' (Shegog, 1981). The demographic trend has prompted fairly crude calculations of the cost to the community of the elderly – from the Department of Health and Social Security's (DHSS) claim that the average cost of care and treatment of a person aged over 75, in health

Table 6.1 Ratios of dependants to workers in the United Kingdom 1841–1980. Data from Thomson (1984).

| Date | Percentage share of the total population | | | |
	0–14 years	65+ years	Total dependants	15–64 years
1841	36	4	40	60
1901	32	5	37	63
1980	21	15	36	64

and personal social services resources, is seven times that of a person of working age (DHSS, 1978), to Treasury estimates that the gross expenditure per capita in England on hospital and community health services in 1981–82 for all groups was £255, but for the 65–75 age group it was £455, and for the over-75s it was £1160 (Maynard, 1985).

Recent government threats to cut the State Earnings Related Pension Scheme (SERPS) were accompanied by similar dire warnings of the consequences of a worsening 'dependency ratio' when a population ages. The 1985 White Paper *The Reform of Social Security* emphasised that the pensioner population would grow from 9.3 million in 1985 to 13.2 million in 2035, and during that period the ratio of those contributing to the state pension scheme to those receiving pensions would change from 2.3:1 to 1.6:1 (DHSS, 1985). If demographic issues create the 'problem', however, they do not dictate the solution (Myles, 1986). Dependency ratios are, indeed, partly determined by policy shifts regarding entry to and exit from the labour market. Thus, a simple dependency ratio, taking no account of the complex shifting patterns of labour-force participation, means virtually nothing and is open to conflicting interpretations. It is true that the ratio of economically active individuals per person of pensionable age in the United Kingdom has fallen from 6.6 in 1901 to 2.6 in 1981, but, on the other hand, it appears that, on a simple age-related division, the mid-Victorian period of unfettered free enterprise capitalism and spectacular economic growth was one in which the ratio of 'active' adults to 'dependent' young and old was extraordinarily low (Table 6.1).

Demographic projections are also meaningless if they fail to take account of future per capita productivity, and it is arguable that this can never be accurately predicted. As recent opponents of the attack on SERPS have pointed out, the 1954 Phillips Committee correctly forecast that by 1979 there would be 9.5 million pensioners; but they went on to make the alarmist declaration that drastic measures would have to be taken to support this burden, such as raising the retirement age (Labour Research Department, 1986). Reddin has likewise cited the illustration that there were 40 per cent of American workers engaged in agriculture in 1900; there are a mere four per cent now, but they produce more food. 'What counts', he argues, 'is the nation's resources and whether we are willing to share them with one group rather than another. The scale of these resources is not a function of the size of the workforce, nor the number of taxpayers' (Reddin and Pilch, 1985). Thus, if dependency is 'a socially rather than a biologically constructed status' (Walker, 1985) we must recognise that social accounting is also a highly political exercise: to the 1985 White Paper's claim that 40 per cent of hospital and community health service costs go to retired people (DHSS, 1985) can be directed the retort that fully three-quarters of NHS expenditure pays the wages and salaries of its employees (DHSS, 1979).

This recent debate echoes uncannily the 'population panic' of fifty years ago, when similar concerns suddenly blossomed. The fall in fertility from the late 1870s had a profound effect on attitudes to the elderly in the 1930s and 1940s. For while the population of Britain was continuing to increase, from 10.5 million in 1801 to 37.0 million in 1901 and 46.6 million in 1941, the rate of increase was diminishing and family size was falling (fertility reaching its low point in 1933). It appeared that the age-structure pyramid would become top heavy, with an increasing proportion of elderly people supported by a decreasing number of producers.

The most notorious projections were by Enid Charles (1935) who made the often quoted calculation that, if the falling trends in fertility and mortality continued, between 1935 and 2035 the proportion of the England and Wales population aged 60 and over would rise from 12.5 to 57.8 per cent. Though this was a purely hypothetical projection, completely unjustifiable on grounds of common sense let alone demography, it was widely accepted by public and political opinion. Duncan Sandys, for example, in a 1937 House of Commons debate on the birth rate, called Enid Charles 'one of the greatest living experts on population problems', and warned that 'the time will sooner or later be reached when a smaller number of productive workers will be called upon to support an increasing number of old people. One aspect of this will be the increased burden to the nation of old age pensions, which at present cost £40m. and in 1965 are likely to have risen to £64m.' (House of Commons, 1937). By the late 1930s there were appearing in the press numerous lurid tales of a future Britain with deserted cities and idle factories while the spa towns were clogged up with pensioners in bath chairs.

The envisaged consequences of an ageing population in the 1930s were even worse than they have been in the 1980s: industrial retardation, spiralling welfare costs, a lack of economic enterprise, higher taxation of the 'producers', and a decline of 'creativity' and energy in the national psyche (Titmuss and Titmuss, 1942). As in the 1980s, it can be seen that concern over an ageing population was actually symptomatic of wider economic and global insecurities – mass unemployment, fiscal retrenchment and the drift towards war – in which the 'burden' of old age was seized upon as a convenient scapegoat. Then as now, the empirical evidence was open to different interpretations: for example, it could be pointed out that, whereas in the mid-Victorian boom year of 1851, 59.8 per cent of the population had been in the 15–64 years 'producers' group, by the recession of 1939 this proportion had actually improved, to 69.7 per cent (owing, of course, to a fall in the child population). Some observers viewed the future increase in the elderly with apprehension but also recognised that a growing proportion of consumers could stimulate aggregate demand and be economically beneficial (Henderson, 1938). Likewise, the 1949 *Report of the Royal Commission on Population*, though also alarmist, had to admit that the changing age-structure of the population over the past 60 years had been 'an important factor making for higher standards of living'. (Royal Commission on Population, 1949). Little wonder that when reviewing these conflicting and contradictory statements, the Registrar General, S.P. Vivian, minuted in 1943 that most of the experts had grossly exaggerated the problem, 'owing, it would seem, to a desire to attract publicity to their work and gain public repute' (Public Record Office, 1943). Crude demographic determinism must thus be treated with great caution. In the current political climate, it is clearly being used as one rationale for across-the-board cuts in welfare services. Proponents of the fashionable cry for 'generational equity' (essentially, a claim that resources are unfairly over-distributed to elderly people and should be reallocated to children) should be aware that the lesson from history is that rarely are such debates politically neutral.

PENSIONERS AND POVERTY

Recently, Jowell and Airey (1984) discovered that the elderly are the least likely of all age groups to acknowledge the existence of contemporary poverty levels. This phenomenon suggests that living standards may be evaluated by reference to past experience, which, for the present generation of pensioners, includes memories of childhood and early adulthood during the Depression. Deprivation has a subjective and relative component, and the problem of internalised low expectations is particularly acute in the case of pensioners. Perhaps the most telling illustration of continuing relative disadvantage is the extent of income maintenance provided in old age. The 1950s and 1960s saw a series of investigations, all of which used National Assistance levels as a standard guide to low income. Cole and Utting (1962) found 27 per cent of Britain's elderly population to be on or below the poverty line; Abel-Smith and Townsend's (1965) analysis of Family Expenditure Survey data revealed that 35 per cent of people in low income households were elderly persons whose primary source of succour was the state retirement pension. Later, Jordan claimed that 23 per cent of all retired people were living at the officially determined subsistence level while 'hundreds of thousands' were below it (Jordan, 1978). Official statistics in the 1980s repeatedly showed that around two-thirds of pensioners lived at or below the 140 per cent supplementary benefit level. These figures differ little, as relative measures, from those collected in the 1890s, when Charles Booth (1894) first clarified the connection between poverty and old age, showing between one-fifth and one-third of all those aged over 65 years as below the breadline. Rowntree's first (1899) and second (1936) studies of York also showed that a third of pensioners were on or below subsistence level (Rowntree, 1901; 1941). In 1947 the latter found that, principally because of the fall in unemployment, old age had become the primary cause of poverty in the population (Rowntree, 1901; 1941; 1947).

In the 1970s and 1980s, however, rising unemployment and economic recession have focused attention on all low-income groups generally, to the benefit of elderly people. Unemployment has in fact revealed the complexity of the old age experience. Firstly, it has accelerated the withdrawal of the elderly from the labour market and from reliance on state welfare such that, as Nicholas Bosanquet puts it, 'to retire is, for many people, to step on a time machine and move backwards in terms of living standards' (Bosanquet, 1978). Yet, on the other hand, high unemployment has encouraged early retirement and has led to what Schuller (1986) has called 'a crumbling of the conventional dividing line between active and retired people', which can only erode simplistic age-related definitions and improve public attitudes to the elderly. Thirdly, unemployment has lifted the *relative* economic position of pensioners: in 1971 over half the families (52%) in the lowest quartile group of incomes were pensioners, but by 1982 the percentage had fallen to 27 (their place being taken by the younger unemployed and one-parent families) (Central Statistical Office, 1986).

Since the Second World War, state pensions have risen in real terms: the basic state retirement pension for a single man rose from 20 per cent of average net male manual earnings in 1951 to 33 per cent in 1981 (Fiegehen, 1986). And in as much as consumer spending is a valid indicator, the absolute improvement in the material status of the elderly has been significant since the 1950s:

the percentage of people aged 65 or over living in households with a washing machine rose from 22 to 70 between 1959 and 1982, and the equivalent figures for refrigerators were 12 to 88; for a telephone, 9 to 64; and for a television set, 42 to 96. Between 1959 and 1982 home ownership among the general population increased from 38 to 59 per cent whilst among those aged 65 or over it rose from 44 to 52 per cent (Abrams, 1983). Thus, the political potential of the elderly has increased, and the growth of 'old age investment' has likewise been impressive, with the share of UK equities owned by pension funds rising from 7 to 29 per cent between 1963 and 1983 (Schuller, 1986).

By the early 1970s, the elderly represented 16 per cent of the UK population whilst the proportion of public expenditure absorbed by their social security, health and welfare costs was 48 per cent (Wroe, 1973). The first half of this century had seen a considerable broadening and redefinition of state provision, and, following the introduction of the new universal pension scheme in 1946, the average person over 65 had resources equal to 83 per cent of those possessed by people of working age (Thane, 1984). This, it has been argued, was a considerably higher proportion than had been granted previously. However, Thomson contends that, since the war, 'the economic position of elderly persons has deteriorated badly (while) the true value of pensions has fallen steadily and unrelentingly'. Whereas the pension has maintained its relative value at around 40 per cent of the mean income of a person of working age, 'the total "package" of incomes which the elderly enjoy ... has had its value eroded' (Thomson, 1983). Using evidence from some 22 family expenditure surveys conducted over the past 150 years, Thomson claims that whilst mid-nineteenth century Poor Law payments to the elderly were equivalent to more than two-thirds of the incomes of the working-aged, it has 'been accepted in the present century that 'the elderly should be given little more than one-third of the resources of other adults' (Thomson, 1984). In 1979, however, the average person over 65 had 68 per cent of the resources of a working-aged adult, some 15 per cent less than in the early 1950s but more than double the proportion suggested by Thomson. The explanation for this apparent inconsistency lies in the fact that, 'the earnings of adult male manual workers, the most common standard by which social security incomes are assessed, have become an increasingly inadequate indicator of the resources of British households'. Increased percentages of men in white-collar occupations, growing numbers of women in paid employment (until recently, at least), tax allowances, fewer children and the exclusion of elderly relatives from the household, have combined to boost the average incomes of those below retirement age. Such factors, however, have remained absent from the standard earnings index used (Thomson, 1984).

Conversely, it can be shown that in 1981 pensioners were receiving 15 per cent of the total national disposable income, more than twice the proportion they received 30 years previously. Clearly the overall rise in numbers was the principal explanation. Nevertheless, in real terms pensioner incomes tripled over the period, the value of the basic pension relative to that of the male manual worker's wage increasing from one-fifth to a third. On the other hand, households headed by persons over 64 years had more to spend or save relative to other households in 1965 than they do today (*New Society*, 1986). Since increasing numbers of older people tend to live alone or in couples, the implications are not favourable.

Relative to all other household incomes among older people, the basic pension has fallen from a mid-nineteenth century level of 70–90 per cent to a postwar twentieth century one of 40–50 per cent (Thomson, 1987). Superficially, such figures may suggest that older people have either become financially more independent or increasingly reliant upon a combination of dwindling state benefits and local welfare services. We should note, however, that intergenerational transfers are notoriously difficult to gauge and that indirect financial support from relatives who do not co-reside may be of considerable account in some cases.

Older people who are single, widowed, divorced or separated have fewer resources than those who are married, whilst those of advanced age are poorer than the 'young old'. Only 13 per cent of supplementary benefit claimants of pensionable age live in married couples. Thirty-five per cent of all pensioners on benefit are widows, an indicator of the greater longevity of women as well as the poverty accruing from their earlier dependent status (Central Statistical Office, 1986).

The belief that an increasing proportion of elderly people live in non-private homes is unfounded: in 1981, approximately three per cent of the pensionable population resided in communal establishments, whereas in 1906 almost six per cent had been living in Poor Law institutions (OPCS, 1984; Anderson, 1983). Thomson has argued that when collective expenditure on the elderly is high, pensioners will be able to maintain their independence in the community, but, when pensions are low, more will be forced into institutions. Such a correlation is perhaps too simplistic. Community care solutions have been advocated as a means of keeping older people in their own homes for as long as possible, yet the closure of local authority residential homes, the abandonment of plans to build new ones and decreases in staffing levels have run in tandem with a failure to expand domiciliary services (Thomson, 1983; Phillipson, 1982). Whilst many old people depend upon indirect subsidies, maintaining some form of 'intimacy at a distance' from their relatives, others rely more directly on the personal social services of family caregivers, predominantly their daughters. Yet, older people will always require a measure of state funding. Whether rising numbers of the very old living institutionally are financed by cuts in the incomes and living standards of those still in the community, or if growing numbers of the latter demand higher subsidies, the fiscal consequences of population ageing are likely to remain considerable.

PENSIONERS AND POLITICS

There are few indications that increased representation by or on behalf of the elderly has had a major impact on policy decisions. This absence of political influence is the outcome of a process of social fragmentation which has three important dimensions: firstly, each cohort of pensioners appears to exhibit a different generational awareness of social change over the life cycle; secondly, the elderly are themselves segregated by pervasive inequalities in income (horizontal divisions); and, finally, as we have seen, the development of age-related classifications, embodied strikingly in the emergence of retirement, has led to an increasing vertical separation between people of working age and those officially disqualified from normal employment.

Organised militancy amongst pensioners first developed in the late 1930s and early 1940s with the rise of the National Federation of Old Age Pensions Associations. The putative causes behind this development include the fact that both the mass literacy and 'trade union habits and organization' acquired by pensioners of this generation were historically unprecedented (Branson and Heinemann, 1971). Not surprisingly, since the beneficiaries of these trends were mostly working people, campaigns for better pensions were fuelled by the economic priorities of the relatively poor. This remains so 50 years later. Campaigns by middle class elders, pressing specific issues, are, meanwhile, conspicuous by their absence, whilst educational groups such as the University of the Third Age, pre-retirement associations and health promotion activities are consciously apolitical. Such heterogeneity of commitment is reflected in voting behaviour: in 1984, for example, 38 per cent of men over 65 and 47 per cent of older women identified with the Conservative Party, whilst 36 and 30 per cent respectively, preferred Labour (Jowell and Airey, 1984). Retirement acts as a form of severance, not only in terms of income and activity, but also as regards social and political exclusion. The absence of industrial muscle renders the non-working population relatively powerless whilst disengagement from the collective focus of the work-place inhibits the growth of new solidarities, a process not helped by the labour movement's tendency to concentrate on trade union struggles. Transport costs and the onset of physical disability further constrain the possibilities for collective activity in later life. Over five million elderly people inhabit households without cars, a disadvantage which increases with age and is greatest for those who live alone (OPCS, 1984).

Such factors alone do not adequately explain the failure of pressure groups to influence decision making. If they did, then we should be forced to conclude that the structured dependence of the elderly plays a larger role than has in fact been the case. When assessing the politics of specific groups strategic considerations also have some bearing. The National Conference on Old Age Pensions, formed in 1916, was instrumental in winning a series of concessions and supplements to the basic pension during and after the First World War. However, they were not successful in achieving their grander aim of a universal pension which abolished the means test. Their key target had been the 'penalty on thrift' which the 1908 pension imposed through income disqualifications, but, in the event, providence was part of a moral language appropriate to the 'labour aristocracy' rather than the mass of working people. The rhetoric of respectability became increasingly unrealistic during the economic depression in which, as was frequently noted, unemployment might disperse the savings of a lifetime overnight. Composed largely of friendly society and labour movement affiliates, the organisation's membership was not one of pensioners themselves.

As already noted, later initiatives did involve older people acting on their own behalf. The localised branch network and fiercely combative attitude of the National Federation, resembling 'the abrasive approach of 1960s pressure groups such as Shelter, rather than the more staid "non-political" approach of the voluntary organisations', acted as a powerful consciousness raiser. Such confrontationalism, hinging on pensions but failing to discuss in depth the inadequacies of medical and social provision, won little favour with Beveridge. He paid scant attention to the pensioners' own lobbying when he introduced his recommendation of a retirement condition for receipt of the state pension through pressure from the Trades Union Congress, who believed that only a retirement condition would enable pensions to be raised without resulting in wage cuts to elderly workers which threatened the entire wage structure (Macnicol and Blaikie, 1989). In contrast, the acquiescence of groups like the National Old People's Welfare Committee helped to facilitate the postwar division of responsibilities whereby, 'central government would be responsible for pensions (and) local authorities would develop residential care. The National Health Service would offer medical services (and) the voluntary organisations would be expected to develop visiting schemes and other services' (Means and Smith, 1985).

In the 1930s and 1940s, therefore, representative organisations of the elderly were relatively impotent in influencing state pensions policy. In the 1950s, a 'pensions lobby' did develop, headed by Richard Titmuss, Brian Abel-Smith and Peter Townsend, and succeeded in keeping the issue to the forefront of policy debates. In the 1960s, however, the claims of the elderly were rather pushed aside as the 'rediscovery of poverty' turned attention to other issues such as child poverty, educational disadvantage, community action, positive discrimination and inner-city deprivation (Banting, 1979). Significantly, no pensioners' lobby was formed equivalent in political influence to the Child Poverty Action Group. In the 1960s, the elderly were not a cause upon which political reputations were made. Ironically, although the Federation's membership rose to 250 000 in the immediate postwar period, it was dissatisfaction with a declining militancy which led to the formation of breakaway regional, trade unions and local groups whose impact was, and is, perhaps more limited in scale. During the 1970s, promotional organisations such as Age Concern and Help the Aged, whilst presenting a broadly popular image, focused upon lobbying policy makers through the presentation of expert advice, rather than petitioning Parliament by means of collective, mass support. And in the 1980s, a rupture has occurred in the all-party consensus over the worthiness of the pensioners' cause. We may soon witness the rise of a less conciliatory politics of concern, although the likelihood of such a strategy delivering higher pensions and better services remains slight. Older people tend to vote as they voted when they first entered work. To date a rootedness in convictions formed in the 1930s and forties may have augured well for Labour; the generation which came of age in the 1950s and '60s is unlikely to think in similar fashion.

The status of older people in modern British society is thus complex and varied, reflecting – if not sharpening – inequalities among those of working age. Running through this complexity, however, is a clear correlation between old age and poverty. Public opinion recognises this, yet fails to provide a sufficiently strong pressure to redirect resources towards the third age, even though, in the long run, most of us can expect to become pensioners. Few have given much serious thought to the desirable distribution of incomes and resources among the elderly: it is a topic that is conspicuously absent from the economic literature, Midwinter (1985) being an honourable exception. Meanwhile, examples abound of our ageism defeating even our long-term self-interest, ranging from woeful under-participation by members in their own private pension schemes to public tolerance of the disgraceful ill-treatment of residents in some old people's homes. We have a long way to go before we can begin to appreciate fully what Simone de Beauvoir (1977) once termed 'the necessity of our contingency'.

It is still too easy and common for those who oppose the redistributive potential of state welfare to portray the elderly as a horrific fiscal burden, with little positive economic or social contribution to make to society. We have, in short, progressed little way since the 1947 Nuffield Survey candidly observed that:

> We are confronted with two co-existent and sometimes incompatible facts. On the one hand there is the natural desire of the community to minister generously to the needs and comfort of old age; on the other hand . . . the burden of maintaining the aged may become so great as to result in a lowering of the national standard of living.   (Rowntree, 1947)

REFERENCES

Abel-Smith, B. and Townsend, P. (1965). *The Poor and the Poorest.* Occasional Paper on Social Administration, No. 17. G. Bell and Sons, London.

Abrams, M. (1983). Changes in the life-styles of the elderly 1959–1982. In *Social Trends 1984*, Central Statistical Office, pp. 11–16. HMSO, London.

Anderson, M. (1983). What is new about the modern family: an historical perspective. *Office of Population Censuses and Surveys Occasional Papers*, **31**, 1–16.

Banting, K. (1979). *Poverty, Politics and Policy: Britain in the 1960s.* Macmillan, London.

Booth, C. (1894). *The Aged Poor in England and Wales.* Macmillan, London.

Bosanquet, N. (1978). *A Future for Old Age.* Temple Smith, London.

Branson, N. and Heinemann, M. (1971). *Britain in the Nineteen Thirties.* Weidenfeld and Nicholson, London.

. Central Statistical Office (1986). *Social Trends 1986*, No. 16. HMSO, London.

Central Statistical Office (1987). *Social Trends 1987*, No. 17. HMSO, London.

Charles, E. (1935). *The Effect of Present Trends in Fertility and Mortality upon the Future Population of England and Wales and upon its Age Composition.* London and Cambridge Economic Service Special Memorandum No. 40, London.

Cole, D. with Utting, J. (1962). *The Economic Circumstances of Old People.* Occasional Paper on Social Administration No. 4. Codicote Press, Welwyn, Hertfordshire.

De Beauvoir, S. (1977). *Old Age.* Penguin, Harmondsworth, Middlesex.

Department of Health and Social Security (DHSS) (1978). *A Happier Old Age. A Discussion Document on Elderly People in Our Society.* HMSO, London.

DHSS (1979). Royal Commission on the National Health Service Report. (Cmnd 7615). HMSO, London.

DHSS (1985). *The Reform of Social Security.* (Cmnd 9517). HMSO, London.

Fiegehen, G.C. (1986). Income after retirement. In *Social Trends 1986*, Central Statistical Office, pp. 13–18. HMSO, London.

Foner, N. (1984). *Ages in Conflict: A Cross-Cultural Perspective on Inequality Between Old and Young.* Columbia University Press, New York.

Francis, D. (1984). *Will You Still Need Me, Will You Still Feed Me, When I'm 84?* Indiana University Press, Bloomington, Indiana.

Graebner, W. (1980). *A History of Retirement. The Meaning and Function of an American Institution, 1885–1978.* Yale University Press, New Haven, Connecticut.

Guillemard, A-M. (1983). Introduction. In *Old Age and the Welfare State*, A-M. Guillemard (Ed.), pp. 3–15. Sage, London.

Hannah, L. (1986). *Inventing Retirement. The Development of Occupational Pensions in Britain.* Cambridge University Press, Cambridge.

Havighurst, R. (1978). Ageing in western society. In *The Social Challenge of Ageing*, D. Hobman (Ed.), pp. 15–44. Croom Helm, London.

Henderson, H.D. (1938). Economic consequences. In *The Population Problem*, T.H. Marshall (Ed.), pp. 84–106. Allen and Unwin, London.

House of Commons (1937). *Debates*, 5s, Vol. 320, 10 Feb. 1937, Cols. 492, 494.

Johnson, P. (1985). *The Economics of Old Age in Britain: A Long-Run View 1881–1981.* Discussion Paper No. 47. Centre for Economic Policy Research, London.

Jordan, D. (1978). Poverty and the elderly. In *An Ageing Population*, V. Carver and P. Liddiard (Eds), pp. 166–78. Hodder & Stoughton, Sevenoaks, Kent.

Jowell, R. and Airey, C. (Eds) (1984) *British Social Attitudes: The 1984 Report.* Gower, London.

Labour Research Department (1986). *Social Insecurity: Callous Plans for Pensions and Benefits.* Labour Research Department, London.

Macnicol, J. and Blaikie, A. (1989). The politics of retirement, 1908–48. In *Growing Old in the Twentieth Century,* M. Jefferys (Ed.). Routledge, London.

Maynard, A. (1985). Policy choices in the health sector. In *Challenges to Social Policy,* R. Berthoud (Ed.), pp. 139–68. Gower, Aldershot, Hampshire.

Means, R. and Smith, R. (1985). *The Development of Welfare Services for Elderly People.* Croom Helm, London.

Midwinter, E. (1985). *The Wage of Retirement: The Case for a New Pensions Policy.* Centre for Policy on Ageing, London.

Myles, J. (1984). *Old Age in the Welfare State: The Political Economy of Public Pensions.* Little, Brown and Co., Boston.

Myles, J. (1986). Why does population aging matter? Paper delivered to 39th Annual Scientific Meeting of the Gerontological Society of America, Chicago.

New Society (1986). Database, 5 December 1986.

Office of Population Censuses and Surveys (OPCS) (1984). *Britain's Elderly Population.* Census Guide 1. HMSO, London.

Phillipson, C. (1982). *Capitalism and the Construction of Old Age.* Macmillan, London.

Phillipson, C. (1983). The state, the economy and retirement. In *Old Age and the Welfare State,* A-M. Guillemard (Ed.), pp. 127–39. Sage, London.

Public Record Office (1943). Memorandum by S.P. Vivian (1943), PRO RG 26/11.

Reddin, M. and Pilch, M. (1985). *Can We Afford Our Future?* Age Concern England, Mitcham, Surrey.

Riddle, S.M. (1984). Age, obsolescence and unemployment: older men in the British industrial system, 1920–1939: a research note. *Ageing and Society,* 4(4), 517–24.

Rowntree, B.S. (1901). *Poverty: A Study of Town Life.* Macmillan, London.

Rowntree, B.S. (1941). *Poverty and Progress. A Second Social Survey of York.* Longman, London.

Rowntree, B.S. (1947). *Old People.* Report of a Survey Committee on the Problems of Ageing and the Care of Old People for The Nuffield Foundation, Oxford University Press, Oxford.

Royal Commission on Population (1949). *Report of the Royal Commission on Population* (Cmnd 7695). HMSO, London.

Schuller, T. (1986). *Age, Capital and Democracy. Member Participation in Pension Schemes.* Gower, Aldershot, Hampshire.

Shegog, R.F.A. (Ed.) (1981). *The Impending Crisis of Old Age.* Oxford University Press/Nuffield Provincial Hospitals Trust, Oxford.

Sheldon, J.H. (1948). *The Social Medicine of Old Age: Report of an Inquiry in Wolverhampton.* Oxford University Press, Oxford.

Taylor, R. and Ford, G. (1983). Inequalities in old age: an examination of age, sex and class differences in a sample of community elderly. *Ageing and Society,* 3(2), 183–208.

Thane, P. (1978). The muddled history of retiring at 60 and 65. *New Society,* 3 August 1978.

Thane, P. (1984). *Ageing and the Economy: Historical Issues.* Discussion Paper No. 16, Centre for Economic Policy Research, London.

Thomson, D. (1983). Workhouse to nursing home: residential care of elderly people in England since 1840. *Ageing and Society*, **3**(1), 43–69.

Thomson, D. (1984). The decline of social welfare: falling state support for the elderly since early Victorian times. *Ageing and Society*, **4**(4), 451–82.

Thomson, D. (1987). The relief of poverty: a forgotten element in English historical demography. Paper presented to ESRC Cambridge Group for the History of Population and Social Structure, February.

Titmuss, R. and Titmuss, K. (1942). *Parents Revolt: A Study in the Declining Birth Rate in Acquisitive Societies.* Secker and Warburg, London.

Townsend, P. (1981). The structured dependency of the elderly: a creation of social policy in the twentieth century. *Ageing and Society*, **1**(1), 5–28.

Walker, A. (1981). Towards a political economy of old age. *Ageing and Society*, **1**(1), 73–94.

Walker, A. (1985). Care of elderly people. In *Challenges to Social Policy*, R. Berthoud (Ed.), pp. 185–209. Gower, Aldershot, Hampshire.

Wroe, D.C.L. (1973). The elderly. In *Social Trends 1973*, Central Statistical Office, pp. 23–33. HMSO, London.

Toni Antonucci

and

James Jackson

Institute for Social Research
The University of Michigan
Ann Arbor, Michigan, USA

7 SUCCESSFUL AGEING AND LIFE COURSE RECIPROCITY

RECIPROCITY AND SUCCESSFUL AGEING

In this paper we propose that the concept of reciprocity is related in complex but important ways to successful ageing. It is hypothesised that individuals who view themselves as having reciprocal relationships with important others in their lives are most likely to achieve a successful adjustment to ageing. The norm of reciprocity is generally considered to be strong in the United States and perhaps in most other western countries (Gouldner, 1960). We believe that the norm of reciprocity affects how the individual accepts, provides and perceives the exchange of social support. It is hypothesised that those people who feel that their interpersonal relationships across the life course have been reciprocal – that they have both given to and received from others – will be the most successful in coping with problems related to individual ageing.

Individuals who feel that they have made a contribution to the world in which they live are likely to feel good about themselves; to feel personally competent; and to feel that they are capable of confronting and coping with problems as they arise. Hence, it is reasonable to assume that these same people are the most likely to adapt successfully to the problems and changes that often accompany the ageing process. People often feel good about making a contribution to the lives of others but we hypothesise that they feel even better about maintaining a reciprocal relationship with others. Reciprocity is considered to be a more attractive option for people than the simple receipt of goods, services, or affection from significant others for two reasons. Firstly, it avoids the feeling of exploitation, and it has clear implications of a long-term relationship. It is difficult to have a relationship in which only one of the two parties is giving. Inevitably a feeling of indebtedness (Greenberg, 1980) emerges on the one hand, or a feeling of exploitation on the other (Hatfield *et al.*, 1978). A sense of reciprocity mitigates this potential problem in the exchange relationship. Secondly, reciprocal relationships, because they involve giving and receiving from both participants, imply temporal duration of the relationship. Admitted-

This research was conducted while the first author held a Research Career Development Award from the United States National Institute on Aging and the second author was a National Research Council/Ford Foundation Senior Postdoctoral Fellow at the Groupe D'Études et de Recherches sur la Science, Études des Hautes Etudes en Sciences Sociales, Paris, France. An earlier version of this paper was presented at the Second European Conference on Developmental Psychology in Rome, Italy, September, 1986. We would like to thank Karin Clissold, Susan Crohan, Halimah Hassan and Linda Shepard for the analyses and tables reported in the chapter, Rose Gibson for her comments on an earlier version and Kay Davis for preparation of the final manuscript.

The data computation upon which this paper is based employed the OSIRIS IV computer software package which was developed by the Institute for Social Research, The University of Michigan, using funds from the Survey Research Center, Inter-University Consortium for Political Research, National Science Foundation, and other sources.

ly, some 'enduring' reciprocal relationships may be temporally restricted (college friends, for example), but others are of long duration such as the relationships between parent and child, or husband and wife.

The concept of reciprocity

Our definition of the term reciprocity is most consistent with that proposed by Gouldner (1960) in his seminal article on the norm of reciprocity. Reciprocity refers to the equal or comparable exchange of tangible aid, emotional affection, advice, or information between individuals or groups. This basic definition of reciprocity is relatively non-controversial. The definition, however, can be considerably more complicated. One's concept of reciprocity may be quite limited in both time and content, or it may be considerably broadened. For example, the framework in the present paper assumes that generalised reciprocity is possible, involving both cognitive mechanisms (expectations) and tangible exchanges across time, individuals and groups (Krebs and Miller, 1985; Trivers, 1971).

On the basis of an anthropological study of older people in the United States, Wentowski (1981) concluded that the norm of reciprocity was quite strong but that it varied depending upon several characteristics of a relationship. These included its nature, duration and function. For example, close relatives have long-term, enduring relationships with each other. Their concept of reciprocity is significantly different from short-term relationships among non-relatives. Relationships can be viewed on a continuum of closeness; the closest having both long duration and emotional closeness, define reciprocity in the most general and non-specific manner. Both members of the dyad feel a general commitment and obligation to the partner for support received in the past, or expected in the future. The commitment is generalised, the obligation enduring. On the other hand, relationships with people at the other end of the continuum of closeness are marked by a limited, specific, and time-bound sense of reciprocity. In these latter situations one member of the dyad receives support of some kind from the other member. It may even be the case that the contact is initiated solely for transacting a specific exchange. For example, a neighbour might introduce a friend in need of a ride to a neighbour who is going to the same place and who can provide transport. In this case, there is no assumption of an enduring relationship, nevertheless, the norm of reciprocity operates. The passenger is likely to seek to repay the felt obligation in a comparable and immediate fashion. She might offer to drive the neighbour's friend to the next meeting, to pay for the gasoline, or she might reciprocate by offering to provide refreshments after the meeting. In this short-term relationship, there is a perceived need to reciprocate immediately. Unlike the case of the family relationship, where each party has confidence in the continuing interaction and future exchanges, this short-term relationship requires a prompt return.

Reciprocity has not held a central place in the social support and ageing literature. Several theorists, however, are beginning to consider seriously its potential implications and applications (e.g. Akiyama et al., in press; Knipscheer, 1985; Lee, 1985; Hinde, 1979; Mitchell and Trickett, 1980; Shinn et al., 1985; Shore, 1985). Lee (1985), in an extension of the work of Dowd (1975; 1980), reconsidered supportive interactions and social networks within the context of social exchange theory. Longino and Lipman (1981) used a life course reciprocity notion to explain their findings of consistent sex differences in the social support networks of men and women. Israel et al. (1984) report that affective reciprocity was the only interactive support variable from an entire battery of social network measures which significantly predicted psycho-logical well-being. Recently, Israel and Antonucci (1987) replicated this finding with a national sample of people 50 years of age and over.

Clark *et al.* (1986) discuss two types of reciprocal relationships in older age: communal and exchange. The first is quite similar to that described by Wentowski (1981) as long-term and enduring. Communal relationships assume a long-term perspective of mutual benefits over time. Exchange relationships, on the other hand, involve a more explicit and immediate form of reciprocity. Dowd (1975; 1980; 1984) employed an extension of exchange theory as an explanatory framework for the interpersonal interactions of older people. His work has been largely confined to issues of broad social policy, the emergence of politicised age consciousness and the potential for conflict among members of different age strata. Dowd assumes that as people age they are at an increasing disadvantage in social exchanges because they possess ever decreas-ing power and prestige. His central thesis is that old age is accompanied by a reduction in the possession of valued exchange commodities. This reduction in valued goods lessens the ability of older people to interact successfully with younger people, since the latter do have valued goods and seek like goods from others. Dowd (1984) stated that, 'rather than reciprocity, our treatment of the very old is based upon the norm of beneficience'.

Dowd's (1984) conceptualisation of exchange in older age is dependent upon a specific, time-circumscribed notion of recriprocity. We agree that immediate reciprocity is a culturally important aspect of social and economic transfer among individuals and groups. In the case of exchanges in older age, however, a broader individual life course perspective may be necessary (Longino and Lipman, 1981).

Two central issues are particularly relevant when examining reciprocity in the context of ageing. One is the continuing or enduring aspect of the relationship. The individual feels confident in these interactions, secure in the knowledge that the relationship itself will continue. Also important is the potential for a long-term or life span accounting system. If a relationship is certain to continue for years, then one can assume that supports provided or received can and will eventually be repaid or provided. There will be confidence that the relationship will endure and that potential exchanges will continue to be available. Similarly, the length of the relationships and the comprehensive accounting of supports given and received, also works in favour of successful ageing. Not to be minimised is the repeated empirical finding that people on average report that they provide more support than they receive (Antonucci and Akiyama, 1987a; Antonucci and Israel, 1986). This lasts well into old age and suggests to us that people build up a reserve of support in case they later find themselves unable to provide support or, perhaps because of functional disability, they require support from others. In a culture where the norm of reciprocity is prevalent, this point is critical. It suggests that older people can receive a great deal of support from close and important others, potentially for an extended period of time, and still feel relatively unindebted. Greenberg (1980) and his colleagues have argued and empirically demonstrated that feelings of indebtedness are noxious and active-ly avoided by individuals. Similarly, individuals also labour to avoid or to reduce situations of exploitation and the concomitant feelings of lowered self-worth and esteem, and reduced tangible resources (Hatfield *et al.*, 1978). We suggest that people go to great lengths to avoid indebtedness in social relationships and that a life course perspective best explains how it is circumvented.

THE SOCIAL SUPPORT BANK

We have proposed the notion of a *Social Support Bank*, that incorporates both a life course perspective and the concept of reciprocity in a unified conceptualisation of long-term social interactions (Antonucci, 1985; Antonucci and Jackson, 1987). We hypothesise that as the individual develops and matures he or she experiences a continuing series of exchanges with significant others. Examples of dyads which might involve these long-term exchanges include parent–child, husband–wife, and perhaps certain long-term friendships. These relationships and the reciprocity exchanges are similar to those described both by Wentowski (1981) as maintaining generalised conceptualisations of reciprocity and by Clark *et al.* (1986) for communal relationships.

The Social Support Bank suggests that individuals continually monitor their support exchanges. They maintain an accounting system which is relatively informal, a cognitive activity conducted with little specifically directed attention. Individuals are hypothesised to have a continuing awareness of what others have done for them and what they have done for others. This cognitive support account might be considered as analogous to a savings' account, an individual's attempt to develop a support reserve in case of need. Individuals attempt to maintain, at minimum, a balance between what is deposited, i.e. what is provided to others, and what is withdrawn, i.e. what is received. The development of a support reserve, where one consistently provides more to others than is received, is, however, optimal since this support reserve can be drawn upon in the future at a time of need. Thus, one is motivated to maintain exchanges that help significant others.

This accounting system is not conceived as either mercenary or uncharitable. On the contrary, it is best viewed as a culturally specific, adaptive mechanism. The Support Bank allows one to have commitments to continuing relationships which can be invested in and relied upon in case of future needs. Similarly, there is no convincing evidence that these accounting systems are necessarily accurate (see, for example, Antonucci and Israel, 1986). The Support Bank concept describes a psychological process, one which may or may not correspond to an objective observer's assessment.

RECIPROCITY AND SOCIAL SUPPORT: RECENT FINDINGS

Our work on the concept of reciprocity has had a large empirical component. For the last ten years we have been involved in several national studies in the United States. Of particular relevance to the concepts in this chapter are the two waves of the Social Supports of the Elderly (SSE) study (Kahn and Antonucci, 1984; 1986), the National Survey of Black Americans (NSBA) (Jackson *et al.*, 1982) and the National Three Generation Family Study (TGFS) (Jackson and Hatchett, 1986). The SSE provides extensive national data on the social networks and social supports of men and women aged fifty years and over in 1980. The NSBA is based upon a national probability sample of non-institutionalised black American citizens over the age of 18 residing in households in the continental United States in 1979–80 (Jackson, in press). The size of the sample (2107) provides a large representative number of blacks over the age of fifty. Similarly, the 1981 TGFS is a survey of three generation family lineages based upon a sample from the NSBA. This sample provides an additional 1006 separate interviews, approximately half of which are from respondents who are over the age of fifty.

Findings from the 1980 SSE study led directly to some of the life course hypotheses outlined above. The collection of a second wave of data four years later from the survivors of the first SSE sample made it possible to begin a preliminary exploration of these hypotheses derived from earlier analyses. Similarly, analyses of the NSBA and TGFS have yielded important findings on social support relationships with direct implications for the reciprocity conceptualisations and hypotheses proposed in this chapter (Taylor *et al.*, 1982; Chatters *et al.*, 1985; 1986; Taylor, 1985; 1986; Taylor and Chatters, 1986a; 1986b). The availability of data on national samples of the general elderly population as well as special populations of blacks, whose social support relationships have been the subject of much speculation (Cantor, 1979; Dressler, 1985), provide a rich source of evidence for the theoretical notions advanced in this chapter.

Relevant findings from each of these data sets can be summarised. The 1980 SSE study represented the first United States national, in-depth examination of the social support of older adults. As a result of our early interest in the concept of reciprocity, a great deal of time was devoted to obtaining detailed information on the exchange of six specific types of social support. After respondents generated their support network, they were asked to name the people to whom they provided and from whom they received each of six types of support. The types of support were: confiding, reassurance, respect, care when sick, talk when upset, and talk about health problems. The NSBA and TGFS were not as systematically conceived to focus on the social support and reciprocity concepts. Many of the questions, however, are relevant for the central themes of this chapter. Parallel analyses were conducted where appropriate and are reported below.

It had initially been hypothesised, consistent with the relevant literature (Dowd, 1980; 1984), that the supportive exchanges of older people would be marked by an excess of receiving and a deficit of providing. Using the life course Support Bank concept outlined above, we hypothesised that older individuals would feel comfortable reporting this lack of current reciprocity. The youngest respondents were aged 50–64, the middle group between 65–74, and the oldest group between 75 and 95 years. For the oldest age group in the SSE sample, it was assumed that people would feel it appropriate to receive more supports and provide fewer.

The results only partially corroborate this hypothesis. Older respondents did report that they provided fewer supports to fewer people than younger respondents, but there were no comparable age differences in the reported amount of support received from others. An analysis of the same age groupings in the NSBA and TGFS data sets yielded nearly identical results as the SSE. The two older age groups of blacks reported very little difference from the younger group in the frequency or amount of help received. In fact, there were no significant age differences across the three age groups. On the other hand, the older two groups, particularly the oldest, reported that they were less likely to provide help to family than the younger age group. It may be that older respondents receive comparable support as in earlier years, but from fewer people (Litwak, 1985; Chatters *et al.*, 1985). Long-term longitudinal data are needed to assess accurately this type of change. Two additional questions were asked in the TGFS on perceived changes over time in the amount of help given and received from adult children. While they are not strictly questions of reciprocity of assistance, they do relate to our concern with changes in age in the amount of support obtained and given. Consistent with our hypotheses, the oldest respondents were the least likely to report providing more help now than in the past to their children, but they were the most likely to report that their children helped them more than than formerly.

We assume, based upon these preliminary analyses, that the norm of reciprocity is so strong that people of all ages strive to maintain it. It has been hypothesised that healthy older people continue to maintain an immediate, temporal reciprocity as long as possible (Dowd, 1984). As noted above it has been a consistent finding (e.g., Israel, 1982) that most people who report non-reciprocal relationships indicate that they give more support than they receive. Maintaining a reciprocal relationship for younger, less frail older people can thus be readily accomplished using current, cross-sectional interactions and exchanges. It is possible that an adaptive technique used by relatively healthy older people is both to deny the receipt of support and to maximise their perception of the support they provide. We suspect that most people readily ignore sizeable discrepancies between their receipts and their contributions. When the discrepancies become too great to ignore, however, the adaptive older person then switches to a longitudinal, life course accounting system. Here, the Support Bank concept is particularly helpful. People who are no longer able to provide support to others draw from a psychological reserve of support. This support reserve only exists, however, within the close, long-term relationships described above, hence the necessity of reducing the number of people from whom one accepts support. Litwak (1985) has discussed the consequences of loss of network members on the provision of support. In our conceptualisation, it is argued that older individuals may reduce the members of the network from which they accept support on a voluntary basis (Chatters *et al.*, 1986). Both views have empirical support.

Other analyses from the SSE study are also relevant to the reciprocity concept. Antonucci and Israel (1986) explored the degree to which principal respondents and members of their support network agreed on the amount of support given and received. Ingersoll-Dayton and Antonucci (1988) examined perceived reciprocal versus non-reciprocal relationships in two types of support: confiding and sick care in spouse, children, and friend relationships. These analyses differ from Antonucci and Israel's (1986), in that they are based completely upon the principal respondent's report with no input from network members.

Antonucci and Israel (1986) found that agreement or overall veridicality was quite low. In the general analyses of agreement between principal and network respondents, veridicality was lowest when specific functions and specific network members were considered. It was highest when veridicality across all support functions was considered. However, when more specific relationships were taken into account, it became clear that veridicality was highest between spouses and the network member mentioned first (usually but not always the spouse). Although there was an average of 89 per cent agreement among spouses, the percentage between other network members was much lower, reaching a low of 30 per cent. It is interesting to note that veridicality was not significantly related to well-being as measured by overall life satisfaction, happiness and negative affect. We view this as further evidence of the importance of the psychological aspects of social support.

Ingersoll-Dayton and Antonucci (1988) found reported reciprocity to be greatest between spouses, less between parents and children, and least among friends. These data involve the respondents' reports of support provided and received. Over all age groups, if a lack of reciprocity was reported, the principal respondents indicated that they provided more support than they received. An examination of age differences indicates that with age, people reporting non-reciprocal confiding relationships with their spouse and children feel that they confide more than their network members confide in them. They also report an increase in the number of non-reciprocal sick care relationships with their children. Particularly noteworthy in the light of our hypothesis, however, is that there were no significant age differences among non-reciprocal relationships with friends. These findings support the hypothesis that people do try to maintain temporal reciprocity but when this is not possible switch to a life course reciprocity assessment. Since this life course reciprocity is more likely to be established with the spouse and children than with friends, the latter relationships are more likely to be terminated or limited when temporal reciprocity cannot be maintained. Some support for this observation was provided by an analysis on the NSBA data set by Chatters *et al.* (1986). These findings indicated that regardless of the type of available helper, older black Americans were more likely than younger respondents to select friend and other non-relative helpers. In the analyses reported by Ingersoll-Dayton and Antonucci, reciprocity was found to be related to well-being, particularly perceptions of the network as too demanding and to negative affect. Although Ingersoll-Dayton and Antonucci's (1988) findings suggest a complex pattern of relationships, it is notable that people who report receiving more sick care from their friends than they provide, experience significantly greater negative affect than those who report reciprocated sick care.

Analyses of the NSBA and TGFS data sets also reveal a complex pattern of relationships among reciprocity and well-being indices. Generally, the reciprocity variables were more likely to be related to happiness and satisfaction than reported frequency of current support. For 'younger' older blacks (50–64 years), those who reported receiving increased help from children in comparison to the past had significantly greater happiness and satisfaction scores than those who reported less or the same amount of help. For the oldest blacks (75 and older), however, those who received *less* help from children now than in the past reported significantly greater happiness and satisfaction scores than those who indicated that they received the same or more help from their children than in the past. Finally, consistent with Ingersoll-Dayton and Antonucci's (1988) analyses of the NSBA and TGFS, reports by the oldest groups (75 and older) of giving children greater help now than formerly were significantly related to increased reports of happiness.

Another suggestive pattern of sex differences has emerged from the 1980 SSE data. The support literature has traditionally suggested that women have larger networks than men and that they both receive and provide more support to others (Antonucci, 1985). Antonucci and Akiyama (1987b) have recently examined sex differences in the relationship between social support and happiness. Of eight quantitative measures of support (network size, spouse in network, number of children in network, number of friends in network, frequency of contact, number of supports received, number of supports provided, and reciprocity) and seven qualitative measures (satisfaction with marriage, satisfaction with family, satisfaction with friends, network too demanding, network gets on nerves, network does not understand, and want more people in network) entered into separate regression analyses for men and women, only reciprocity emerged as a significant predictor of happiness in both analyses. For both men and women, providing more than one receives is positively related to happiness.

In summary, all the analyses suggested important factors associated with the concept of reciprocity. As the life course reciprocity hypotheses were developed, it was particularly limiting that the 1980 SSE data only assessed current reciprocity, and did not provide the details on the reciprocity of either each type of support or each network relationship of the 1984 SSE study. It was possible, however, to assess perceptions of both current and long-term reciprocity for the person nominated as most important, as well as aggregated data for both family and friends. These results, along with analyses of the age and reciprocity items for family in the NSBA and TGFS, are now considered.

In the 1984 SSE study the question was asked, 'In general, do you feel others have provided more support, is it about equal, or you have provided more? This question was asked of: (a) the person most important in the network; (b) family; and (c) friends. The series of questions were asked for the present and over most of the duration of the relationship(s). This was an attempt to assess the differences between the feelings of reciprocity at the present time and over the life of the social interaction. The results suggested a new aspect of the hypothesis consistent with our general framework.

There were no age or sex differences in the balance of reciprocity reported either contemporaneously or over time with the most important person or friends, but both varied by age and sex for the relationship with family members. The oldest people and men were the most likely to report that they received more support than they provided both at the present and over the life course. The male–female difference is consistent with the complex pattern of results suggested by our analyses of the 1980 SSE data and requires a separate and lengthy consideration (see Antonucci and Akiyama, 1987b). For the age differences, both the lack of a distinction between lifetime and contemporaneous reciprocity and the finding that the older age group reported receiving more support, initially appeared disappointing and somewhat contradictory. As indicated earlier, however, our life course hypothesis is not necessarily linked to age *per se*, but rather to the frequent but age-independent concomitant of ageing, namely the onset of functional disability. It is supposed that healthy people of any age use 'exchange' types of reciprocity, but that they switch to the life course approach to reciprocity when they begin to experience disabilities (Clark *et al.*, 1986). To test this notion, further analyses of reciprocity perceptions have been conducted separating those who reported functional limitations from those who did not.

Table 7.1 shows reported reciprocity of support with family, contemporaneously and over the individual life course, by age and functional limitations. Consistent with the hypothesis presented above, at all ages there were small differences in lifetime reciprocity exchanges between individuals with functional limitations and those without. This applied to relationships with both the important person, usually a spouse, or for other family members. On the other hand, across all ages, people with functional limitations reported that they received more support now from other family members than people without functional limitations. These results support the hypothesis that on the basis of their physical functioning, people differentiate between current and life course recriprocity. This cognitive distinction may be a useful coping mechanism for successful ageing. Our interpretation of these preliminary findings is that age alone does not require an individual to adopt a life course reciprocity accounting system.

Analyses of the NSBA and TGFS for black Americans indicate, however, that significant differences among age groups exist in the perceptions of the differences between the present and previous levels of help given to children. Smaller changes over time were reported in help received from children (see Table 7.2 (a) and (b)). Black older people also reported giving less help and receiving more help in the present than in the past to and from their adult

Table 7.1 Age, functional limitations and reciprocity of support. Data from USA Social Supports of the Elderly National Survey.

Functional limitations	50–64 years			65–74 years			75 years and over			All ages		
	None	Some	Total	None	Some	Total	None	Some	Total	None	Some	Total
(a) Extent of perceived reciprocity of support with family now (per cent)												
Received more	7.1	17.6	8.3	5.3	21.7	8.5	11.1	28.9	18.5	7.3	24.4	10.9
Same	65.7	47.1	63.7	81.1	73.9	79.7	79.6	65.8	73.9	73.4	64.1	71.4
Received less	27.1	35.3	28.0	13.7	4.3	11.9	9.3	5.3	7.6	19.4	11.5	17.7
N	17	140	157	23	95	118	38	54	92	78	289	367
(b) Extent of perceived reciprocity of support with family over lifetime (per cent)												
Received more	5.0	0.0	4.4	5.1	16.7	7.4	12.7	7.9	10.8	6.5	8.8	7.0
Same	62.9	72.2	63.9	72.4	75.0	73.0	69.1	81.6	74.2	67.2	77.5	69.4
Received less	32.1	27.8	31.6	22.4	8.3	19.7	10.2	10.5	15.1	26.3	13.8	23.6
N	18	140	158	24	98	122	38	55	93	80	293	373

Table 7.2 Age, functional limitations and frequency of support. Data from USA National Survey of Black Americans; USA Three-Generation Family Study.

Functional limitations	50–64 years				65–74 years				75 years and over				All ages			
	Low	Med	High	Total	Low	Med	High	Total	Low	Med	High	Total	Low	Med	High	Total
(a) Frequency respondent helps child(ren) now (per cent)																
Not too often/never	21.2	30.0	33.9	25.8	49.0	52.1	48.6	49.7	61.6	48.7	60.7	58.3	40.1	44.4	47.6	43.0
Fairly often	28.5	22.0	25.4	26.5	14.5	9.9	14.3	13.3	9.6	17.9	10.7	11.9	19.2	15.6	16.8	17.8
Very often	50.3	48.0	40.7	47.7	36.6	38.0	37.1	37.1	28.8	33.3	28.6	29.8	40.7	40.0	35.7	39.2
N	151	50	59	260	145	71	70	286	73	39	56	168	369	160	185	714
(b) Frequency family helps respondent now (per cent)																
Not too often/never	56.0	53.6	60.8	56.7	60.5	57.6	54.5	58.1	52.3	47.2	53.3	51.5	56.9	53.7	56.4	56.1
Fairly often	21.3	16.7	17.6	19.3	14.2	16.3	15.2	15.0	13.8	26.4	17.3	17.7	17.0	18.8	16.6	17.3
Very often	22.7	29.8	21.6	23.9	25.3	26.1	30.4	26.9	33.9	26.4	29.3	30.8	26.1	27.5	27.0	26.7
N	207	84	102	393	190	92	112	394	109	53	75	237	506	229	289	1024
(c) Respondent helps child(ren) more, less or same as past (per cent)																
More often	14.6	17.0	11.3	14.3	13.8	5.1	7.1	10.1	8.2	8.9	8.2	8.4	12.9	9.7	8.8	11.2
Same	56.3	47.2	46.8	52.4	47.2	42.3	50.0	46.6	51.8	51.1	34.3	46.1	51.7	46.0	44.0	48.5
Less often	29.1	35.8	41.9	33.3	39.0	52.6	42.9	43.3	40.0	40.0	57.4	45.5	35.4	44.3	47.2	40.3
N	158	53	62	273	159	78	70	307	85	45	61	191	402	176	193	771
(d) Child(ren) helps respondent more, less or same as past (per cent)																
More often	18.7	28.8	33.3	24.0	21.4	14.7	31.0	22.0	29.4	35.6	39.3	34.0	22.1	24.4	34.4	25.7
Same	58.1	55.8	38.3	53.2	55.8	65.3	49.3	56.7	61.2	55.6	34.4	51.3	57.9	59.9	41.1	54.1
Less often	23.2	15.4	28.3	22.8	22.7	20.0	19.7	21.3	9.4	8.9	26.2	14.7	20.1	15.7	24.5	20.2
N	155	52	60	267	154	75	71	300	85	45	61	191	394	172	192	758

children (see Table 7.2(c)). Functional limitations do not have clear effects as found from the SSE (see Table 7.2(d)). Black Americans report helping less as they age; and their perceptions of temporal change in receiving and giving help are related to functional limitations. While consistent with analyses on the SSE, the pattern of results for age and functional limitations are more complex. Race and socio-economic status (not explored here) may play important mediating roles in how age and functional limitations affect help given, help received and reciprocity, and, by extension, well-being and successful ageing.

The relationships between functional limitation and reciprocity revealed by the 1984 SSE data set illuminate the overall reciprocity hypothesis in two important ways. Firstly, they suggest that individuals in the general older population do distinguish between life course and current reciprocity in their interpersonal relationships; and secondly, by implication, they suggest that this distinction may be used to optimise successful ageing. The NSBA/TGFS data also suggest that blacks may maintain a life course accounting system and distinguish between immediate and long-term instrumental exchanges. The data have indicated that blacks with functional disabilities report levels of life course reciprocity similar to those of people who are not currently functionally disabled, although both age and its interaction with functional limitations may be more important than in the general population. We are in the process of conducting additional analyses of these national data sets to explore further these complex relationships.

CONCLUSIONS

In the present paper we have argued that notions of social exchange, particularly reciprocity, should be considered in a life course, life span framework. We have assumed that successful ageing is predicated upon the receipt and provision of social support, an assumption that has been widely reported in theoretical and empirical literature. While agreeing with the basic propositions of other researchers on the utility of a social exchange perspective on ageing (Dowd, 1984; Lee, 1985; Clark *et al.*, 1986), we have added for consideration the theoretical outline of a Social Support Bank. We have conceptualised this bank as a social support accounting framework constituting a lifetime of net investments and interest for the older individual. These investments can take the form of exchanges provided for others, as well as the avoidance of the receipt of goods and services from others, early in the life course. We believe that generalised reciprocity is also important. In this sense, credited support may be obtained from others than those involved in the original exchange.

It was our intent in formulating this Social Support Bank to account for different findings in the empirical social support ageing literature. In a wide variety of scientific, anecdotal and mass-media sources, one finds accounts of elderly individuals so self-sufficient that they will not accept help, even if not to do so results in their severe decrement. Other findings document cases of over-dependent elderly people who accept help from nearly every conceivable source, much to the detriment of others. Finally, the literature has described elderly people who accept support, but only from a very limited set of helpers, often disparaging assistance from family and friends who are willing to help. While some (e.g., Dowd, 1984) may account for these observed behaviours as a reduction in the possession of valued goods for exchange, and others (e.g., Litwak, 1985) point to the reduction in the availability of individuals in the supportive networks due to loss, none adequately account for all of these documented patterns of observed behaviours in old age. We feel that an adult development framework that includes a conception of reciprocity over the life course in social and economic exchanges can provide a basic theoretical foundation.

We have reviewed the preliminary findings from two stages of a major national study, Social Supports of the Elderly, as well as two national studies on elderly blacks, the National Survey of Black Americans and the Three Generation Family Study. Although these studies were not designed to assess directly the Social Support Bank concept, they contain data which provide some support for the notion of a Social Support Bank. However, they also suggest some revisions in our original thinking, indicating the importance of temporal reciprocity in old age (Dowd, 1984). Particularly important are the findings that individuals can and do distinguish between a life course and a contemporaneous process of reciprocity, and that while the need for functional care clearly distinguishes immediate reciprocity levels, it does not distinguish life span reciprocity perceptions. Finally, the complex findings by age and functional limitations for black Americans suggest the importance of race and possibly class differences in reciprocity and successful ageing over the individual life course.

We believe that the Social Support Bank concept holds considerable promise as a model for social support exchanges in old age and for resolving many of the ambiguous and contrasting accounts in the literature. In addition, the concept of reciprocity may have more general utility as a mediator of successful ageing. The data that we have presented provide preliminary positive support for the proposed theoretical framework. New and better data addressed directly to the concept are now needed to advance our understanding of these important relationships. Particularly helpful would be large longitudinal panel data sets that included relevant measures of actual and perceived social support exchanges across adult individual life courses.

REFERENCES

Akiyama, H., Antonucci, T.C. and Campbell, R. (in press). Rules of support exchange among two generations of Japanese and American women. In *Growing Old in Different Societies*, J. Sokolovsky (Ed.). Wadsworth Publishing Company, Belmont, California.

Antonucci, T.C. (1985). Personal characteristics, social networks and social behavior. In *Handbook of Aging and the Social Sciences*, 2nd edition, R.H. Binstock and E. Shanas (Eds), pp. 94–128. Van Nostrand Reinhold, New York.

Antonucci, T.C. and Akiyama, H. (1987a). Social networks in adult life and a preliminary examination of the convoy model. *Journal of Gerontology*, **42**, 519–27.

Antonucci, T.C. and Akiyama, H. (1987b). An examination of sex differences in social support among older men and women. *Sex Roles*, **17**(11/12), 737–49.

Antonucci, T.C. and Israel, B. (1986). Veridicality of social support: A comparison of principal and network members' responses. *Journal of Consulting and Clinical Psychology*, **54**(4), 432–7.

Antonucci, T.C. and Jackson, J.S. (1987). Social support, interpersonal efficacy and health. In *Handbook of Clinical Gerontology*, L. Carstensen and B.A. Edelstein (Eds), pp. 291–311. Pergamon Press, New York.

Cantor, M.H. (1979). Neighbors and friends: An overlooked resource in the informal support system. *Research on Aging*, **1**, 434–63.

Chatters, L.C., Taylor, R.J. and Jackson, J.S. (1985). Aged blacks' choices for an informal helper network. *Journal of Gerontology*, **41**, 94–100.

Chatters, L.C., Taylor, R.J. and Jackson, J.S. (1986). Size and composition of the informal helper networks of elderly blacks. *Journal of Gerontology*, **40**, 605–14.

Clark, M.S., Mills, J. and Powell, M.C. (1986). Keeping track of needs in communal and exchange relationships. *Journal of Personality and Social Psychology*, **51**, 333–8.

Dowd, J.J. (1975). Aging as exchange: a preface to theory. *Journal of Gerontology*, **15**, 303–17.

Dowd, J.J. (1980). *Stratification Among the Aged*. Brooks/Cole Publishing Co., Monterey, California.

Dowd, J.J. (1984), Beneficence and the aged. *Journal of Gerontology*, **39**, 102–8.

Dressler, W.W. (1985). Extended family relationships, social support, and mental health in a southern black community. *Journal of Health and Social Behavior*, **26**, 39–48.

Gouldner, A.W. (1960). The norm of reciprocity: a preliminary statement. *American Sociological Review*, **25**(2), 161–78.

Greenberg, M.S. (1980). A theory of indebtedness. In *Social Exchange: Advances in Theory and Research*, K.J. Gergen, M.S. Greenberg and R.S. Willis (Eds). Plenum Press, New York.

Hatfield, E., Walster, G.W. and Pilivan, A.J. (1978). Equity theory and helping relationships. In *Altruism, Sympathy and Helping*, L. Wispe (Ed.). Academic Press, New York.

Hinde, R.A. (1979). *Towards Understanding Relationships*. Academic Press, London.

Ingersoll-Dayton, B. and Antonucci, T.C. (1988). Reciprocal and non-reciprocal social support: contrasting sides of intimate relationships. *Journal of Gerontology*, **43**(3), S65–S73.

Israel, B.A. (1982). Social networks and health status: linking theory, research and practice. *Patient Counseling and Health Education*, **4**(2), 65–79.

Israel, B.A. and Antonucci, T.C. (1987). Social network characteristics and psychological well-being: a replication and extension. *Health Education Quarterly*, **14**(4), 461–81.

Israel, B.A., Hogue, C.C. and Gorton, T.A. (1984). Social networks among elderly women: implications for health education practice. *Health Education Quarterly*, **10**(3/4), 173–203.

Jackson, J.S. (in press). The program for research on black Americans. In *Advances in Black Psychology*, R. Jones (Ed.). Cobb and Henry Publishers, Richmond, California.

Jackson, J.S. and Hatchett, S.J. (1986). Intergenerational research: methodological considerations. In *Intergenerational Networks: Families in Context*, N. Datan, A.L. Green and H.W. Reese (Eds). Erlbaum Associates Inc., Hillsdale, New Jersey.

Jackson, J.S., Tucker, M.B. and Bowman, P.J. (1982). Conceptual and methodological problems in survey research on black Americans. In *Methodological Problems in Minority Research*, T. Liu (Ed.). Pacific/Asian American Mental Health Center, Chicago.

Kahn, R.L. and Antonucci, T.C. (1984). *Social Supports of the Elderly: Family/Friends/Professionals*. Final report to the National Institute on Aging, Hyattsville, Maryland.

Kahn, R.L. and Antonucci, T.C. (1986). *Cancer Symptoms in the Elderly: Support and Responses*. Final Report to the National Cancer Institute, Bethesda, Maryland.

Knipscheer, K. (1985). Social support in the relationship between older parents and their adult children: questions and suggestions. Unpublished manuscript.

Krebs, D. and Miller, D.T. (1985). Altruism and aggression. In *The Handbook of Social Psychology*, 2nd edition, G. Lindzey and E. Aronson (Eds). Random House, New York.

Lee, G.R. (1985). Kinship and social support of the elderly: the case of the United States. *Ageing and Society*, **5**(1), 19–38.

Litwak, E. (1985). *Helping the Elderly*. Guilford Press, New York.

Longino, C.F. Jr. and Lipman, A. (1981). Married and spouseless men and women in planned retirement communities: support network differentials. *Journal of Marriage and the Family*, **43**, 169–77.

Mitchell, R.E. and Trickett, E.J. (1980). Task force report – social networks as mediators of social support: an analysis of the effects and determinants of social networks. *Community Mental Health Journal*, **16**(2), 27–44.

Shinn, M. Lehmann, S. and Wong, N.W. (1985). Social interaction and social support. *Journal of Social Issues*, **40**(4), 55–76.

Shore, B. (1985). Extended kin as helping networks. In *Social Support Networks and the Care of the Elderly: Theory, Research, Practice and Policy*, W. Sauer and R. Coward (Eds), pp. 108–20. Springer Publishing Company, New York.

Taylor, R.J. (1985). The extended family as a source of support to elderly blacks. *The Gerontologist*, **25**, 488–95.

Taylor, R.J. (1986). Receipt of support from family among black Americans: demographic and familial differences. *Journal of Marriage and the Family*, **48**, 67–77.

Taylor, R.J. and Chatters, L.M. (1986a). Church-based informal support among elderly blacks. *The Gerontologist*, **26**, 637–42.

Taylor, R.J. and Chatters, L.M. (1986b). Patterns of informal support to elderly black adults: family, friends, and church members. *Social Work*, **31**, 432–8.

Taylor, J.R., Jackson, J.S. and Quick, A. (1982). The frequency of social support among black Americans: preliminary findings from the National Survey of Black Americans. *Urban Research Review*, **8**, 1–4.

Trivers, R.L. (1971). The revolution of reciprocal altruism. *Quarterly Review of Biology*, **46**, 35–7.

Wentowski, G.J. (1981). Reciprocity and the coping strategies of older people: cultural dimensions of network building. *The Gerontologist*, **21**, 600–9.

Emily Grundy

Age Concern Institute of Gerontology
King's College
University of London

8 LIVING ARRANGEMENTS AND SOCIAL SUPPORT IN LATER LIFE

INTRODUCTION

The domestic environment is of great importance in most people's lives as the home is generally the focus of intimate relationships and, to an increasing extent, of leisure activities, as well as a place to eat and sleep. Although earlier in the century it seems that, at least in some urban working class districts, housekeeping arrangements sometimes involved groups of relatives who had separate dwellings (Sheldon, 1948; Young and Willmott, 1957; Townsend, 1957), in modern Britain households are generally discrete units of consumption. Trends in household composition and size are therefore relevant to all concerned with the production and distribution of goods and services. Some of these trends, and their possible implications for the support of the elderly, are reviewed here.

For a number of reasons the housing and household circumstances of elderly people are likely to be particularly important, both for them and for policy makers and planners. The elderly tend to spend longer at home than those in younger age groups (with the possible exception of mothers of young children and the unemployed). In 1977 a survey of elderly people living in four urban areas of England found that those aged 65–74 years had spent on average seven hours, and those aged 75 years or more nearly eight hours, of the preceding day watching television, listening to the radio, reading or resting (Abrams, 1980) – activities generally pursued at home. Nearly half the respondents had not been out at all during the previous weekend.

Apart from the fact that elderly people often spend so much time at home, the domestic environment may be especially important in other ways. Although most elderly people, certainly in age groups under 80, are relatively fit and well, the ageing process is associated with biological changes which increase the risk of ill health and functional decline. It has been estimated from data collected in the 1980 *General Household Survey* (GHS) that 25 per cent of women and 17 per cent of men aged 80 or over and living outside institutions have severe functional health disabilities (Evandrou *et al.*, 1986). Housing of poor quality or unsuitable design may exacerbate health problems and inhibit the capacity of the less fit to preserve functional capabilities and autonomy. Even more important for the welfare of the elderly, particularly the very old, may be the availability of support and help within the household.

HOUSING AND AMENITIES

As a group, the elderly are relatively disadvantaged in housing terms, although in this respect as in all others the older population is extremely heterogeneous.

For historic reasons the elderly, particularly the very old, are more likely to be living in the privately rented sector and less likely to be owner occupiers than the population as a whole. In 1984 in Great Britain, for example, 11 per cent of households headed by someone aged 70 years or over were in privately rented, unfurnished accommodation compared with five per cent of all households (Office of Population Censuses and Surveys (OPCS), 1986a). It has been shown elsewhere that those who were in this sector, which is associated with poor housing conditions, in 1971 were more likely than others of the same age and marital status to be in institutions ten years later (Grundy, 1989a).

The elderly population are also more likely than those in younger age groups to live in housing lacking amenities or convenient heating systems. The 1984 GHS showed that 44 per cent of households consisting of one adult aged 60 years or over lacked central heating, compared with 34 per cent of all households (OPCS, 1986a). In 1981 one in twenty of 75–84 year olds and six per cent of those aged 85 years and over lived in accommodation lacking a bath compared with one per cent of the whole population (OPCS, 1983). Those in households with a head who has retired are also less likely than those in other households to have access to consumer durables, such as washing machines, as shown in Table 8.1.

Table 8.1 Possession of consumer durables by whether the head of household was economically active or retired: Great Britain, 1980. Data from 1980 General Household Survey.

Head of household	Percentage in households possessing:				
	Refrigerator	Washing machine	Tele-phone	Car or van	Central heating
Economically active	95	84	78	73	61
Retired	88	61	62	35	48

These age variations in the proportions lacking amenities are indicative of the generally poorer housing standards that the old as a group have when compared with the rest of the population, and may be regarded as an example of the 'inverse care law' as those in the greatest need of comfort in the home are the least likely to have it (Hart, 1971). Age differences in housing standards or access to consumer durables reflect cohort effects and also the poverty experienced by a proportion of the elderly population; for some this poverty may have been lifelong. Victor and Vetter's (1986) analyses of 1980 GHS data showed that half the elderly population had an income below 140 per cent of supplementary pension level and that the proportion of elderly people living in poverty increased with both age and level of disability.

HOUSEHOLD COMPOSITION

The post-war decades in Britain, other north west European countries, North America and elsewhere, have been marked by a trend towards smaller, simpler households and an increase in the propensity to live alone (Burch, 1985; Kobrin, 1976). One aspect of this has been a substantial increase in the proportion of elderly people living on their own, illustrated for Britain in Table 8.2. The proportion living alone among those aged 65 years and over in the private household population (not in institutions) increased by over half from 22 per cent in 1962 to 35 per cent in 1984. Conversely, the proportion of elderly

Table 8.2 Percentage of elderly people in private households living alone: Great Britain, 1962–1984. Data from the 1971, 1976, 1981 and 1984 General Household Surveys.

Year	Age (years)	
	65+	75+
1962[1]	22	28
1971[2]	27	35
1976[3]	32	43
1981	34	45
1984	35	47

1 Derived from data presented in Townsend, 'The structure of the family', and Stehower, 'The household and family relations of old people', in Shanas *et al.* (1968).
2 Figure for the 75+ age group taken from a Census sample.
3 Figure for the 75+ age group relates to 1977.

Table 8.3 Elderly people living alone in selected countries for various dates during 1976–1984. Data from national census reports; Havlik *et al.* (1987) and Wall (1985).

Country	Year	% living alone
Belgium	1981	26
Denmark	1977	35
Eire	1979	18
England and Wales	1981	34
Finland	1976	30
France	1983	32
W Germany	1982	39
Hungary	1980	20
Norway	1981	35
Poland	1978	21
Portugal	1981	18
Switzerland	1980	29
USA	1984	33

Not all the figures shown are exactly comparable as some show the elderly living alone as a percentage of the whole elderly population and others as a percentage of the elderly private household population. The extent of this discrepancy has been assessed and is slight. Where both figures can be derived the former has been used in preference to the latter.

people living with relatives other than a spouse has fallen. In 1971, for example, 27 per cent of women and 16 per cent of men aged 65 and over in England and Wales were lone parents living with a child who had never married, or were not part of a nuclear family but lived with other people – generally relatives – compared with 20 per cent and 10 per cent respectively in 1981 (Grundy, 1987).

These recent changes do not represent the continuation of a long-term secular trend from more complex to simpler households. Wall (1984) has suggested that the extent of change in the living arrangements of the elderly between 1962 and 1981 may be greater than the difference between 1962 and pre-industrial England. He has also shown that the proportion of elderly people not currently married who headed their own households was lower in 1951 than in the pre-industrial period, and that the number of relatives other than spouses and unmarried children in the household was at its maximum, not in the pre-industrial era, but shortly after the Second World War (Wall, 1984; 1985). Neither is Britain alone in having a large proportion of elderly people living alone. As Table 8.3 shows, in several north European countries the proportion is also high.

Table 8.4   Family/household type of those aged 65 years and over in 1981, England and Wales. Data from OPCS Longitudinal Study presented in Grundy (1987).

		Family/household type (%)					
		In families		Not in families			
		Married couple	Lone parent	Solitary	With others	Non-private household	All
65–69	M	77	2	12	7	2	100
	F	54	5	30	9	2	100
	P	64	3	22	8	2	100
70–74	M	72	2	16	7	3	100
	F	41	5	39	12	3	100
	P	54	4	29	10	3	100
75–79	M	65	2	19	9	4	100
	F	26	6	48	15	6	100
	P	40	4	38	13	5	100
80–84	M	50	4	26	12	8	100
	F	15	7	49	19	11	100
	P	26	6	42	17	10	100
85–89	M	40	4	28	17	11	100
	F	7	8	44	25	17	100
	P	15	7	40	23	16	100
90+	M	22	6	27	25	21	100
	F	2	9	32	26	31	100
	P	6	8	31	26	29	100
65+	M	69	2	16	8	4	100
	F	36	6	39	14	6	100
	P	49	4	30	12	5	100

The proportion of elderly people living alone may be a useful summary indicator of a nation's general patterns of household structure and the availability of domestic support for the elderly population, but it reveals little about age-related changes in living arrangements. Recent changes in household structure have been variously attributed to rising real incomes, more homogeneous age and gender roles influencing perceived needs for space and privacy, increases in housing supply, and decreases in the availability of relatives with whom to live (Michael et al., 1980; Burch, 1985; Ermisch, 1985; Kobrin, 1976). For the individual elderly person, while general changes in attitudes or housing supply may influence decisions about living arrangements, the chief constraints are likely to reflect their stage in the family life cycle and their health status, both of which are strongly age related.

Age and sex variations in the household circumstances of the elderly in England Wales in 1981 are shown in Table 8.4. The data are drawn from the OPCS Longitudinal Study (LS), a prospective record linkage study based on a one per cent sample of the population of England and Wales enumerated in the 1971 Census. The 1981 Census records for sample members have been linked to the 1971 information, and losses by death or emigration have been compensated for by adding in one per cent of births and immigrants. In Table 8.4 this 1981 information has been used to show cross-sectional variations in living arrangements for one point in time. A strictly nuclear definition of a family has been used in the classification and only those living with a spouse (with or without children and other people) or a never-married child (with or without others) are counted as living in a family. Most of those categorized as living 'not in a family, with others' co-resided with other relatives, such as married children or siblings.

Table 8.4 shows that among women aged 75 years or over, living alone was the most usual domestic situation, while most men under 85 years were in married couple type households. The proportion living alone was highest in the 80–84 year old age group as, although the proportions living with a spouse continue to decline in extreme old age, living in an institution or with relatives becomes more common. These two groups together accounted for over half of the extreme aged – those aged 90 years or more.

AGE-RELATED CHANGES IN LIVING ARRANGEMENTS

The age and sex differences in domestic circumstances shown in Table 8.4 largely reflect variations in the incidence of widowhood or the onset of frailty, which are likely to precipitate a change in living arrangements. Fillenbaum and Wallman (1984), in a 30 month follow up study of some 280 older Americans, found that changes in household composition were associated both with changes in marital status and with changes in the amount of help available. As men have higher age-specific mortality rates than women, and tend to have wives younger than themselves, at older ages larger proportions of men than women are in married couple households. The higher proportion of spinsters among very old women than of bachelors among men in the same age group – a difference reflecting the shortage of eligible men earlier in the century – and the higher remarriage rates of widowers compared with widows also contribute to this differential.

It is evident from these age variations that household circumstances are highly changeable in later life and need to be viewed dynamically. Previous analyses of longitudinal data in the OPCS LS showed that over a third of those aged 65–74 years in 1971 and nearly two-thirds of those aged 85 or over who

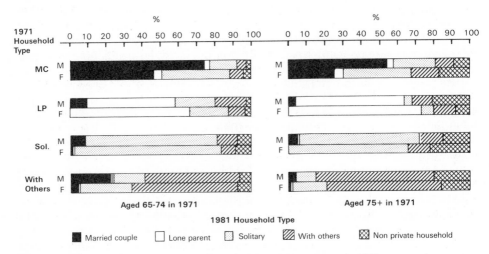

Fig. 8.1 Family/household type in 1971 by family/household type in 1981: men and women aged 65 years and over in 1971, England and Wales. Adapted from Office of Population Censuses and Surveys Longitudinal Study data presented in Grundy (1987).

survived to 1981 were by then living in a different family/household type (Grundy, 1989b). Among women aged 65–74 and elderly men, whether aged less or more than 75 years in 1971, half of these shifts in broad household type were a change from living in a married couple household to living alone. For women who were 75 or over in 1971, transitions to living alone from living in a married couple accounted for a third of all changes, while changes from living alone to living with others or from living alone to living in an institution each accounted for over a fifth of all household type transitions (Grundy, 1987). Figure 8.1 illustrates these changes and shows for the sample members alive in 1981 their family/household type in that year and in 1971. Both among those aged 65–74 years in 1971 and among those aged 75 or over, the majority of those living alone were still in single person households ten years later, indicating that for many this residential arrangement is of long duration. Among those living in different family/household types in 1971 and 1981, 45 per cent of men and 51 per cent of women aged 65–74 in 1971 and 48 per cent of men and 70 per cent of women aged 75 and over had also changed their address (Grundy, 1989b).

LIVING ARRANGEMENTS AND SOCIAL SUPPORT

Although recent increases in the proportion of elderly people living alone have been considerable, this does not imply a rejection of the elderly by their younger relatives. As we have seen (Table 8.4), a quarter of the very old, aged 85 years or more, do live in the households of relatives. Complex extended family households have never been the norm in Britain (Laslett, 1972) and it is extremely rare for modern families to reject elderly relatives (Isaacs et al., 1972).

There is little indication that many of those elderly people who have close surviving kin but live alone would prefer to live with relatives. In a study of 104 arthritis and rheumatism patients reported by Thompson and West (1984), respondents were asked whether, if unable to continue at home, they would move to live with a relative, to sheltered housing or to residential care. Sheltered housing was by far the preferred choice and over three-quarters said the least likely option would be to move in with relatives. A recent poll on the attitudes of elderly people in Britain and four other anglophone countries found that only nine per cent of respondents said they would choose to live with relatives or friends if they became unable to care for themselves (Louis Harris, 1982).

Higher rates of co-residence in Britain in the past, and elsewhere in Europe now, may reflect constraints rather than positive choices. In Poland, for example, 35 per cent of elderly people were living with offspring in 1985, but large proportions of elderly people in this situation complained of poor relationships with other household members (Synak, 1987). This was particularly true of elderly people who had joined their children in urban areas, where housing shortages are more likely to constrain choices about domestic arrangements.

Living alone does not necessarily imply a lack of familial support. Familial relationships extend beyond households and those elderly people who need help with domestic or personal care tasks and have close relatives tend to turn to them for help, whether co-resident or not. Among the elderly living alone in Britain in 1980, for example, 55 per cent of those needing help with cooking, 56 per cent of those needing help with shopping and 42 per cent of those needing help with bathing, relied on relatives (Evandrou et al., 1986).

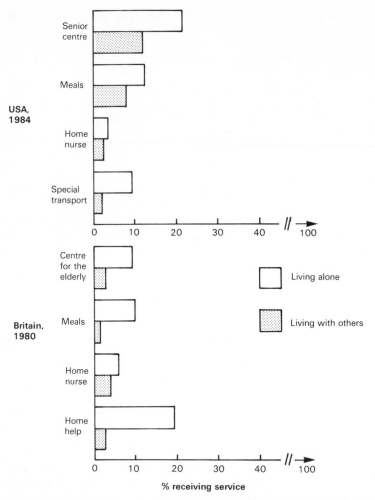

Fig. 8.2 Percentage of the private household population aged 65 years and over using certain community services by whether living alone or with others: Great Britain, 1980 and the USA, 1984. Data from *1980 General Household Survey*, reported in Evandrou *et al.* (1986) and *1984 National Health Interview Supplement on Aging*, reported in Havlik *et al.* (1987).

The trend towards residential independence among the elderly does, however, have some important policy implications, particularly as the number of people aged 75 years and over is now increasing rapidly (OPCS, 1986b). Elderly people living alone make greater use of most welfare services than others of the same age, including their peers with a similar level of functional health (Evandrou *et al.*, 1986). Figure 8.2 shows for Britain and the United States the use of various services among elderly people either living alone or with others. In both countries those living alone made greater use of the services shown than elderly people living with others. Furthermore, as indicated in Fig. 8.1, elderly people living alone in England and Wales in 1971 were the most likely to be in institutions ten years later. It should be noted that these differences are influenced by the inclusion of a selected subgroup lacking any close relatives within the wider group of elderly people living alone, and by the policies of some welfare agencies which tend to give those living alone priority over those with co-resident carers.

Family and friends are of importance, not just because of the practical help they may provide, but also because the formation and maintenance of relationships are necessary aspects of well-being and health. Berkman and Syme (1979), in a Californian study, found that among those in their sixties at the start of a nine year follow-up period, the risk of dying among the most socially isolated females was three times that of those with most connections: the comparative rate of mortality among males was 1.8. Welin *et al.* (1985) reported an association between social networks and mortality in a Scandinavian follow-up study of two cohorts of men in their fifties and sixties. They also found a negative association between household size and mortality risk. Evidence from other studies also supports the hypothesis of a relationship between social networks and health (House *et al.*, 1982).

The elderly population would seem to be at particular risk of social isolation and a lack of close relationships. Among women, widows and divorcées outnumber the currently married from the age of 73 years and, as shown earlier, large proportions live alone. Higher rates of celibacy and childless marriage in the past also mean that large proportions of the very old lack children. Abrams (1978) found that a third of those aged 75 years or over in his 1977 study had had no children.

However, there is some evidence to suggest that among those living alone, it is only in subgroups with special characteristics that there is a serious risk of isolation and poor psychosocial health. While Brown and Harris (1978) found that among young women the lack of an intimate confiding relationship with a husband increased the chance of developing depression following a serious life event or a major difficulty, Murphy (1982) has shown that among the elderly, having a close relationship with someone seen only every two or three weeks seems just as 'protective' as having a confidant in the same household. It was those who had no close relationship – most of whom had *never* had such a relationship – who were at risk. The results of surveys conducted by Wenger (1984) and Hunt (1978) both suggested that those not currently married tended to compensate by having more friends than other elderly people of the same age. Taylor *et al.* (1983) also found that although the elderly living alone included in a survey in Aberdeen had, as expected, fewer confidants or intimates available to them than other elderly people, they tended to have more friends and as a group were not characterised by low levels of psychological functioning.

Other studies, however, do suggest poorer psychosocial health among those living alone, particularly among men. Results from the *1987 Health and Lifestyle Survey* (Huppert *et al.*, 1987) showed that among men aged 65 years or over, living alone was associated with a higher number of psychiatric symptoms as measured by scores on the General Health Questionnaire (GHQ), a well validated psychiatric screening instrument (Goldberg, 1972). Forty per cent of men living alone scored five or more on the GHQ compared with 27 per cent of men living with a spouse and/or other adults. Calculations based on these results show that this difference was statistically significant at a level of confidence of one in twenty ($p < 0.05$). Huppert *et al.* (1987) suggested that a cut-off between four and five, although found in other studies to be a useful first stage screen for possible minor psychiatric disorder, would seem to be too low a discriminator in this kind of survey. Be this as it may, the difference between men living alone and other men would still suggest that the former, as a group, had poorer psychological health. Differences between women living alone and other women in the proportions with GHQ scores of five or more were much smaller and not statistically significant.

The *Health and Lifestyle Survey* also included another measure of psycho-social health: a malaise score, which has been used in other studies but not validated. Among those aged 60 years or over, larger proportions of those living alone had high scores on this compared with those living with a spouse and/or other adults; the differences were greatest among men (Stark, 1987). The proportion of high scorers among women living alone with high levels of contact with friends was similar to that among women living with a spouse but with low friend contact. This suggestion of compensation, which would be consistent with the findings of Taylor *et al.* (1983), was not evident among men.

The implications of the trend towards solitary living for the well-being of the elderly population as a whole needs to be considered with care, particularly in the light of the results of these studies which in some respects conflict. It would seem that there is a relationship between social networks – of which domestic arrangements are an important aspect – and health, and that some groups of elderly people are better able than others to compensate for a lack of company inside the home through contacts with others outside the home. Selection factors are undoubtedly important in influencing associations between domestic status and health. Thus, elderly men who live alone are a more selected group than women living alone; both because widowerhood is less usual than widowhood and is more prevalent in socio-economically disadvantaged groups (Helsing *et al.*, 1981), and because remarriage rates are higher for elderly widowers than widows. Remarriage is itself associated with better health (Helsing *et al.*, 1981), higher social status (Grundy, 1989a) and probably better psychological adjustment. Further work is needed to identify both the subgroups at particular risk (and events associated with entering such subgroups), and the individual, socio-economic and environmental factors which promote or inhibit the development of social relationships which partly compensate for the lack of a co-resident.

REFERENCES

Abrams, M. (1978). *Beyond Three Score and Ten: A First Report on a Survey of the Elderly.* Age Concern England, Mitcham, Surrey.

Abrams, M. (1980). *Beyond Three Score and Ten: A Second Report on a Survey of the Elderly.* Age Concern England, Mitcham, Surrey.

Berkman, L.F. and Syme, S.L. (1979). Social networks, host resistance and mortality: a nine year follow up of Alameda County residents. *American Journal of Epidemiology*, **109**, 186–204.

Brown, G.W. and Harris, T.O. (1978). *Social Origins of Depression.* Tavistock, London.

Burch, T.K. (1985). Changing age sex roles and household crowding: a theoretical note. Proceedings of XXth International Population Conference. International Union for the Scientific Study of Population, Liège.

Ermisch, J. (1985). *Economic Implications of Demographic Change*, Discussion Paper 44. Centre for Economic Policy Research, London.

Evandrou, M., Arber, S., Dale, A. and Gilbert, N. (1986). Who cares for the elderly?: family care provision and receipt of statutory services. In *Dependency and Interdependency in Old Age*, C. Phillipson, M. Bernard and P. Strang (Eds), pp. 150–66. Croom Helm, Beckenham.

Fillenbaum, G.G. and Wallman, L.M. (1984). Change in household composition of the elderly: a preliminary investigation. *Journal of Gerontology*, **39**, 342–9.

Goldberg, D.P. (1972). *The Detection of Psychiatric Illness by Questionnaire.* Oxford University Press, Oxford.

Grundy, E. (1987). Household change and migration among the elderly in England and Wales. *Espace, Populations, Sociétés*, **1**, 109–23.

Grundy, E. (1989a). Longitudinal perspectives on the living arrangements of the elderly. In *Growing Old in the Twentieth Century*, M. Jefferys (Ed.). Routledge, London.

Grundy, E. (1989b). Ageing: age-related change in later life. In *Population Research in Britain*, J. Hobcraft and M.J. Murphy (Eds). Oxford University Press, Oxford.

Hart, J.T. (1971). The inverse care law. *The Lancet*, **(i)**, 405–12.

Havlik, R.J., Liu, B.M., Kovar, M.G. *et al.* (1987). *Health Statistics on Older Persons.* Vital and Health Statistics Series 3, No. 25. Department of Health and Human Services, Pub. No. (PHS) 87–1409. US Government Printing Office, Washington D.C.

Helsing, K.J., Szklo, M. and Comstock, G.W. (1981). Factors associated with mortality after widowhood. *American Journal of Public Health*, **71**, 802–9.

House, J.J., Robbins, C. and Metzner, H.L. (1982). The association of social relationships and activities with mortality: prospective evidence from the Tecamseh Community Health Study. *American Journal of Epidemiology*, **116**, 123–40.

Hunt, A. (1978). *The Elderly at Home.* HMSO, London.

Huppert, F.A., Roth, M. and Gore, M. (1987). Psychological factors. In *The Health and Lifestyle Survey*, B.D. Cox, M. Blaxter, A.L.J. Buckle *et al.* (Eds), pp. 51–8. Health Promotion Research Trust, London.

Isaacs, B., Livingstone, M. and Neville, Y. (1972). *Survival of the Unfittest.* Routledge & Kegan Paul, London.

Kobrin, F.E. (1976). The fall of household size and the rise of the primary individual in the United States. *Demography*, **13**, 127–38.

Laslett, P. (1972). Introduction: the history of the family. In *Household and Family in Past Time*, P. Laslett and R. Wall (Eds). Cambridge University Press, Cambridge.

Louis Harris and Associates Inc. (1982). *Priorities and Expectations for Health and Living Circumstances: A Survey of the Elderly in Five English-Speaking Countries.* Louis Harris and Associates Inc., New York.

Michael, R., Fuchs, V. and Scott, C. (1980). Changes in the propensity to live alone. *Demography*, **17**, 39–53.

Murphy, E. (1982). The social origins of depression in old age. *British Journal of Psychiatry*, **141**, 135–42.

Office of Population Censuses and Surveys (OPCS) (1983). Great Britain Census 1981, *National Report*, Part 1. HMSO, London.

OPCS (1986a). *General Household Survey 1984.* HMSO, London.

OPCS (1986b). *Population Projections, Mid-1985 Based.* OPCS Monitor PP2 86/1, OPCS, London.

Shanas, E., Townsend, P., Wedderburn, D., Friis, H., Milhøj, P. and Stehower, J. (1968). *Old People in Three Industrial Societies.* Routledge & Kegan Paul, London.

Sheldon, J.H. (1948). *The Social Medicine of Old Age.* Oxford University Press, Oxford.

Stark, J. (1987). Health and social contacts. In *The Health and Lifestyle Survey*, B.D. Cox, M. Blaxter, A.L.J. Buckle *et al.* (Eds), pp. 59–66. Health Promotion Research Trust, London.

Synak, B. (1987). The elderly in Poland: an overview of selected problems and changes. In *Social Gerontology: New Directions*, S. di Gregorio (Ed.), pp. 131–51. Croom Helm, Beckenham.

Taylor, R., Ford, G. and Barber, H. (1983). *The Elderly at Risk.* Age Concern Research Unit, Mitcham, Surrey.

Thompson, C. and West, P. (1984). The public appeal of sheltered housing. *Ageing and Society*, **4**, 305–26.

Townsend, P. (1957). *The Family Life of Old People.* Routledge & Kegan Paul, London.

Victor, C.R. and Vetter, N.J. (1986). Poverty, disability and use of services by the elderly: analyses of the 1980 General Household Survey. *Social Science and Medicine*, **22**, 1087–91.

Wall, R. (1984). Residential isolation of the elderly: a comparison over time. *Ageing and Society*, **4**, 483–503.

Wall, R. (1985). The living arrangements of the elderly in Europe in the 1980s. Revised version of a paper presented at the International Union for the Scientific Study of Population workshop on Later Stages of the Life Cycle. Cambridge Group for the History of Population and Social Structure, Cambridge.

Welin, L., Svardsudd, K., Ander-Peciva, S., Tibblin, G., Tibblin, B., Larrson, B. and Wilhelmsen, L. (1985). Prospective study of social influences on mortality. *The Lancet*, **(i)**, 915–18.

Wenger, C. (1984). *The Supportive Network: Coping with Old Age.* Allen & Unwin, London.

Young, M. and Willmott, P. (1957). *Family and Kinship in East London.* Routledge & Kegan Paul, London.

Janet Askham

Age Concern Institute of Gerontology
King's College
University of London

9 THE NEED FOR SUPPORT

INTRODUCTION

Through illness, disability or frailty, many elderly people are unable to carry out for themselves all the activities necessary to enable them to live independent lives in their own homes. But the receipt of help or assistance depends upon socially determined definitions: about whether a person is ill, disabled or frail rather than merely idle; about what activities are 'necessary' rather than optional, about what constitutes 'independence' and at what point the costs of such independence become too high; and about what sort of services are appropriate, and what quality adequate, to sustain people at home. This chapter reviews some of these definitions, from the point of view of elderly people themselves, their relatives (who form the majority of their informal carers), and some of their service providers. The aim of the chapter is not only to expose assumptions which are sometimes taken for granted but also to demonstrate the wide variety of perceptions, attitudes and beliefs about the care needs of elderly people.

THE VIEWS OF ELDERLY PEOPLE THEMSELVES

Elderly people of course have their own definitions of need; they will decide for themselves whether they want help. However, only limited research evidence on this topic exists; many studies tell us how many elderly people receive assistance, and with what tasks, but they less frequently address the more complex question of how elderly people feel about the receipt or non-receipt of help. For example, secondary analysis of the *1980 General Household Survey*, carried out by Evandrou *et al.* (1986), shows that, 'the majority of older people do not have any limitations on their physical mobility and can easily perform tasks such as getting in and out of bed, walking indoors, cooking main meals and washing laundry'. For example, only 12 per cent of those aged 65 and over either required help or could not manage to go out of doors and walk down the road, and only eight per cent needed help or could not manage to bath, shower or wash themselves all over.

It has to be borne in mind, however, that perceptions of need for help by elderly people may bear only limited relation to their reported inability to carry out certain care tasks: some without these inabilities may see themselves as needing help, some with them may deny a need for assistance. Interestingly, the GHS data show that all those identified as requiring assistance received it in some form (overwhelmingly from kin); needs therefore appear to be defined in terms of receipt. Other studies show a similar picture, with a small proportion of elderly people reporting that they are unable to manage, or need help to carry out, day-to-day tasks. For example, a 1974 study (Age Concern, 1974) of a sample of people of retirement age and over, concluded that, 'for most household tasks four out of five people cope for themselves or have a spouse who does these jobs. For those who need help with, say, shopping, cleaning, laundry and gardening, their own children are most likely to help out (in about 15 per cent of cases). Most, even those in the poorest health, cope with cooking for themselves. As far as personal help is concerned, cutting toenails presents the greatest difficulty with 22 per cent unable to do so without help; two per cent are unable to dress themselves without help, and seven per cent unable to bath themselves' (see also Hunt, 1978; Jones et al., 1983).

But examining data on how many elderly people say they are unable to achieve certain daily activities on their own does not go far towards determining whether and how elderly people perceive a need for help. Neither is the answer provided through information about how many elderly people actually receive help, though studies which take that as their starting point (rather than the starting point of inability) provide an interesting and different perspective on the issue. For example, Salvage (1986) in a South Glamorgan study of a sample of 251 people aged 75 and over, shows the fairly small proportion of even this more elderly sample who made use of health or social services – apart from the general practitioner; 87 per cent of the sample had used this service within the past year, and 42 per cent within the past month. Leaving aside this service, the most widely used was (non-private) chiropody, by 13 per cent of the sample within the past month. For the services more generally associated with dependence and frailty, an expected low proportion of users was found. For example, in the past month nine per cent had used the district nursing service, two per cent a day hospital, one per cent a bath attendant, four per cent a social worker, 18 per cent a home help, seven per cent meals-on-wheels, and six per cent a day centre. Other evidence comes from Age Concern's somewhat younger but less recent sample, among whom one in ten were receiving a home help; and from the latest GHS, which found that eight per cent were in receipt of the district nursing or health visitor service, ten per cent a home help, three per cent meals-on-wheels and five per cent a day centre. But receipt of service does not necessarily imply a perceived need for that service, nor non-receipt an absence of such perception. We still know very little about the self-perceived need for help by elderly people, their willingness or unwillingness to receive it, their beliefs about their eligibility, their feelings about particular services, or about whose responsibility it is to look after them.

Help will be felt to be needed for a variety of different reasons; it will not always be perceived as required because of illness or disability. For some people it will be because they feel they deserve help: 'I've done my part, now its the turn of others to help me'. For some because of accepted gender roles: 'I'm a man and therefore I need someone to do my housework' or 'I'm a woman and therefore I need someone to dig my garden and deal with my finances'. Sometimes it will be because of age itself and the respect felt due to age: 'people ought to help me because I'm an elderly person'. But sometimes, of course, the perceived basis of need for help will be that of illness, disability or frailty. Even where this is the case it may often be difficult for elderly people to recognise a point at which they feel they need help. One of the reasons is that illness itself is not a clearly recognisable objective fact; it has to be perceived. Nor is it a condition which is either present or totally absent, but a continuum along which the need for help at some point may occur. This is particularly true, of course, with so many of the diseases of old age, slowly accumulating disabilities and chronic illnesses, such as some forms of dementia or arthritis, where onset is not sudden as with acute illness episodes or accidents. How can the elderly know when they have reached a stage at which they might expect help?

Strongly held values of independence are likely to accompany an unwillingness to accept help. These may well change with increasing age, but there is also likely to be a cohort as well as an age effect; those who grew up under the welfare state may be readier to accept help than those who did not. When people do accept a need for assistance, what sort and whose help do they want or expect to receive? Do they prefer to purchase help, or to have it provided by their spouses, children or other relatives, or by voluntary agencies or statutory services? The data suggest a mixed picture, but all studies concur that elderly people value their independence and are reluctant to accept help from anyone. For example, the Age Concern study (1974) summarised its findings: 'independence in old age is clearly sought after; only about a quarter of the elderly are not upset by being helped with tasks they used to do themselves'. But studies show the elderly as divided about accepting help from their children.

Salvage (1986) found that just over half of her sample were in agreement with the statement that, 'families should be prepared to make sacrifices to look after us as we get older'. Age Concern found that 'the expectation that children will look after elderly parents is not accepted to any great extent; 67 per cent feel that "old people should not expect their children to look after them"'. Wenger (1984) says that while the elderly may turn to their children for help, this is not without reluctance, for being dependent on children can lead to loneliness and demoralisation (see also Blau, 1973; Stevenson, 1981). She adds, however, that 'the elderly are reluctant to talk about the negative aspects of dependency on children. The nature of the adult child–parent relationship is, perhaps for this reason, not a well researched field despite being a frequent fictional topic'. Indeed, one can see from the studies it has been possible to cite, how meagre is the research on this issue. For instance, we know little about what distinguishes those who are willing to accept or who expect help from their relatives, from those who do not; nor do we know what distinguishes those who would prefer to accept help from the state or other agencies, from those who would see such assistance in negative terms such as 'charity'.

Willingness to receive help from statutory social services depends not only upon general feelings about receiving such help but also upon such factors as awareness of the existence, nature and cost of services. It would be useful to compare people's perceptions of the receipt of health and social services; the recognition of the need for social services support may be a much more difficult one to make. It is not recognised as a 'normal' need at younger ages, as is consulting a doctor. If we are sick we visit a doctor, a non-stigmatising action, whereas if we are inadequate, criminal or disabled we visit social services, which is stigmatising. How can people in later life, therefore, be expected to see the use of social services as normal?

Awareness of services also has been shown to be relatively low. Salvage (1986), for example, found that whilst the overwhelming majority of her sample had heard of meals-on-wheels or home helps, a quarter were unaware of social workers and day centres, and three-quarters unaware of luncheon clubs. As far as health services were concerned, the majority were unaware of bath attendants, incontinence laundries and day hospitals, though almost everyone was aware of general practitioners, district nurses, chiropodists and outpatients' departments. There is much more to knowledge than awareness; people may not ask for help or may refuse it if they think, for example, that only the poor receive home helps, or that they will have to pay a good deal for the service, or, again, that old people's homes are depressing places where residents sit doing nothing all day. Salvage found that, 'of those who felt able to give a definite response, twice as many agreed as disagreed with the statement that "those living in residential homes/geriatric hospitals have lives which are too restricted"'. Willcocks *et al.* (1987) similarly state that, 'the prospect of moving into an old people's home is seldom viewed with pleasure ... The impressions that old people have of residential life, if not entirely coloured by images of the workhouse tradition of the past, are often based upon some knowledge of the restrictions that will be placed upon them'.

Unfortunately, the only major conclusion which can be drawn is that we know very little indeed about the complexities of the attitudes of elderly people towards the receipt of help. We know, of course, that the vast majority (like the rest of the population) are able to look after themselves, but this becomes less true as people become more elderly. In line with this finding, we know that only a small proportion of the elderly actually receive help with personal and household care (but again increasing with age). It is important to recognise that our knowledge extends very little further. For example, it may be that much dissatisfaction or reluctance to accept help could be allayed by a greater understanding of older people's reactions and of the circumstances in which they find assistance most acceptable; it may be that over time people's attitudes towards the receipt of help are changing. Perhaps more recent cohorts are less reluctant and more demanding than their predecessors with less experience of the modern welfare state. If we do not discover their attitudes and expectations we shall not be prepared for change. Even with the lack of data, however, one can see a good deal of variation and some uncertainties for elderly people in recognising a need for help, and in perceiving whose or what sort of help they need. But it is not necessarily the older person's recognitions which determine what happens, partly *because* of their variation and uncertainty, but also partly because others too have an interest, and want their views to prevail. Most elderly people prefer to remain at home, independent for as long as possible, and if not quite independent at least with the minimum of domiciliary care. Yet what are the perceptions and values of others about the care of the frail elderly? For the elderly, though by no means as passive as is sometimes suggested, are not the only people involved in making decisions about their support.

RELATIVES' ATTITUDES AND WILLINGNESS TO CARE

Relatives have always been the providers of the majority of help and support which elderly people have required. Evandrou *et al.* (1986) found that the pattern of care for that small proportion of elderly people who needed such care was as follows:

> Community care is an euphemism for family care ... The view of the 'community' caring for its elderly members is only supported by our research with respect to a particular household type: elderly people living alone. For elderly persons in other household units it is kin who are the main care providers. The support by formal agencies is generally limited and where it was provided, usually in the form of 'health care', it was found to be influenced by the household structure in which the elderly person lived rather than whether they were able to carry out various activities of daily living without help.

This finding accords with many others. Abrams' (1978) survey of 1600 people aged 65 and over living in four urban areas concluded that only a small minority of the third of the sample with some physical difficulty in carrying out household tasks, 'received any help with them, and this help usually came from relatives and was largely given to those elderly persons who live with others' (see also Hunt, 1978; Isaacs et al., 1972; Levin et al., 1983; Nissel and Bonnerjea, 1982; Shanas et al., 1968). It should also be remembered that much of this family care is care provided by the elderly themselves. As Wenger (1984) concludes from her study of the rural elderly, 'there are more elderly providing help of one sort or another than there are receiving help'. One in ten of her sample was caring for a dependent relative, and one in three helping out their neighbours in a regular way. She also found that help from formal sources was minimal. When the attitudes of family carers are discussed, it is often assumed that they themselves are not elderly; the perceptions of elderly carers are seldom the focus of attention.

Whatever their age, what motivates these family carers to help? Do they see it as their duty, do they do it because they enjoy it, or out of love, because they are under pressure to do it, or just because there simply is no-one else to do it? Studies show that carers take on the tasks willingly and voluntarily (see Blenkner, 1965; Brody 1981; Equal Opportunities Commission, 1980). But what brings them to this state of readiness? An American study suggests that external pressures are of great importance, i.e. that people do it because it is expected of them (Doty, 1986). A British study, examining only the internal pressures, suggests the importance of both reciprocity and of emotional closeness or 'affect' (Qureshi, 1986). This study, carried out in Sheffield among 299 elderly people and their 58 carers not living in the elderly person's home, found that most carers felt an obligation to help, partly through a feeling that the relationship between them and the older person was reciprocal: 'she does things for me just as I do things for her'. Reciprocal expectation was also expressed when past and present were taken into account, i.e. 'she's been a good mother to me, and now its my turn to help her'. Only 16 per cent said they thought the relationship had always been one-sided. Again, 72 per cent of the children carers (the question was not applicable in the same way to neighbour or friend carers) said that they felt emotionally close to their elderly parent, and, indeed, expressed their willingness to form a joint household with the elderly person if he or she could no longer cope with living alone. It should not be forgotten, however, that a substantial minority of the carers did not feel emotionally close to the elderly person, and Qureshi goes on to discuss a number of ways in which potential conflict can be controlled, for example, by the carer threatening to withdraw his or her support, or by an assertion of parental authority on the part of the recipient of the care. Although this is another under-researched area, one can suggest other possible sources of motivation for relatives to come to the assistance of elderly people. For example, it may be seen as a duty imposed by consanguinity: 'blood's thicker than water; he's my father, its my job to look after him'. Sometimes the motivation may not be moral but arise primarily from propinquity: 'well, I'm in the house, it's obviously convenient for me to do it'. The motive may be the lack of an alternative solution: 'there's no-one to do it if I don't, and I can't let him starve, can I? The lack of research is understandable given the sensitive nature of the topic, but many convincing findings have been produced on other sensitive topics, and there is no reason why the same should not be true of family care of the elderly (Ungerson, 1987). It is important to further the understanding of caring motivations, in order to understand the dynamics of the relationships involved and to provide the appropriate kinds of support for both carers and clients.

Even though those family members who provide care to elderly people have been shown to do it willingly and lovingly, there are limits to willingness, and some constraints which make it harder to provide care however willing people may be. Willingness to continue caring for a dependent relative is influenced by factors such as the nature and symptoms of the illness or disability. Chronic double incontinence is hard to tolerate for long, as is night-wakefulness (Sanford, 1975). The nature of the relationship before the illness or frailty began is also very important. As Gilhooly (1986) concludes from her Scottish study of 48 carers of dementia sufferers, 'both the blood/role relationship and the quality of that relationship prior to the development of dementia were significantly associated with the preference for institutional care. Many of the spouses in the sample took their marriage vows quite literally, and said they would continue with home care "until death do us part"'.

Other factors found by Gilhooly to associate significantly with a preference for *institutional* care were: the age of the supporter (younger people were less willing to go on caring); supporter's contact with friends (those with more contact were less willing); satisfaction with help from relatives (those dissatisfied with the amount of help given by other relatives were less willing); whether the carer was in paid employment (with those employed full-time most likely to favour institutional care); and whether or not the carer had another dependant to look after (as one would expect those with more than one dependant were more likely to advocate institutional care). One cannot generalise from one study to other groups of elderly dependent people and their carers. Gilhooly, for example, did not find significant correlations between willingness to care and the elderly person's sex, age or mental impairment, the *amount* of help given by other informal carers, the length of time the supporter had been caring for the elderly person, nor the amount of help received from the domiciliary services. The last finding was unexpected and differed from the findings of a similar London study (Levin *et al.*, 1983), possibly because of the uniformity of the Scottish home care services. Other types of dependants, or supporters or different geographical areas, may show different findings. It seems likely, for example, that in some cases the length of time the carers have been supporting the elderly person contributes to their feelings about continuing to care, or whether there are others to share some of the care. The local availability of formal community services may also be important. Such information is vital to the understanding of the problems of home care and to the planning of levels of formal service provision.

Some people are constrained from contributing to the support of an elderly relative, however willing they may be. Obvious factors are geographical separation, or the lack of skill or ability to provide the necessary support. It is sometimes assumed that *anyone* can provide the kind of care elderly frail people require. Of course this is not the case, but it is consistent with the way that the elderly are often treated. Similarly, when frail elderly people live at home they cannot necessarily be cared for by a family member. The supporter may need considerable physical strength, knowledge about medication, understanding of the course of an illness, or an informed sensitivity to mental frailty. Not everyone can provide these. We hear a good deal about the injustice of the burdens of care borne by daughters and wives, but little about the fact that they may not always be very good at caring. Yet they do provide an immense amount of support. Do their expectations of their role in caring accord with the expectations of those they support? Again we know very little. What proportion of carers, for instance, provide more support than they think they ought to appease a demanding parent? (Qureshi, 1986). And how many provide less than they think they ought because their parent refuses their help?

Relatives' perceptions of what kinds of services are available to elderly people is also an important factor in determining their feelings about the care which *they* provide. Again, we know very little about this, or about the acceptability to relatives of medical and nursing care, social services support, and income support. We know that there is considerable resistance to psychiatric hospital care but a more favourable attitude towards elderly people's homes. A Scottish study (West *et al.*, 1984) found that there was only limited support for informal care without professional involvement. Respondents did not seem inclined to allocate the major responsibility for care of the elderly to family and close kin, but 'preferred a partnership'. Sheltered housing is also strongly favoured, which accords with the public attitude that elderly people ought to be able to remain in the community but receive all the support which they need (Thompson and West, 1984). More specifically, we know little about the attitudes of relatives to particular services or about their knowledge of precisely what they do or who is eligible. Do relatives have interests which conflict with their acceptance of certain kinds of service? For instance, occasionally encountered are cases of children who resist their parent's entry to residential care if it means the sale of the parental house and a consequent loss of assets.

A final important factor in influencing the part which relatives play in the care of older people is the more basic one of their perceptions and understanding of elderly people's needs and of the ageing process. In many cases their perceptions will differ from those of their parents; in other cases, and for a variety of reasons (for example, the stage they have reached in the life cycle, their own health, and the degree of contact they have with elderly people), they will be similar, and the relatives will be ready to assist and/or to acknowledge parental need for support. There has been such a dearth of research on the psychology and sociology of parent–child relationships in later life that all one can do is point to their relevance but bemoan the absence of research findings, as has been the case throughout this section. Relatives help to make decisions about the care of the frail elderly; they provide the bulk of the care which the elderly receive and they provide it willingly; but we still know little about those who do not fall into this pattern, about the details of their perceptions and attitudes, and of their relationships and problems with the elderly people for whom they care.

SUPPORT AGENCIES AND THEIR IDEOLOGIES OF CARE

The provision of support services to elderly people is a large industry; the ideologies of care propounded by such agencies a broad topic. Not only could one address the formal assumptions and values of organisations as enshrined in legal or agreed documentation, but also the formal assumptions and values of the various professional groups who work within those organisations. There are also the informal values, perceptions, beliefs, goals and norms of the individuals working within the agencies, and both national and local perspectives have to be taken into account. The whole of this field cannot be reviewed here; it will perhaps be sufficient to indicate how complex it is, and to draw some conclusions from the recognition of this complexity. It is in the nature of ideologies that they are used in a taken-for-granted fashion; it may be useful to start by describing some current tenets, since this unquestioning acceptance tends to prohibit reflection on them and the drawing out of their implications.

As an example, consider the current explicit adherence to the value of *collaboration* (see Audit Commission, 1986). This is a comparatively recent issue although collaboration in the delivery of care, particularly in rural areas, was probably as prevalent in the past as now. Today it is under constant discussion by service agencies as exemplified in the field of mental health (New Directions, 1987):

> Collaboration in mental health services is essential at all levels but increasingly in service planning. The environment is an extremely complex one. No profession or agency has a monopoly on services, skills or answers. Those with a legitimate stake in services have to be included in negotiations: those who use services, carers and the wider community. Resources are scarce in mental health, so working together makes better use of what is available. Collaboration also ensures the sharing of skills and different perspectives.

The collaboration bandwagon is beginning to roll with very little prior research or analysis of its implications. There are good financial and other reasons for collaboration, but what difference does it make for clients? How, for example, will it fit in with the perceptions, wants and needs of elderly people and their relatives?

Turning to the intra-agency values which concern elderly people, the first and most obvious is the pervasive proclamations of the merits of community care. It is justifiably believed that this is what elderly people want, for, as noted above, the vast majority *do* want it. It is also believed that it is the best option for their mental and physical health, and, at least until recently, it was believed that it was cheaper than institutional care. This strong movement has inevitably understated the circumstances in which community care is neither best nor preferred. A debate on its appropriate application is, however, proceeding, despite the force of less critical advocacy for community care. Recent research has shown, for example, that certain dementia sufferers are hard to sustain at home, and that from certain perspectives they could be better off in institutional care. Some are very expensive to support at home, some prefer to live with other people rather than on their own, some need specialised nursing or medical care not available at home, and some are a health or safety risk to others when they are at home (Askham and Thompson, 1987).

Another emphasis is on maintaining the independence of elderly people, by helping them to maintain or restoring their ability to look after themselves. This harmonises with one widely argued benefit of community care, and is a tenet of good practice in residential care. Its variable application in institutions has been well expressed:

> ... local authorities often voice an ideal philosophy of care as one in which residents retain control of their private world yet at the same time receive care and protection. But the experiential reality for old people may be far removed from this ideal balance, and residential life can become something of a battleground between individual and organisational needs.

(Willcocks *et al.*, 1987)

So it is not an immutable principle. Indeed it should be added that independence does not necessarily mean autonomy or freedom to make one's own choices: paradoxically, restoration to independence may well be forced upon people who do not want it. Independence is only fostered to a point: at some stage or in some circumstances, when, for example, either people's own wishes or a cost-effectiveness principle is put into operation, people may not be rehabilitated or resuscitated, but allowed to die. As is the case for the implementation of community care and collaboration, much research is needed on the perceptions and wishes of older people and their relatives.

Another assumption about elderly people is that they are a separable group, in the sense that they have distinct needs for treatment or support that distinguish them from other sectors of the population. This view supports the development of geriatric medicine, geriatric wards, social work specialists in the elderly, elderly people's voluntary organisations, and old people's homes. Undoubtedly there are good organisational reasons for this segregation, just as there are good reasons for children's homes and paediatricians. But it is rarely emphasised that such separation is not inevitable. Alongside the organisational, scientific and attitudinal reasons for separation is a political argument: only if underprivileged groups have their own pressure groups and protagonists are they likely to achieve a larger share of scarce resources. Yet, while accepting that good reasons prevail, it is worth examining the less constructive implications of separation. It reinforces separation in images of ageing and the elderly, discourages social interaction between different age groups, encourages the confinement of social interaction within other age groups, and perhaps supports ageist attitudes. We also need to know whether separation meets the needs of the elderly and their relatives.

Institutions, agencies and their staff develop attitudes not only towards elderly people, but also about the services to be provided for them. Four characteristics of provision are worth comment, for they are often accepted unthinkingly. One is that services provided for elderly people tend to be *demand led*; that is, the service agencies rarely seek their customers, clients or patients, they wait for them to come. This should mean that the services respond to elderly people's perceptions of their needs. But whereas the identification of need may be left to elderly people, it is the service provider who usually (a) defines or redefines that need, and (b) decides how it should be treated or met. It should be added that not all services are demand led. Some general practices, for example, provide a regular visiting service for everyone on their register over a certain age, but there are few screening services for the elderly (Taylor *et al.*, 1983; Barker, 1986). In other words, needs are often initially left to be defined by the client or patient, but the provision is decided by the services. In what sense, therefore, can one assess whether services meet needs?

A second and related feature of services is that there is very little *consumer choice*. While people are permitted to choose, there is an inadequate range of services from which they may select. People cannot choose, for example, what kind of home help service to have, although, of course, careful attention is given to provide people with the range of services that they are assessed to need. But 'need' is defined narrowly, usually in terms of the illness or disability rather than in terms of tastes or preferences. The traditional model of paternalistic care prevails, perhaps more because of the scarcity of resources than through a belief that people should not have the freedom to choose for themselves.

Thirdly, services are *localised*: for health and social service provision there is nothing equivalent to the planned national core curriculum for schools. An increasing number of local authorities are, however, agreeing basic principles of care for elderly people, which many would like to see adhered to by all. Local control does mean that services for elderly people, as for other groups, vary from one area to another, not only among local government or health authority territories, but also among the areas or patches of particular and partially autonomous social service or nursing *teams.* This makes it extremely difficult to generalise about whether needs are being met. It also means that any one elderly person may be being served by a variety of semi-autonomous service providers, each of whom may be handling his or her needs in different ways.

Finally, most agencies (except for some voluntary ones) deal with other groups as well as the elderly. So the resources available for the care of the elderly are in competition with other potential client groups. It is hard for the service providers to achieve the goal of fulfilling all the perceived major needs of the elderly. These have to be viewed in a context in which the elderly's needs are set against those of children, the acutely ill and accident victims. Although the elderly are often treated as a distinct group, at another level they are competing for scarce resources with other groups. In some ways their separation probably does not help gain maximum resources, unless, as is sometimes but not always the case, they are seen by resource allocators as a priority group.

The agencies which provide services for elderly people often do so on the basis of assumptions which are implicit, changing, unclear and conflicting. Managers and staff handle mainly demand led services but they define needs in their own ways and sometimes meet these needs according to their own definitions. Overall, these services are in competition with other sectors of public life for resources; since they always want to increase their share, they can never say that they are meeting needs.

CONCLUSIONS

Are the needs for health and social care of the elderly being met? In the light of the present waiting lists for hospital treatment, residential care, day care, sheltered housing, and home helps, the answer is undoubtedly 'no'. This chapter has tried to elucidate the complexity of the question, and thereby to define what would be involved in attempting to achieve a different answer. We are a long way from such change. Of course, there are vast areas of unmet need; anyone can hold a Utopian vision of a society in which no one is lonely, in discomfort or pain, and all live a contented long life in the kind of environment which is most suitable. The important questions are not whether overall needs are being met; we should be examining most closely where new policies are being implemented as well as those which are most resistant to change. It should also be remembered that needs and support are socially determined concepts, and for this reason they vary, and are understood and perceived differently. In this brief survey the variation has been a consistent theme, and the discussion has directed attention to the importance of far more incisive questions about whether or not needs are being met, and whether elderly people are adequately supported.

REFERENCES

Abrams, M. (1978). *Three Score Years and Ten*, vol. I. Age Concern England, Mitcham, Surrey.

Age Concern (1974). *The Attitudes of the Retired and Elderly.* Age Concern England, Mitcham, Surrey.

Askham, J. and Thompson, C. (1987). *Enhanced Home Support for Dementia Sufferers.* Age Concern Institute of Gerontology, King's College, London.

Audit Commission for Local Authorities in England and Wales (1986). *Making a Reality of Community Care.* HMSO, London.

Barker, J. (1986). *Primary Health Care for Older People.* Age Concern Institute of Gerontology, King's College, London.

Blau, Z.S. (1973). *Old Age in a Changing Society.* Franklin Watts, New York.

Blenkner, M. (1965). Social work and family relationships in later life, with some thoughts on filial maturity. In *Social Structure and the Family: Generational Relations,* E. Shanas and G. Streib (Eds). Prentice Hall, Englewood Cliffs, New Jersey.

Brody, E.M. (1981). Women in the middle and family help to older people. *The Gerontologist,* **21**(5), 471–80.

Doty, P. (1986). Family care of the elderly: the role of public policy. *The Milbank Quarterly,* **64**(1), 34–75.

Equal Opportunities Commission (1980). *The Experience of Caring for Elderly and Handicapped Dependants.* Equal Opportunities Commission, Manchester.

Evandrou, M., Arber, S., Dale, A. and Gilbert, G.N. (1986). Who cares for the elderly? In *Dependency and Interdependency in Old Age: Theoretical Perspectives and Policy Alternatives,* C. Phillipson, M. Bernard and P. Strang (Eds). Croom Helm, London.

Gilhooly, M. (1986). Senile dementia: factors associated with caregivers' preference for institutional care. *British Journal of Medical Psychology,* **59**, 165–71.

Hunt, A. (1978). *The Elderly at Home: A Study of People Aged 65 and Over Living in the Community in England in 1976.* HMSO, London.

Isaacs, B., Livingstone, M. and Neville, Y. (1972). *Survival of the Unfittest: A Study of Geriatric Patients in Glasgow.* Routledge & Kegan Paul, London.

Jones, D.A., Victor, C.R. and Vetter, N.J. (1983). Carers of the elderly in the community. *Journal of the Royal College of General Practitioners,* **33**, 707–11.

Levin, E., Sinclair, I. and Gorbach, P. (1983). *The Supporters of the Confused Elderly at Home.* National Institute of Social Work, London.

New Directions (1987). Editorial in Newsletter, Summer Issue. Good Practices in Mental Health, London.

Nissel, M. and Bonnerjea, L. (1982). *Family Care of the Handicapped Elderly: Who Pays?* Policy Studies Institute, London.

Office of Population Censuses and Surveys (1986). *General Household Survey.* HMSO, London.

Qureshi, H. (1986). Responses to dependency: reciprocity, affect and power in family relationships. In *Dependency and Interdependency in Old Age: Theoretical Perspectives and Policy Alternatives,* C. Phillipson, M. Bernard and P. Strang (Eds), pp. 167–71. Croom Helm, London.

Salvage, A. (1986). *Attitudes of the Over-75s to Health and Social Services.* Research Team for Care of the Elderly, University of Wales College of Medicine, Cardiff.

Sanford, J. (1975). Tolerance of debility in elderly dependants by supporters at home. *British Medical Journal,* **3**, 471–3.

Shanas, E., Townsend, P., Wedderburn, D., Friis, H., Milhøj, P. and Stehower, J. (1968). *Old People in Three Industrial Societies.* Routledge & Kegan Paul, London.

Stevenson, O. (1981). Caring and dependency. In *The Impact of Ageing,*

D. Hobman (Ed.). Croom Helm, London.

Taylor, R., Ford, G. and Barber, H. (1983). *The Elderly at Risk*, Research Perspectives on Ageing 6. Age Concern Research Unit, Mitcham, Surrey.

Thomson, C. and West, P. (1984). The public appeal of sheltered housing. *Ageing and Society*, 4(3), 305–26.

Ungerson, C. (1987). *Policy is Personal: Sex, Gender and Informal Care.* Tavistock, London.

Wenger, C.G. (1984). *The Supportive Network.* Allen & Unwin, London.

West, P., Illsley, R. and Kelman, H. (1984). Public preferences for the care of dependency groups. *Social Science and Medicine*, 18(4), 287–95.

Willcocks, D., Peace, S. and Kelleher, L. (1987). *Private Lives in Public Places.* Tavistock, London.

James McEwen
Department of Community Medicine
University of Glasgow

10 PLANNING HEALTH CARE: THE COMMUNITY APPROACH

INTRODUCTION

The differences in approach between those who provide care to individuals and those who have responsibility for planning services is becoming more evident with increasing competition for scarce resources and little funding for new developments. Both planners and health professionals might use the word 'need': doctors might refer to their right to prescribe treatment according to their patient's need, as assessed by the doctor, irrespective of cost; while the health planner might cite the necessity to take account of all aspects of the needs of the community, not even just the groups of the elderly, based on routinely available statistics and local strategy documents. Neither are likely to have a comprehensive picture of need, or have good evidence as to the expected outcome of various forms of intervention. Despite the frequent conflicts between the champions of clinical freedom who insist on meeting patients' needs and those who support the concept of the greatest good for the greatest number with the assessment of priorities, the individual doctor is more likely to be able to provide the best care for an elderly patient in a district health authority which has undertaken a meticulous and comprehensive approach to the planning of health needs of its elderly population.

This chapter will review briefly the current position with regard to the planning of health care for the elderly; the general principles of planning health care will be summarised and the rationale for the 'needs derived' approach will be examined. These will be used to illustrate the ways in which a local planning system, such as exists in a district health authority, can examine the needs of the elderly in their local community and proceed to determine priorities and plan programmes which can be evaluated subsequently. Such evaluation will, in turn, lead to a re-examination of priorities, policies and plans, thus ensuring a service which is flexible and capable of adapting to the changing needs of the local community. The community approach involves a single, comprehensive planning system that covers all aspects of health service care: inpatient (short and long stay); day hospital; outpatient; accident and emergency; and services for those who are living in their own home by family practitioner services and the community health services.

THE PRESENT POSITION

There is much discussion about an 'impending crisis' associated with the increasing numbers of the elderly, the lack of resources to meet the accepted government philosophy of 'care in the community', and the resulting gaps and inequalities in service provision. Everyone knows of sad stories of individual suffering and hardship and the burdens that are placed on family and friends who try and provide the necessary care, love and attention.

In a review of all aspects of community care, including care for the elderly, the Audit Commission (1986) summarises the present position:

(i) *There are serious grounds for concern* about the lack of progress in shifting the balance of services towards community care. Progress has been slow and uneven across the country, and the near-term prospects are not promising. In short, the community care policy is in danger of failing to achieve its potential.

(ii) *Fundamental underlying problems need to be tackled* if community care is to be translated from an attractive policy to reality throughout England and Wales. The major underlying problems are:
  – The pattern of distribution of finance is out of step with community care policies. Local authorities cannot be expected to play their full part given the loss of grant incurred for expanding services under current arrangements.
  – There is considerable organisational fragmentation and confusion, with responsibility for the introduction of community care divided between a variety of separately funded organisations who often fail to work together effectively.
  – There are inadequate arrangements for training and providing opportunities in community services for existing staff in long stay hospitals, and for training sufficient numbers of community based staff.

(iii) *Radical steps will be necessary* if the underlying problems are to be solved. Fine-tuning the existing arrangements, or treating the symptoms, will not meet the needs of the situation. Despite the difficulties outlined above, progress is being made. Such progress can usually be attributed to individuals with enough determination to manœuvre their way around the system; they are succeeding in spite of and not because of the present organisation and financing arrangements.

The Audit Commission concludes that, 'The purpose of this report is to convince all the interests concerned that at present, community care is far from a reality for many of the very people it is intended to help'.

It might be assumed that the detailed planning of any category of services would depend on the related pillars of a philosophy of care and identified need. Sadly, this seldom occurs in the field of health care at either the national or the local level.

HEALTH SERVICE PLANNING: INFORMATION AND POLICY

In health service planning, resources traditionally were allocated to sustain and improve existing established services, and such services were usually under the control of powerful and senior doctors well able to organise their case. Inevitably, there was and still is conflict over priorities. Conflicts arise between hospital and community health professionals, between planners and administrators and within community pressure groups. Policies, politics, power and prejudice are all involved. Conflict often remains unresolved because of a lack of data, a failure to use data, or because the information is of poor quality.

As O'Neill (1983) points out, the technological advances which have produced marked benefits to patients have added to the chaos that exists in health services planning in both developed and developing countries.

> Increased knowledge has often led to too much specialisation in medicine and to the large uncontrolled proliferation and fragmentation of health services. This, in turn, has led many countries to develop what amounts to distintegrated systems of health care dominated entirely by specialists.... Coverage of people's health needs has suffered and resources and manpower have been wasted. Worse, the public's expectations have constantly grown, influenced often by considerations far removed from those of good health care.... This has meant that health systems have been too much characterised by a hit and run approach ... There are no clear health policies, no effective structures for health planning and no adequate system for assessing the real value of new development plans or how they are put into effect.
>
> (O'Neill, 1983)

It is salutory to be reminded of the scale and implications of this lack of information. As the World Health Organization (WHO) recently commented, 'Vital statistics, including death registration and census information, have been available in many countries for more than a century. However, very little work has been done on the health, social conditions, needs and problems of the elderly' (WHO, 1983). The problems are elaborated later in the report, with emphasis placed on the dearth of epidemiological studies of the health status of the elderly in representative population samples. The interpretation of data is rendered difficult by inconsistency in diagnostic methods and reporting, and there is 'difficulty in distinguishing between the manifestation of normal ageing and pathological conditions'.

The WHO's review of the situation of elderly people in 11 countries and the response of medical services points out that,

> Two major approaches are used in the estimation of health needs. The medical approach is based primarily on the International Classification of Diseases, and diagnostic procedures are selected and developed for that purpose. This approach is often criticised for over-specialisation and insensitivity to the psycho-social dimensions of health and disease. Another approach is based on the assessment of functional abilities in order to discover what limits a person's capacity to cope with the activities and stresses of everyday life. Subjective assessment of functional ability is regarded as a valuable indicator both of health and the need for services, and this can be complemented by objective measures of functional ability. The diagnostic procedures for the medical approach are rich and well advanced, whereas fewer tools are available for the assessment of functional abilities.
>
> (WHO, 1983)

As Alderson (1986) has shown, routine statistics can be used to indicate the overall national demographic and health trends that have occurred during this century, thus providing an excellent basis for further detailed studies. Despite this lack of detailed and accurate information, new philosophies and new directions for care have been advanced and accepted by the government in the United Kingdom. However, as the Audit Commission (1986) has commented, 'guidance on the development of community-based services for elderly people is far less specific than it is for the mentally handicapped and mentally ill people. There are no indications of how the balance of care should change'.

In 1981 the government published *Care in Action* (DHSS, 1981). This enumerated the social and health care services, set out objectives for health authorities and local government social service departments, but failed to give a clear lead for the future. The principal recommendations were as follows.

(a) The primary health care and community care services should be strengthened, including those provided by the voluntary sector, in order to support elderly people living in their own homes. It made clear that sheltered housing provision was regarded as an option for a small minority.

(b) A more active approach should be taken to the hospital treatment of elderly people and their rehabilitation, to encourage wherever possible their return to the community. This recommendation thereby gave approval for the development of acute geriatric units in general hospitals, which are seen as centres of expertise for the paramedical and social service groups involved in the care of elderly people.

(c) Capacity in the hospital acute sector should be maintained to deal with the increasing number of elderly patients. Presently two-thirds of all non-psychiatric inpatients aged 75 years or more are treated in general acute beds. It is among this age group that treatment needs are most complex, because often there are multiple conditions requiring simultaneous treatment and because of the special difficulties of rehabilitation.

(d) Provision for the minority of elderly people requiring long-term care in hospital or residential homes should be maintained.

The general principles of planning health care are no different for the elderly than for any other age category or defined population group. Although at national level there are vague policies and major problems in funding and management, there are exciting examples of schemes and policies at local levels, and it is encouraging that whether in voluntary or statutory organisations, the emphasis is now being shifted to local responsibility and local decisions based on involvement by public, patients and providers.

A FRAMEWORK FOR PLANNING

The main barriers to effective community care have been identified. While solutions are readily apparent, it is equally obvious that there are difficulties in achieving the desired objectives. Among the problems are the complexities of achieving:

(i) a spectrum of care provision involving a range of options and a variety of different settings;

(ii) increased emphasis on community care with the necessary redistribution of staff and resources ensuring quality of care;

(iii) services which provide flexibility and facilitate an individual to move according to changing individual requirements; and

(iv) services which are adaptable to the changing needs of the community and sensitive to local conditions such as the special needs of ethnic groups.

As the Audit Commission (1986) has concluded, 'the change to a community-based service involves much more than a change to the pattern of service provision. It involves a change of approach, with emphasis and priority placed on encouraging patients and clients to do as much for themselves as possible'. In practice this can only be achieved satisfactorily by a subtle combination of formal, informal and self-care. Formal care will always be needed for some people, but even the most severely handicapped can be encouraged to live more independently, to realise their full potential within services that combine practical support with caring. 'To provide the necessary framework for such an approach, a wide range of services that complement each other is required' (Audit Commission, 1986). The range of these services is reviewed in the following paragraphs. Although the subheadings will be familiar, the nature, emphasis and priority accorded to these services can be radically changed.

Information

Information needs go well beyond the Natural Health Service's established routine statistics and the newly expanded but still minimal tables reported by DHSS which will become available with the implementation in 1987 and 1988 of Körner information systems. A comprehensive package is needed of qualitative and quantitative data, which are locally relevant and up to date. They should result from a planned programme of routine and special studies designed by the community teams, both those with responsibility for planning and those who provide the services being involved in the generation and use of such information. Information about the clients becomes the driving force identifying the *needs* of the population. This in turn can lead to the determination of the *tasks* that are appropriate which will indicate the *skills* that are required. This may result in a re-examination of the work of the existing professionals with either the establishment of a new category of health worker or retraining of existing categories to provide the appropriate mix of skills in community based professionals. Thus the service provided becomes 'needs-derived' rather than one based on the narrow constraints of existing professionalism (Backett, 1980).

A vital ingredient will be information on clients and carers. This will involve both estimates of satisfaction and measures of health status. The lack of appropriate health measures has been mentioned, but recent research in several countries has developed a variety of useful health measures, indicators or profiles, in the determination of need and the evaluation of outcome. By 1981 Culyer was able to produce a comprehensive review of these health indicators. He suggested that they could be grouped into three main categories:

1. Indicators of health status of individuals in a community, for example, mortality, morbidity, disability and perceived health.
2. Indicators of the work, scope and efficiency of health care services, for example, episodes of illness, bed days and clinic attendances.
3. Indicators of social and environmental status of the community, for example, environmental pollution, housing conditions and leisure facilities.

The majority of these indicators are available routinely, although insufficient use is made of them. Most effort is presently devoted to identifying the overall requirements for funding, often with an emphasis on the problems of inner-city areas (Golding *et al.*, 1986). Most health authority and local authority information and planning departments can provide data by relevant local small areas (see examples in Figs 10.1 and 10.2). The creation of composite indices such as ACORN, *A Classification of Residential Neighbourhoods* (CACI, undated), appears to offer a valuable tool which may be linked to other measures in health services planning and resource allocation (Lowe and McEwen, 1987).

In small local community surveys routine mortality and morbidity statistics are insufficiently sensitive measures. For this purpose and for the evaluation of different forms of clinical care, attempts have been made to find a measure of health status which is relatively easy to administer, cheap, reliable, valid and

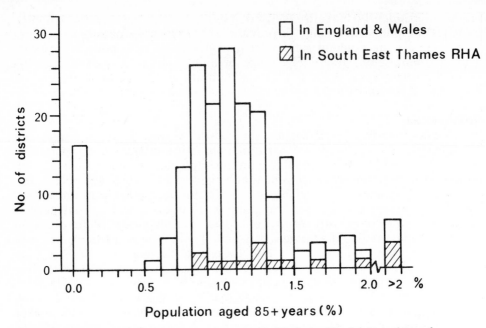

Fig. 10.1 The frequency distribution of District Health Authorities by their share of population aged 85+ years: England and Wales, 1981. Prepared by John Yates.

acceptable to the population in general. As far as health status is concerned, professional descriptions based on physical or biological departures from normal and the professional estimates of the effects that such departures have on individuals, must be compared with the individual's own view of feeling and function. Magi and Allander (1981) propose that statements on need should be classified on the basis of who makes them. They propose a primary classification of:

(i) self assessed need (an individual's assessment of his own situation); and
(ii) other assessed need (the assessor and the assessed are not the same person).

They suggest both that congruence between the two is unusual because of the unique and introspective character of self-assessed need, and that the greatest disparities occur in health measures because of the special position, knowledge and responsibility of health professionals. *Activities of Daily Living* indices have a long and proven tradition in the category of professional assessments, while more recent measures of subjective health include the *Sickness Impact Profile* and the *Nottingham Health Profile* (Hunt *et al.*, 1986).

An example of the use of the Nottingham Health Profile is shown in Fig. 10.3 which illustrates how the different levels of function and feeling can be identified in different groups. Although this was a preliminary study, it was concluded that there was evidence that self-assessment of health status appears to reflect functional status, is sensitive to group differences, and to a large extent reflects existing health problems (Hunt *et al.*, 1986).

There is great variation in the knowledge of and beliefs about the health of the elderly. Professionals and the public tend to underestimate the health

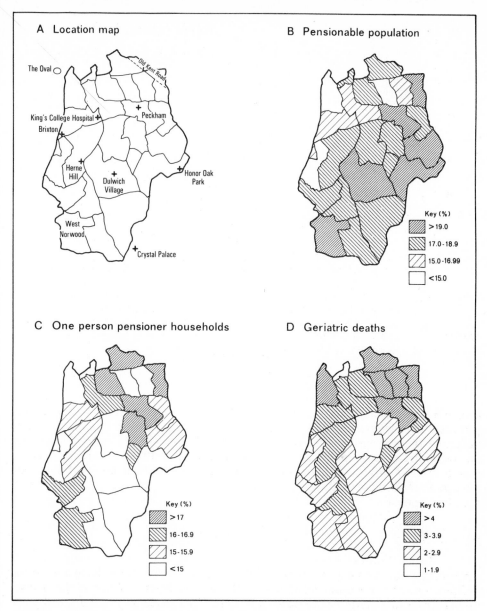

Fig. 10.2 Elderly population profiles in the Camberwell Health District, south London. **A** Key to locations; **B** Percentage of population of pensionable age, 1981; **C** One-person pensioner households as a percentage of all households, 1981; **D** Geriatric deaths and discharges in 1982 as a percentage of the pensionable population.

status of the elderly and overestimate the number that require institutional care. It is interesting to note that the elderly themselves do the same for other elderly. Quite a different picture emerges when the elderly are asked to rate their own health, although there are differences of detail between studies which may reflect variations in research and social inequalities. Often 80 per cent or more judge themselves to be in fair, good or excellent health: this

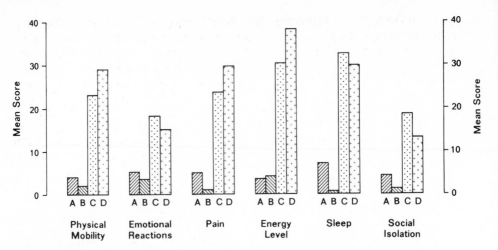

Fig. 10.3 Average health scores under the Nottingham Health Profile of four groups of elderly people: the higher the score the greater the health problems. **A** Men participating in a research programme on physical exercises for elderly people described as fit on the basis of their exercise heart rates; **B** Sample of patients from general practice with no known chronic disease and who had not contacted their general practitioner for at least two months; **C** Group attending a luncheon club run by a Social Services Department and with varying health and social problems; **D** Group of patients from general practice records described as chronically ill. See text for further explanation.

usually accords with professional estimates and with survival (Hunt, 1978; Maddox and Douglas, 1973; La Rue *et al.*, 1979). It must be noted that a different picture emerges for the very elderly, emphasising the importance of definition in all research. In an Age Concern survey in 1977, of those aged 75 or more who were living in their own homes, only ten per cent said that they had no physical problems, while 41 per cent had one or two (Abrams, 1985).

The importance of self-definition of health in determining the use of professional health care has been demonstrated. (Robinson, 1971). Several factors, such as self-image, life satisfaction, amount of physical activity and attitudes to retirement are interrelated with actual and perceived health status (Linn, 1976). Self-estimates of health have been found to account for the majority of the variance in ratings of life satisfaction by the elderly and these self-estimates were found to be closely related to both functional status and physicians' judgements of the patients' health (Palmore and Luikart, 1972). It can be concluded that elderly people's perception of themselves and the world may be more important determinants of adjustment than their actual condition.

While detailed research studies and routine statistics can form a useful backcloth, the local picture requires detailed knowledge of local statistics and the illumination of regular, efficient local studies. In attempting to describe the health of the elderly in a particular community, recognition should be given to the possibility of great variation within a health district – particularly in urban areas, and the fact that no single approach will be sufficient. A selection of indicators will be required. Indeed, even within a particular category, different indicators can provide separate but equally valid measures.

The team planning and evaluating the health care provided will require to co-ordinate epidemiological, sociological, statistical and economic skills to ensure comprehensive information, but there is more to information than the presentation to planners of sophisticated packages of statistics. Clients also welcome quantitative and qualitative information which covers voluntary and statutory services, their times, places, telephone numbers, types of care and names of those in charge. Many district health education officers, independently or in collaboration with local authorities, have produced publications on the services for the over-sixties in their areas. Co-ordination between general practitioners, family practitioner committees, local authorities, voluntary organisations and health authorities can be co-ordinated and publicised through a planning team or care group for the elderly. Such publications often prove equally informative to professionals as well as members of the public.

The 'patch'

Although there has been discussion over many years about the most appropriate size of area for planning health services, this has received new impetus with the publication of the Cumberledge Report (DHSS, 1986b) which suggests that a population of 10–25 000 may be the best size for the provision of community nursing services. Published almost at the same time as the discussion paper on primary health care (DHSS, 1986a), these reports encouraged further examination of the opportunities for collaboration at the level of primary and community care.

Unfortunately, at present there is often no easily identifiable 'patch' which would be accepted by all the relevant organisations providing care, and if locally relevant data are required the position is complicated. Although there may be similarities between a local authority ward and an identifiable community, there is unlikely to be co-terminosity with social services areas or the health districts, clinics and community nursing and health visitor boundaries. While in rural areas it may not be too difficult to relate to general practitioner populations as the focus, in urban areas this is a major problem. Aggregations of enumeration districts into the patch, if possible, will ensure the availability of routine data, but natural boundaries such as railway lines or bus routes may render this difficult. As there still seems to be uncertainty about the most appropriate size for the planning of health care, district health authorities may wish to undertake pilot studies to determine what appears to be the best local solution.

Targets and evaluation

The concept of setting measurable targets is one which has been developed by the World Health Organization in its commitment to *Targets for Health for All by the Year 2000* with particular reference to health promotion. European Region of WHO (1985) has specified 38 targets and, although their importance will vary from one country to another, they can be set out as four dimensions of action in relation to health outcomes:

(i) ensure equality in health by reducing the present gap in health status between countries and among groups within countries;
(ii) add life to years by ensuring the full development and use of peoples' integral or residual physical and mental capacity to derive full benefit from and to cope with life in a healthy way;
(iii) add health to life by reducing disease and disabilities; and
(iv) add years to life by reducing premature deaths and thereby increasing life expectancy.

Throughout these proposals there is an emphasis on health promotion and primary health care, with health being achieved through active participation by people themselves within their communities. This must be accompanied by multisectoral co-operation as health authorities can deal with only a portion of the problems to be solved. As far as care is concerned, the emphases are upon appropriateness, the integration of prevention and care, and the promotion of health.

Virtually all the specific targets can lead directly or indirectly to improved health for the elderly. The Faculty of Community Medicine (1986) has begun to identify responsibility for achieving these targets for central government, local government, health authorities and individuals. Within the suggested framework, district health authorities and local planning teams can identify their own specific targets for the elderly, establish baseline data, using the skills available, and then set targets, which can be measured for five, ten and fifteen years.

Promotion of health

Health promotion is a major theme of *Targets for Health for All by the Year 2000*, but it has grown out of a larger and rather uncertain past of health education activities and screening programmes for the elderly. Traditionally, health education concentrated on young people, special groups such as pregnant women and unhealthy personal behaviour such as smoking and drugs. Gradually, the development in educational theory associated with health education programmes in schools indicated the relevance of education throughout life and special programmes were designed for adult populations including those at work, often including pre-retirement programmes. In 1984, The Health Education Council for England (HEC), Wales and Northern Ireland issued a consultation document *A Programme of Education for Health in Old Age* (HEC, 1984). As they point out, the title is not age specific since, 'quite simply education for health in old age demonstrably should begin among the young'. Repeated evidence of unrecognised and recognised untreated health problems prompted the establishment of screening programmes by general practitioners or health authorities. Although few of these studies have indicated long-term benefits in changed outcome, they have shown that this approach is valued by old people, and may improve contact and communication with health professionals.

With the commitment by the Royal College of General Practitioners (1981) to 'anticipatory care', care with an eye to the future, it has been suggested that:

Anticipatory care as a planned procedure during normal patient/doctor contact is a logical development of screening and makes the best use of manpower in primary care. It is particularly suitable in the elderly population, most of whom are seen regularly. There are no practical obstacles to it becoming standard practice in family medicine.

(Williams, 1985)

The importance of health promotion and prevention of disease is acknowledged in the UK government's White Paper, *Promoting Better Health*, as is the key role of the family doctor in encouraging people to use the available services, and in their provision (DHSS, 1987).

The potential in primary care for making a significant contribution to the promotion of health, through screening and health education in the elderly, and indeed at all ages, will only be achieved once there is information available on the defined practice population. One needs to identify who may be at risk and who has received particular health promotion packages. This may be achieved by the computerisation of records which in turn will be enhanced when linked to a comprehensive district based information system. As well as this essentially personally based aspect of health promotion, the district health authorities, local authorities and voluntary bodies will be pushing for a health promotion element in social, environmental, financial and other policies.

The team: planning and responsibility

The breadth and diversity of concerned organisations are summarised in Fig. 10.4 and Table 10.1, and demonstrate clearly the problems of providing a co-ordinated and integrated service. A radical proposition which would achieve considerable unification has been put forward by the Audit Commission (1986). It proposes a single budget in an area, established by contributions from the NHS and local authorities. This budget would be under the control of a single manager who will purchase from a public or private agency, the appropriate services for elderly people in the community in the areas for which he or she is responsible. The manager's activities should be overseen by a small joint board of National Health Service and local authority representatives. If

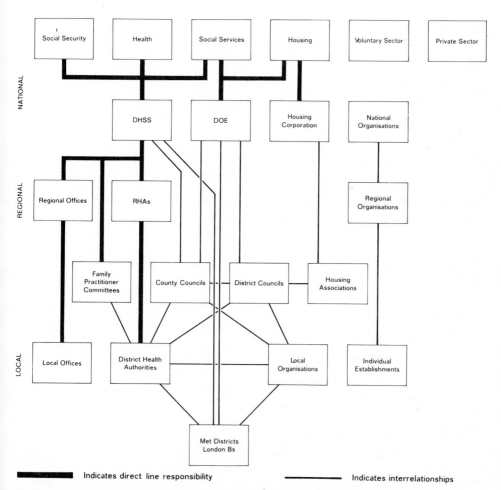

Fig. 10.4 Principal agencies involved in community care. Data from Audit Commission (1986).

Table 10.1 Main care and accommodation services in England and Wales. Data from Audit Commission (1986).

Agency	Form of care	Service	Variations
Health authorities	Hospitals	Inpatients	Long-stay Short-stay/respite
	Residential	Day Community units Nursing homes	
	Community services	Nurses	Qualified Auxiliary
		Health visitors Therapists	Physiotherapists Chiropody
Family practitioner committees	Primary health care	GPs Nurses Dental and ophthalmic services	
Social services	Residential	Residential homes	Long-stay Short-stay/respite
	Accommodation	Staffed group homes Unstaffed group homes Sheltered lodgings	
	Day care	Workshops Day centres Training centres Drop-in centres	
	Domiciliary	Social workers Good neighbours Home helps Therapists	Occupational
Housing authorities	Housing	Sheltered housing	Wardens Alarm systems
		Hostels Group homes Flats/houses	Improvement grants
Education	Training facilities for adults		
Voluntary sector and housing associations	Residential Housing	Residential homes Group homes Sheltered housing Flats/houses	For special needs
	Day care	Luncheon clubs Drop-in centres	
	Domiciliary	Care attendant schemes Volunteers/good neighbours	
Private sector	Residential	Nursing homes Residential homes	
	Housing Domiciliary	Sheltered housing Domestic agencies	

this cannot be achieved, there does need to be a comprehensive team with responsibility for planning, involving representatives of statutory and voluntary organisations, as well as the consumer voice – both elderly people and patient representatives. Although for the purpose of this chapter the teams of planners and providers of service have been distinguished, those who provide the services must be involved either directly or through representatives on the planning teams.

In practice, it is likely that the three main bodies – health authorities, family practitioner services and local authorities – will have the major responsibility, and their effective collaboration is vital. At present, in most parts of the country, the district health authorities are likely to assume the initiative in co-ordination and planning as they have better resources and support for the planning function, although they must recognise that the majority of old people live at home and that the maximum effort is required in the provision of services designed to support people in the community. Horrocks (1986), in his view of the components of a comprehensive district health service for elderly people, notes that, 'no one Health District currently offers the whole range of provision envisaged in this paper. Nevertheless, with few exceptions, each component cited does already exist in one District or another in England and Wales'.

The team: providers

Community care implies to some an increasing burden on those who care for the elderly, with patchy and inadequate support from official services, and the belief that the state is failing in its responsibility. Elderly people, their immediate carers and the professionals involved directly in care, have all expressed feelings of frustration, anger or disappointment. The burden on carers, themselves often elderly, was described well by Isaacs *et al.* (1972), while many studies point to the difficulties faced by professionals and their potential for causing problems of morale and high staff turnover (Squires and Livesley, 1984; DHSS, 1986b). It is believed that one theme of current health service philosophy, the encouragement of decision-making by those who provide care accompanied by the creation of local teams, will lead to easier working relationships, more effective care and less isolation between different types of provider. Members of the team with special skills, such as a patients' placement officer, can be employed to tackle specific issues, while sufficient time for continuing education and staff meetings may do much to help morale (Jones and Golding, 1987).

While the emphasis in the planning team may be on the roles of the three large organisations, in the providing team it is likely to be on the professionals' tasks of enabling individuals, the individuals' carers and the voluntary organisations to achieve their maximum potential. There is unlikely to be any hierarchy of importance attached to the tasks of the professionals and the lay members of the team. Blood pressure checks, the dressing of wounds, transport to a day centre, cleaning the house or friendship, all rate equally in their contribution to improving the quality of life. Although there are many studies showing the need to provide support, relief and respite to immediate carers, there is also evidence of the value of involving elderly people as providers of care with benefit to those who are fit enough to provide care and to those who are recipients (Bowles, 1976).

ACTION

The change-over to community care is, therefore, a fundamental shift, not only in the location of services, but also in the type and range of services provided and in organisational attitudes and skills of staff involved. It thus presents a considerable challenge to management. Any failure to meet the challenge of community care will result in a lower quality service and reduced value for money.

(Audit Commission, 1986)

Many health authorities are now facing up to this challenge and are seeking to improve their care for the elderly in the community. International and national guidelines and targets are available, as are outstanding examples of good practice in different statutory and voluntary organisations throughout the country. It is suggested that what is required primarily is the continuing application of existing techniques and forms of care. However, there needs to be a renewed commitment both to provide and manage those services so that they are responsive to changing community need (the needs derived approach), and to provide a spectrum of care with a shift towards the client and away from the requirements of the provider or the system. While in this review, the importance of the team in the planning and the provision of care has been described, the general practitioner is likely to assume major responsibility for health care along with other members of the primary care team. The White Paper, *Promoting Better Health*, proposes increased remuneration to enable the general practitioner to provide such comprehensive care, and encourages the establishment of multidisciplinary teams in the community (DHSS, 1987).

However, it is also necessary to look to the future and to relate the planning of health care for the elderly to the wider aspects of planning for health in the next century. Advances in diagnosis and care will lead to reduced hospitalisation, less invasive investigation techniques, better quality of life for those with chronic disease, and more people living to a greater age. Public and patients will have higher expectations. New methods of community care, especially in nursing care, linked to flexibility in residential accommodation, are likely to be required. The decisions made now will determine the quality of care provided in the next century.

REFERENCES

Abrams, M. (1985). The health of the very elderly. In *Recent Advances in Geriatric Medicine*, B. Isaacs (Ed.), pp. 217–26. Churchill Livingstone, Edinburgh.

Alderson, M. (1986). An ageing population – Some demographic and health trends. *Public Health*, **100**, 263–77.

Audit Commission (1986). *Making a Reality of Community Care*. The Audit Commission for Local Authorities in England and Wales. HMSO, London.

Backett, E.M. (1980). The needs derived approach. Personal communication.

Bowles, E. (1976). Older persons as providers of services: three federal programs. *Social Policy*, **7**, 81–8.

CACI (1975). *Database Systems: A Practical Reference*. CACI INC-International, London.

CACI (undated). *A Classification of Residential Neighbourhoods*. CACI INC-International Market Analysis Division, London.

Culyer, A.J. (1981). Health and Health Indicators. Proceedings of a European

Workshop. Report to the British Social Sciences Research Council and the European Science Foundation, University of York.

Department of Health and Social Security (DHSS) (1981). *Care in Action: A Handbook of Policies and Priorities for the Health and Personal Social Services in England.* Her Majesty's Stationery Office, London.

DHSS, Scottish Office, Welsh Office and Northern Ireland Office (1981). *Growing Older* (Cmnd 8173). HMSO, London.

DHSS (1986a). *Primary Health Care: An Agenda for Discussion* (Cmnd 9771). HMSO, London.

DHSS (1986b). *Neighbourhood Nursing – A Focus for Care.* Report of the Community Nursing Review. HMSO, London.

DHSS (1987). *Promoting Better Health: The Government's Programme for Improving Primary Health Care.* HMSO, London.

Faculty of Community Medicine (1986). *Charter for Action.* Faculty of Community Medicine, London.

Golding, A.M.B., Hunt, S.M. and McEwen, J. (1986). Health needs in a London district. *Health Policy*, **6**, 175–84.

Health Education Council (1984). *A Programme of Education for Health in Old Age: A Consultative Document.* Health Education Council, London.

Horrocks, P. (1986). The components of a comprehensive district health service for elderly people – a personal view. *Age and Ageing*, **15**, 321–42.

Hunt, A. (1978). *The Elderly at Home.* HMSO, London.

Hunt, S.M., McEwen, J. and McKenna, S. (1986). *Measuring Health Status.* Croom Helm, London.

Isaacs, B., Livingstone, M. and Neville, Y. (1972). *Survival of the Unfittest.* Routledge & Kegan Paul, London.

Jones, M.E.B. and Golding, A.M.B. (1987). Placing long-stay patients. *Public Health*, **101**, 169–71.

La Rue, A., Bank, L., Jarvik, L. and Hetland, M. (1979). Health in old age: how do physicians' ratings and self-ratings compare? *Journal of Gerontology*, **34**, 687–91.

Linn, M.N. (1976). Studies in rating the physical, mental and social dysfunction of the chronically ill aged. *Medical Care*, **14**(5), 19–125.

Lowe, D. and McEwen, J. (1987). ACORN: Perceived Health and the Definition of Health Needs. Unpublished MS, Academic Department of Community Medicine, School of Medicine, King's College, London.

Maddox, G.L. and Douglas, E.B. (1973). Self-assessment of health: a longitudinal study of elderly subjects. *Journal of Health and Social Behaviour*, **14**, 87–93.

Magi, M. and Allander, E. (1981). Towards a theory of perceived and mentally defined needs. *Sociology of Health and Illness*, **3**, 49–71.

O'Neill, P. (1983). *Health Crisis 2000.* Heinemann Medical Books, London.

Palmore, E. and Luikart, C. (1972). Health and social factors related to life satisfaction. *Journal of Health and Social Behaviour*, **13**, 68–73.

Robinson, D. (1971). *The Process of Becoming Ill.* Routledge & Kegan Paul, London.

Royal College of General Practitioners (1981). *Health and Prevention in Primary Care*, Report No. 18. Royal College of General Practitioners, London.

Squires, A. and Livesley, B. (1984). Beware of burnout. *Physiotherapy*, **70**(6), 235–8.

Williams, E.I. (1985). Anticipatory care for the elderly in general practice. In *Recent Advances in Geriatric Medicine 3*, B. Isaacs (Ed.), pp. 255–64. Churchill Livingstone, Edinburgh.

World Health Organization (1983). *The Elderly in Eleven Countries: A Sociomedical Survey*, Public Health in Europe No. 21. WHO, Copenhagen.
World Health Organization (1985). *Targets for Health for All by the Year 2000.* WHO, Regional Office for Europe, Copenhagen.

Cameron Swift

School of Medicine and Dentistry
King's College
University of London

11 HEALTH CARE OF THE ELDERLY: THE CONCEPT OF PROGRESS

INTRODUCTION

In considering the effectiveness or otherwise of any form of health care provision, it is necessary not only to define its objectives, but also to retain an historical perspective – a view of the way things were. The intention of this chapter is to direct the reader's attention to some of the important issues in addressing the questions, 'Has the health care of elderly people (in particular the medicine of old age) progressed in recent years?' and, 'If so, what critical lessons have been learned and what outstanding deficiencies can be readily identified?'. Such a stocktaking view is of great importance, since there are few branches of medical care where theories are embraced and stated with greater emotion and dogmatism and where hard facts are more difficult to come by. There is, nevertheless, historical documentation of some fifty years standing as well as a massive clinical and scientific literature which continues to grow exponentially. The views expressed here are personal and will reflect a bias towards experience in the United Kingdom. This is partly because organisational aspects have, to some extent, been facilitated by the country's particular State system of care.

If the situation is viewed from the point of view of the consumer, it is immediately apparent that there are no grounds for complacency. This most important viewpoint has often in the past been the least vocalised and the last to be perceived. 'The geriatric problem' has been rightly defined as 'the difficulty experienced by older people in obtaining the high standard of medical care they require' (Evans, 1987).

Perhaps the ultimate overall objective is to provide a system of health care which every citizen approaching old age should be able to view with confidence instead of with fear. It is important to recognise, however, that some progress in this respect can be identified over the last half century. Standards have begun to be set, but remain rather patchily represented. Regrettably, the entitlement of older people to such standards has still sometimes to be argued. The phrase 'Cinderella service' is a contradiction in terms, since if a job is worth doing it is worth doing well. Such attitudes are also extremely short-sighted, since they lead to the squandering of resources on second-rate provision, which in turn perpetuates need by its ineffectiveness.

DEFINING THE OBJECTIVES

Progress in medicine rightly originates in scientific advance. This results in new options for investigation or treatment which, when they become accepted practice, are subsequently identified as patient necessities. This process is one of the fundamental problems of the economy of health care provision. Modern health care of the elderly found its origin paradoxically in the sheer volume of patient necessity uncovered in the overcrowded workhouse infirmaries of the 1930s and 1940s. The graphic description provided by Thomson (1947) of the Western Road Infirmary in Birmingham is a well known example cited by Brocklehurst (1985). This hospital contained 1083 patients, of whom 983 were confined to bed and 49 per cent had major incontinence problems. The mean length of stay was of the order of three years. Staffing consisted of six doctors who also had responsibility for 300 further beds and a venereal disease clinic. The average nurse to patient ratio at the time was 1:35, in spite of which only nine pressure sores were found. There were long waiting lists for admission, both in the community and in the related acute hospital, where a substantial proportion of beds were blocked by the waiting process. Ill older patients were accordingly accepted by the acute hospitals with great reluctance.

It was in such a context that the new option of a positive, organised and interventional approach to the management of older patients was pioneered by the originators of modern geriatric medicine, such as Warren, Amulrie, Sheldon, Woodford-Williams and Anderson. By the application of first principles of care in diagnosis, systematic problem identification, judicious medical intervention and the involvement of multidisciplinary teams in management, many older people achieved an excellent response to treatment and were enabled to regain acceptable levels of function and a realistic return to community living. Substantial numbers were also removed from waiting lists.

In consequence, the need for a specifically organised discipline of health care of the elderly, staffed by trained, committed and accountable physicians, was developed and subsequently recognised by the Royal College of Physicians (1977) as a distinct specialist area of medicine. Irrespective of clinical specialisation, it is, however, important to extract certain key principles from the historical perspective, which have been strengthened by subsequent wider experience:

1. Diagnosis in the elderly may present particular problems because of insidious or atypical disease presentation and the existence of concurrent disorders. It is, however, indispensable to proper health care.
2. Assessment of function – physical, mental and social – should *always* occur in parallel with clinical diagnosis and treatment.
3. The above procedures require specialist skills supported by the availability of sophisticated diagnostic and treatment techniques.
4. Organised professional teamwork with linkage to other informal and formal agencies is necessary at all stages.
5. Problem identification and multidisciplinary 'management by objective' are of equal importance to the skills of traditional diagnosis and prescription.
6. The capacity of older people to recover from illness and regain complete or partial functional independence should never be underestimated.
7. The organisation and delivery of care should eliminate delay, minimise personal disruption and achieve continuity of information and professional contact.

If one accepts the importance of these historical lessons, it will be immediately apparent that progress, so far as the elderly are concerned, depends not only on technical sophistication (much of which is of specific benefit to older people), but also on how this, together with the necessary specialist professional skills and other services, is deployed and organised to ensure that the care is delivered in the right way and at the right time. To achieve these objectives in terms of service and to ensure that the accompanying body of knowledge is both taught and researched is the challenge facing modern academic Departments of Health Care of the Elderly. The remainder of this chapter will consider firstly, progress in both the technical and organisational aspects of service provision, and secondly, developments in teaching and research.

SERVICE PROVISION: TECHNICAL ASPECTS

Diagnostic problems

As already implied, diagnosis may present particular difficulties in the elderly. Important interactions exist between normal ageing processes and the manifestation of 'classical' symptoms and signs, which for many conditions significantly alter clinical presentation.

Pain thresholds, for example, have been shown to rise with age (Woodrow *et al.*, 1972), so that the usual symptoms of conditions such as myocardial infarction, appendicitis and even fracture of the femoral neck may be masked (Pathy, 1967). The interpretation of classical physical signs may have to be modified, particularly in neurological disorders (Stern, 1985). The diagnostic boundaries of otherwise reasonably defined clinical syndromes may become blurred (for example, depressive illness) (Post, 1978). There is a marked tendency for ill health to have its initial presentation in the form of functional problems, particularly those of mobility, mentation and micturition, with the associated social sequelae. Precise diagnosis may be further compounded by the co-existence of multiple conditions. A further problem is that of low expectation on the part of older people, their relatives and carers, so that stereotypical disabilities or disorders are readily attributed to old age rather than identified as indicators of medical need. Similar inhibition of diagnostic incentive has adversely affected much decision making by clinicians in the past.

Recognition and documentation of these important areas has now advanced considerably, and the various phenomena are well known to clinicians specialising in the field and increasingly to many others involved with older patients. It is, nevertheless, true that much remediable disease in the elderly continues to be missed in many cases and steps should be taken to heighten the index of suspicion.

The facilities available to reach a diagnosis have also improved greatly. Where relevant, modified ranges of biochemical and other investigational data to take account of advanced age, have been derived and published to give the clinician a better basis for the interpretation of abnormal findings (e.g., Hodkinson, 1985). The enormous progress in non-invasive techniques of organ-imaging has significantly expanded the potential for more accurate and earlier diagnosis available to older patients, where previously the hazards or discomfort of more invasive techniques would have been difficult to justify. In an era of cost-consciousness, considerable skill and judgement are required to ensure that such expensive resources are not used wastefully. While stressing the importance of diagnosis, it is imperative that these tools are judiciously utilised in the context of an overall plan of clinical management for each patient, rather than primarily to satisfy professional curiosity.

An important point is that the most sophisticated and expensive technique does not invariably yield superior evidence to that which can be obtained from longer established and less costly methods. The place of each individual procedure can, of course, only be determined with wide use. Clinicians, radiologists and their colleagues need to collaborate closely to ensure that these resources are well stewarded.

For example, the demonstration of diffuse or multifocal abnormalities in the EEG (electroencephalogram) may often obviate the need for further investigations, such as CT (computerised tomography) scans. Radio-isotope techniques may still be of value in some circumstances; for example, the three-phase dynamic bone scan in predicting the likelihood of avascular necrosis in fracture of the femoral neck. The application of more advanced procedures, such as magnetic resonance imaging will require extensive research evaluation before their true place in clinical practice can be established. In the meantime, techniques which are widely available in most district general hospitals already have a great deal to offer older patients, provided skilled clinical judgement regulates their use. This is one of the reasons why multidisciplinary assessment procedures should be instituted at the outset of acute illness to achieve a clear perspective on the options open to individual patients in terms of likely outcome and quality of life.

Treatment possibilities

There are now many new developments in operative and non-operative interventions and in therapeutics, which have specifically widened the possibilities for treatment open to older people. Well known examples include the removal of gallstones from the biliary tree using endoscopic techniques and the increasing applications of balloon angioplasty for occlusive atheromatous vascular disease in various sites. These procedures are remarkably atraumatic and may be carried out without general anaesthesia. They are particularly applicable in the treatment of certain elderly patients who for various reasons are considered unfit for surgery. Equally, techniques in anaesthesia have greatly improved and age alone (as distinct from medical fitness) is in many cases no contraindication to major surgery, including procedures such as coronary bypass surgery. The literature on pre- and post-operative management of elderly patients is growing and constitutes a fruitful area for collaborative research involving surgeons, physicians with specialist commitment to the elderly, anaesthetists and other professionals. Improved hip replacement techniques, with early weight-bearing regimes, have greatly improved the quality of life of many elderly people with major degenerative hip joint disease.

The principles and practice of drug therapy in the elderly are much better understood and have generated an extensive literature. It is now well known that the mechanisms of drug handling (pharmacokinetics) and response (pharmacodynamics) show changes with advancing age, and that these factors have contributed in the past to the unacceptably high occurrence of iatrogenic morbidity amongst elderly people.

Dosage modifications for a number of drugs are now known to be appropriate because of reduction in the rate of renal glomerular filtration or tubular secretion; examples include digoxin, lithium and the aminoglycoside antibiotics. The rate of oxidative metabolic breakdown of other compounds in the liver microsomes has similarly been shown to be reduced; examples include a number of psychotropic drugs, such as the tricyclic antidepressants. In the case of drug metabolism, however, variability between subjects is greater than with changes in renal elimination (Swift and Triggs, 1987). The rate of clearance of these compounds from the plasma is generally reduced in the elderly; in the past the prescription of standard adult doses therefore resulted in the accumulation of unacceptably high steady-state concentrations, with accompanying side-effects and iatrogenic morbidity.

Other, more subtle, mechanisms may be involved. Some orally administered drugs undergo rapid metabolism within the gut wall or portal circulation before they even reach the systemic blood stream. One example is the compound levodopa used in the treatment of Parkinsonism. This compound is extensively decarboxylated by the enzyme dopa decarboxylase within the stomach before entry into the absorptive areas of the proximal duodenum and small intestine. The incidence of adverse drug reactions when this compound was initially administered to elderly sufferers was extremely high and the compound was said to be unsuitable for use in the elderly. It is now known, however, that a marked reduction in gastric dopa decarboxylase activity occurs with advancing age, so that in older patients, approximately three times the amount of unchanged levodopa per administered dose is absorbed into the circulation than in younger recipients (Evans *et al.*, 1980). The correspondingly high levels of circulating levodopa clearly accounted for most, if not all, of the unexpected toxicity in older recipients.

For other drugs it has been found that the sensitivity of the target organ or system is greater in the elderly. The best known examples include warfarin and the benzodiazepines (Shepherd *et al.*, 1979; Swift, 1986). Corresponding adjustments in dosage for the elderly with both of these compounds are known to be necessary in order to avoid significant adverse effects.

There is thus, in general, a much better body of information to enable clinicians to individualise and tailor drug therapy more closely to the needs of individual older patients. There is also a greater awareness of the scale of the problem, of the risks of unreviewed repeat prescribing and of the extent to which problems of drug compliance increase with the number of drugs prescribed and the complexity of the dosage schedule. Methods have been introduced to enable clinicians to be more readily aware of drug interaction risks, notably computer-based systems (Gosney and Tallis, 1984). There are grounds for optimism that the excessive amount of prescribing and iatrogenic morbidity amongst the elderly may be decreasing, but far too many problems are still encountered. Therapeutics in old age remains a major challenge to undergraduate and postgraduate medical education, to the involvement of other professional workers, and to public education in general.

In relation to new drugs, the UK Committee on Safety of Medicines requires specific data sheet recommendations for use in the elderly where this is at all clinically relevant. Such recommendations are required to be based on sound factual evidence, usually clinical trials and/or experimental data. This undoubtedly constitutes an important safeguard for the elderly, but there is a risk that additional prolongation of the pre-marketing process may lead to correspondingly aggressive marketing techniques after the granting of a product licence, with resulting pressures to over prescribe.

Disease prevention
This important, but conceptually very difficult, aspect of health care of the elderly is technically at a very early stage. Issues concerning health promotion are further considered in Chapter 10. Definition of objectives is particularly important in considering this topic, and there is now probably a consensus that we aim for the prevention of avoidable morbidity in old age, rather than set explicit goals for longevity.

There is evidence that the combined effects of social and medical advances (including advances in geriatric medicine) have joined to produce a 'rectangularisation' of survival curves, postponing the effects and onset of disabling disease to a later age (Fries, 1980), although the extent to which this has taken place with some conditions, particularly arthritis and dementia, is strongly questioned (Schneider and Brody, 1983). Data of this kind also emphasise the difficulties of measurement involved (a topic also addressed in Chapters 5 and 10).

This epidemiological phenomenon clearly cannot be attributed in a simple way to defined preventative initiatives. *Primary* prevention of pathology may entail anything from genetic engineering to the economics of the tobacco industry, and at present it is difficult to identify defined targets for such initiatives amongst the elderly population. *Secondary* prevention (the early detection of disease or its precursors in asymptomatic individuals) also presents many conceptual, logistic and economic problems as far as the elderly are concerned. The best efforts so far have been rightly directed at the problem of non-reporting of early established health problems by means of case-finding, which has been described as a form of *tertiary* prevention (Williamson, 1981). Even at this level, the methodological difficulties of defining those at risk have been well illustrated (Taylor *et al.*, 1983).

Benefits from such initatives have consisted mainly of detecting and addressing a number of unmet care delivery needs (mainly contact with available services and active health symptoms requiring treatment). To what extent the need for acute interventions, including hospital admission, may be prevented as distinct from postponed is still in need of demonstration.

There are also potential pitfalls, in that the importance of technical sophistication in the diagnosis of ill health in the elderly is readily underestimated, and delay in access to such facilities might have a negative rather than a positive effect. Perhaps the most tangible example of prevention to date has been the reduction in long-term institutional morbidity achieved by those specialist medical services for the elderly which have eliminated waiting lists, delays in treatment and problems of access to mainstream medical attention. This topic will be considered further in the next section.

If unjustified morbidity amongst elderly people results from fundamental deficiencies in the availability to them of known forms of investigation, treatment and clinical management, then it is fallacious to try to compensate for such uncorrected deficiencies under a euphemistic label of 'prevention'. This is in no way to detract from the importance of new approaches to prevention and primary health care. The latter are clearly vital areas for collaborative research.

SERVICE PROVISION: ORGANISATIONAL ASPECTS

It is perhaps in relation to the delivery of medical care that progress over the last 30–50 years in the United Kingdom can be most clearly identified. Indeed, the potential to identify population needs and to organise services for the elderly in an equitable, efficient and economical way may prove to have been one of the most important achievements of the National Health Service. Such progress has regrettably been patchy, and there are major challenges ahead in catering for the needs of different types of population, particularly those in rural areas. Nevertheless, the value of *specialist departments* based centrally in District General Hospitals and staffed by physicians and professional co-workers with specific accountability for the care of older patients, has been set out in several published studies (Bagnall *et al.*, 1977; Evans, 1983; Hodkinson and Jeffreys, 1972; Horrocks, 1986; Mitchell *et al.*, 1987; Rai *et al.*, 1985).

The *outcome measures* needed to assess the impact of such services on elderly people are, as yet, crude (see Chapter 10), and consist mainly of an analysis of hospital activity. There is a strong need for improved 'performance indicators' which are able to chart benefits for patients and their relatives longitudinally over periods of time. In comparison with the 'workhouse infirmary' phenomenon of earlier years, there is no doubt, however, that the available data from reported studies paint a picture of measurable progress. Total numbers of hospital beds per head of elderly population have been dramatically reduced, waiting lists and bed blockage abolished, the through-put of patients greatly increased (typically 12 or more patients per bed per year, some 10–15 per cent only of beds at any one time being occupied by patients staying in hospital more then 6 months), and overall average durations of stay reduced to 20–30 days. These departments have usually been characterised by a clearly defined role in the acute medical care of the elderly (e.g., responsibility for those aged over 75 years), by efficient liaison with the community and with other hospital services, and by effective policies of rehabilitation and discharge, with well-developed multidisciplinary teamwork. Thus, problems of access to hospital treatment without delay have been removed, together with the fears of many patients about hospitalisation. Relatives and other carers retain an involvement, sustained by organised support and the knowledge that rescue in a crisis or planned relief are available without delay. In an important way, the hospital/community interface is bridged by communication and access. Paradoxically, such ostensibly hospital-based approaches, by virtue of their accessibility, have made the reality of community care a genuine prospect, providing a foundation for the definition of quality indices and a starting point for preventive initiatives. There is a strong sense of teamwork, involving general practitioners, district nurses, informal carers and other community-based agencies. Respite admissions and day hospital activity feature prominently. In addition, recruitment and morale present no problems, and the scope for training and research is obvious.

Such services have also provided an operational focus to reverse the *fragmentation* of care. Fragmentation is a fundamental problem in health care of the elderly, because of the multiple and recurring problems which have to be addressed by several agencies. Left to a system-specialised medical service, disjointed community support and the absence of planned co-ordination, the overall system of care can easily break down completely. One of the major challenges facing community and primary health care initiatives for the elderly is to determine how such defragmentation can be effectively achieved with reasonable economy, whilst retaining a proper partnership with hospital-based services.

Delay has also been a besetting problem for elderly people in the past. It is probably wise to err towards the assumption that all presenting problems of significance in elderly people are urgent, especially if there is any unexplained decline in function. To reflect again on the historical situation, illness in elderly people is prone to be characterised by delay in presentation, delay in recognition of a problem, delay in referral and specialist assessment and delay in intervention and organised management. In the context of medical illness, delay at any point is almost invariably deleterious. Waiting lists are usually symptoms of a deficient service. Even in the case of elective surgical procedures, such as hip replacements or cataract removal, it is generally possible on clinical criteria to define an optimum time for surgery, beyond which further postponement is harmful.

The impact made by modern departments and services, such as those cited above, on long-term institutional morbidity has defined a new set of standards, against which all future patterns of care must be measured, even if alternative models are adopted. The activities of planners must take into account not only the identification of existing population need (see Chapter 10), but also the demonstrable efficiency or otherwise of established systems of care.

A final point relates to the question of *accountability*. The longstanding discussion about whether we should have 'geriatricians or physicians with an interest' will not be addressed here. However the workload is divided, those undertaking it must be seen to be clearly accountable for ensuring that future standards more than match the achievements of the past. It is insufficient simply to say, 'We are all geriatricians now', without also accepting responsibility for the overall outcome of services for the elderly measured by objective criteria.

The foregoing discussion emphasises that progress in health care of the elderly, to a greater extent than many other branches of medicine, depends not only on the development of new techniques, but on defined and effective strategies to ensure that these are made available to patients in the correct proportion, in the right way, in the proper context and, above all, at the right time.

EDUCATION IN HEALTH CARE OF THE ELDERLY

Progress in any valid discipline of medicine requires not only evidence of benefit to patients, but also a defined theoretical content to provide the basis for continued education and training. There is now a fully classified literature on the medicine of old age, and the establishment of academic Departments of Health Care of the Elderly or Geriatric Medicine in all the major UK medical schools, either autonomously or within academic Departments of Medicine, has enabled considerable strides to be made in the education of undergraduate medical students. Progress has also occurred to a varying extent in medical schools in the United States, Canada, Australasia and Europe.

A degree of worldwide consensus on the training content of Health Care of the Elderly is reflected in the learning objectives of the World Health Organization (WHO, 1982). However, it is evident that a sound clinical service base is indispensable if the main areas of concern are to be successfully covered.

There has been expansion in the postgraduate education of clinicians. The Royal College of Physicians and the General Medical Council have both recognised the importance of specific exposure to the Medicine of Old Age as part of general professional training programmes for intending specialists in internal medicine, so that rotational appointments between both specialities at preregistration house physician, senior house officer and registrar level are well developed features of progressive medical schools and district general hospitals. Academic departments have an important role to play in the further development of such trainee rotations. Senior house officer posts in Health Care of the Elderly also form a common component of vocational training programmes for general practice. The recently inaugurated Diploma in Geriatric Medicine of the Royal College of Physicians, primarily a Diploma for general practitioners, has been heavily subscribed and is established as a successful, registrable higher qualification.

Higher medical training for specialists in Health Care of the Elderly is monitored closely by the Standing Advisory Committee in Geriatric Medicine of the Joint Committee on Higher Medical Training of the Royal College of Physicians. Senior registrar and registrar appointments, a number of which are rotational with General Internal Medicine, aim to provide all the necessary training requirements for whole-time specialists in Health Care of the Elderly, and for general physicians with special responsibility in the field. The value of participation in such rotations for physicians specialising in other branches of medicine has been widely recognised.

Professions allied to medicine have also become committed to ensuring adequate experience in health care of the elderly in both pre- and post-qualification training. True specialisms have probably developed in most disciplines, including nursing, physiotherapy, occupational therapy, clinical psychology and social work, though the extent to which these are given formal structures varies.

The need to draw together in a more formal way the academic activities and expertise of the many professions involved in health care of the elderly and to achieve multidisciplinarianism in both teaching and research has never been more urgent. The Age Concern Institute of Gerontology at King's College, with a truly multifaculty university institution (incorporating the School of Medicine and Dentistry) as its base, constitutes a unique opportunity to move the subject forward. The planned Masters' Course in Gerontology gives structured expression to this concept and will, it is hoped, through its various options, equip gerontologists of academic standing to contribute more effectively along with professional colleagues in their chosen areas of practice.

Perhaps the greatest challenge ahead lies in the need for wide public education to alter traditional attitudes and prejudices, to make expectation more informed and positive, and to encourage the widest possible community involvement. To date, most progress in this area has been substantially due to the committed work of voluntary organisations, in particular Age Concern, whose active community services have given strong credence to a growing effectiveness in political influence, a substantial output of consumer orientated information and a major and still expanding involvement in research. Long-held attitudes change slowly. Nevertheless, it would be short-sighted of any profession committed to this field to expect anything other than a much more informed public, aware of the rights of older people as well as their vulnerability, 20 years from now.

Returning to the education of professionals, it is still true that far too many 'discover' the rewards and fascination of this field of health care by accident, often having to run the gauntlet of negative reactions from their teachers and peers. Once involved, the compelling challenge of the discipline commonly makes its workers totally unwilling to countenance any other option. It is the job of education to swell the growing tide of those coming into health care of the elderly as a matter of first choice.

RESEARCH ISSUES

There is almost limitless scope for research into the phenomena of human old age, quite apart from wider biological investigation into ageing processes in other organisms. This is reflected in the massive growth in the literature on human gerontology over the last two decades in particular. It is, however, important to scrutinise the output critically at some stage in order to define the contribution which has been made to progress in health care of the elderly.

Perhaps the biggest dangers confronting the field are those of sterile empiricism and inappropriate compartmentalisation. In a time of financial stringency, it is important to formulate hypotheses, carry out reliable observations and evaluate interventions that may be seen to carry some realistic prospect of benefit for older people. Equally, error and fallacy both in observation and inference may well take place if the necessary range of skills is not applied to a given problem. For example, an investigation of falls in the elderly in the community might properly involve not only clinicians, but epidemiologists, gait physiologists, social scientists with particular expertise in housing, pharmacologists and biochemists. In order words, the best research in health care of the elderly would commonly be both experimental in outlook and collaborative in execution. A potential hazard of the current 'market economy' approach to research is the discouragement of collaboration between departments, each concerned for its own economic survival.

Some of the suggested key areas for further investigation in Health Care of the Elderly are outlined below.

1. *Applied general medicine of old age* This includes the continued study of altered disease presentation, the effectiveness of treatment in relation to the modified clinical objectives of old age medicine, the study of disorders of high prevalence in the elderly, the study of interacting disorders (e.g., depressive illness and Parkinsonism), the evaluation of therapeutic agents in clinical trials or of therapeutic monitoring, the study of iatrogenic disease, and factors influencing the outcome.
2. *Clinical gerontology* Including, for example, reference ranges in diagnosis, and controlled studies of the pharmacokinetics and pharmacodynamics of drugs and of basic pharmacological mechanisms in ageing man.
3. *Special clinical problems of the elderly* For example disorders presenting with postural imbalance, confusional states, problems of continence and disorders of mobility.
4. *Assessment disciplines* The study of general and specific measures of function, of psychological, social and environmental factors in disease states, the ascertainment of at risk groups in preventive medicine.
5. *Practical management* The study of therapeutic regimens, rehabilitation procedures and corporate decision making.
6. *Service structure and resources* The measurement of need and the evaluation of different forms of service provision.
7. *Basic human gerontology* Biological, psychological, social and demographic.

There is now a sufficient knowledge-base in most of these areas, together with many others unmentioned, to enable some form of structured research planning to take place. The usefulness and quality of further research in the field will almost certainly depend on the extent to which interdisciplinary linkage can be made to work towards objectives agreed and held in common.

REFERENCES

Age Concern Research Unit (1983). *The Elderly at Risk*, Research Perspectives on Ageing, 6. Age Concern, Mitcham, Surrey.

Bagnall, W.E., Datta, S.R., Knox, J. and Horrocks, P. (1977). Geriatric medicine in Hull: a comprehensive service. *British Medical Journal*, **2**, 102–4.

Brocklehurst, J.C. (1985). The geriatric service and the day hospital. In *Textbook of Geriatric Medicine and Gerontology*, 3rd edition, J.C. Brocklehurst (Ed.), pp. 982–95. Churchill Livingstone, Edinburgh.

Evans, J.G. (1983). Integration of geriatric with general medical services in Newcastle. *The Lancet*, **(i)**, 1430–3.

Evans, J.G. (1987). Personal communication.

Evans, M.A., Triggs, R.J., Broe, J.A. and Saines, N. (1980). Systemic availability of orally administered L-Dopa in the elderly Parkinsonian patient. *European Journal of Clinical Pharmacology*, **17**, 215–21.

Fries, J.F. (1980). Aging, natural death and the compression of morbidity. *New England Journal of Medicine*, **303**, 130–4.

Gosney, M. and Tallis, R.C. (1984). Prescription of contraindicated and interacting drugs in elderly patients admitted to hospital. *The Lancet*, **2**, 564–7.

Hodkinson, H.M. (1985). Interpretation of biochemical data. In *Principles and Practice of Geriatric Medicine*, M.S.J. Pathy (Ed.). John Wiley & Sons, Chichester.

Hodkinson, H.M. and Jeffreys, P.M. (1972). Making hospital geriatrics work. *British Medical Journal*, **4**, 536–9.

Horrocks, P. (1986). The components of a comprehensive district health service for elderly people: a personal view. *Age and Ageing*, **15**, 321–42.

Mitchell, J., Kafety, K. and Rossiter, B. (1987). Benefits of effective hospital services for elderly people. *British Medical Journal*, **295**, 980–3.

Pathy, M.S. (1967). Clinical presentation of myocardial infarction in the elderly. *British Heart Journal*, **29**, 190–9.

Post, F. (1978). The functional psychoses. In *Studies in Geriatric Psychiatry*, A.D. Isaacs and F. Post (Eds). John Wiley & Sons, New York.

Rai, G.S., Murphy, P. and Pluck, R.A. (1985). Who should provide hospital care of elderly people? *The Lancet*, **(i)**, 683–5.

Royal College of Physicians (1977). *Working Party Report on Care of the Elderly*. Royal College of Physicians, London.

Schneider, E.L. and Brody, J.A. (1983). Ageing, natural death and the comparison of morbidity: another view. *New England Journal of Medicine*, **309** 854–5.

Shepherd, A.M.M., Hewick, D.S., Moreland, T.A. and Stevenson, I.H. (1979). Age as a determinant of sensitivity to warfarin. *British Journal of Clinical Pharmacology*, **4**, 315–20.

Sterm, G. (1985). Normals of neurology in old age. In *Neurological Problems in the Elderly*, M. Hildick-Smith (Ed.), pp. 1–6. Bailliere Tindall, Eastbourne.

Swift, C.G. (1986). Benzodiazepine pharmacodynamics in the elderly. In *Clinical Pharmacology and Therapeutics in the Elderly*, K. O'Malley and J. Waddington (Eds). Elsevier, Amsterdam.

Swift, C.G. and Triggs, E.J. (1987). Clinical pharmacokinetics in the elderly. In *Clinical Pharmacology in the Elderly*, C.G. Swift (Ed.), pp. 31–82. Marcel Dekker, New York.

Taylor, R., Ford, G. and Barber, H. (1983). *The Elderly at Risk: A Critical Review of Problems and Progress in Screening and Case Finding.* Research Perspectives on Ageing, No. 6. Age Concern England, Mitcham, Surrey.

Thomson, A.P. (1947). Problems of ageing and chronic sickness. *British Medical Journal*, **(ii)**, 243–50, 300–5.

Williamson, J. (1981). Screening, surveillance and case-finding. In *Health Care of the Elderly*, T. Arie (Ed.). Croom Helm, London.

Woodrow, K.M., Friedman, G.D., Siegchant, A. and Cohen, M.F. (1972). Pain tolerance: differences according to age, sex and race. *Psychosomatic Medicine*, **34**, 548–56.

World Health Organization (1982). *Teaching Gerontology and Geriatric Medicine.* Report on a Workshop, Edinburgh, 5–7 April, Publication ICP/ADR 045(2), WHO, Copenhagen.

Sally Redfern*

Department of Nursing Studies
King's College
London

12 KEY ISSUES IN NURSING ELDERLY PEOPLE

The choice of 'key issues' focuses on those aspects of nursing which are related to the quality of care, and on nurses' interpersonal communication skills with elderly patients. In pursuing these topics, the chapter will examine the organisation of nursing care of old people, the reasons why nurses choose not to work with old people, and the difficulties nurses have in communicating effectively with patients.

On the organisation of nursing care, the emphasis is on that research carried out in geriatric wards which shows that old people have not achieved the quality of life we would wish for ourselves. The argument for a move to nurse-managed units outside the hospital environment for old people who require continuing nursing care, is made with the proviso that the nurses in charge give priority to enabling their clients to achieve self-determination and autonomy. This requires a new kind of nurse, one who sees the curing emphasis of acute medicine as inappropriate to the continuing care of long-stay patients. Unfortunately, the unpopularity of geriatric nursing means that it is rarely a first career choice.

Nurses have tremendous difficulties in communicating effectively with their patients, particularly if they have not received training in interpersonal skills. Some of the research which highlights these difficulties and emphasises the need for appropriate training will be assessed. The chapter ends with a summary of a study, being undertaken with Andrée Le May, which focuses on nurse–patient communication through touch. Although still in progress, the findings reveal shortcomings in nurses' interaction with patients, and underline the need for training in interpersonal communication skills.

THE ORGANISATION OF NURSING CARE OF THE ELDERLY

The organisation of geriatric nursing is inextricably linked to that of geriatric medicine. Nursing has followed the lead of geriatric medicine, and accords higher status to the high turnover acute geriatric service than to long-stay continuing care which many old people require. As with acute medical nursing, geriatric nursing supports the energetic 'diagnosis-treatment-cure-discharge' approach of medicine, and so accords low priority to the continuing care needs of the long-stay patient. The published research on the organisation

I am indebted to my co-worker in the touch study, Andrée Le May, who is funded by a Department of Health and Social Security Nursing Research Studentship. We are grateful to the nursing and medical management of the hospitals and nursing home for allowing us access, and to the elderly people and the nurses who participated in the study.

of nursing care in geriatric wards presents a dismal picture. Three studies carried out in the 1970s revealed similar findings (Clarke, 1978; Wells, 1980; Baker, 1983). Although nurses in geriatric wards often had positive attitudes towards old people, they tended both to be patronising and to put higher priority on getting tasks completed than on planning individualised care to meet the needs of each elderly person. Nursing care followed a 'routine geriatric' style (Baker, 1983), and was organised to suit the ward routine of mealtimes, medicine rounds, doctors' rounds, toileting or changing wet pads, getting up and going to bed. Little was done for the patients outside these physical tasks, and the demeaning characteristics of institutions predominated, such as rigid lines of authority, batch processing, lack of privacy, and submissive patients lacking dignity, choice and a sense of purpose.

More recent research is no more encouraging. Evers (1981a; 1981b) found that care in geriatric wards continued to follow a 'warehousing' or batch processing approach, particularly for long-stay patients. The 'acute-career' patient, who responded to active medical and rehabilitative intervention, was seen as a success, but not so the patient who failed to respond so promptly to conventional cure objectives. The priority needs of the long-stay patient are no longer medical ones. Important to these old people is the retention of as much independence as possible, and engagement in purposeful activity which ensures self-esteem and a reasonable quality of life. The geriatrician retains control of long-stay patients, but normally accords them low priority because they do not respond to medical treatment. It is left to nurses to take charge by default. They too fail to meet the psychosocial needs of these old people: their commitment to the primacy of cure work over care work makes them as ill-equipped as geriatricians to enhance elderly people's quality of life.

With a few notable exceptions, for example, the Nursing Development Unit at Burford Cottage Hospital near Oxford, nurses working in geriatric wards tend to accept both the role of doctor's assistant and the medical emphasis on cure work. The nurse is unlikely to have had the training or the experience to modify nursing objectives for long-stay patients, for whom psychosocial needs at least match physical needs. The routinised, task-orientated, traditional approach to nursing has not been compatible with the development of an effective and mutually satisfying relationship between nurse and patient. Introducing planned individualised nursing care is likely to improve this relationship and enhance patient well-being. Unfortunately, efforts by nurses to introduce change in the organisation of nursing have met with resistance from the medical profession (Bolt, 1983; Mitchell, 1984). Many doctors deny the need for change and have challenged nurses to produce evidence for the effectiveness of the 'nursing process'.

In the case of elderly people, however, this evidence does exist for patients who have been in geriatric wards for more than one month (Miller, 1984; 1985a; 1985b). Audrey Miller showed clearly that, for these patients, being nursed in traditional task-orientated wards was positively unhealthy. Though not the case for short-stay elderly patients, the longer stay patients in traditional wards were more dependent, and had higher levels of urinary and faecal incontinence than those nursed in wards in which care was individually planned for each patient. Discharge rates were lower and death rates were higher in the traditional wards. The style of nursing in the traditional wards was highly routinised and put priority on getting through the work. Speed and convenience took precedence over individual needs. This meant that nurses discouraged slow self-care, spoon-feeding slow eaters was not unusual, and catheters were the solution to urinary incontinence. Miller's research shows that the organisation of nursing in traditional geriatric wards has changed little from that found in the earlier research of May Clarke (1978), Thelma Wells (1980), Dorothy Baker (1983) and Helen Evers (1981a; 1981b).

In marked contrast the style of nursing in Miller's individualised care wards followed a more supportive-educative approach, which encouraged self-care and the promotion of independence. Nurses in these wards spent more time talking with the patients, although the amount of physical nursing given was not significantly different from that in the traditional wards.

It is encouraging that sufficient change has occurred in the nursing care of old people in some hospitals to enable Miller to find a few geriatric wards which met her criteria for individualised care. These were the existence of: written care plans; continuity and coordination of care; accountability for care; and an absence of fragmented care. Other examples exist where nurses have taken the lead to provide an environment which is less clinical and more homely (Storrs, 1982; Pearson, 1983). Pearson's initiatives at Burford Cottage Hospital have led to the establishment of nurse-controlled beds; the care is individualised, planned and evaluated, and the nurses receive continuing education and support in introducing change.

These developments are exciting, and show the challenge and scope for change which nurses can initiate. However, it takes a unique mix of determination, hope, resources and leadership skills for nurses to succeed in achieving change within the complex bureaucracy of a large hospital. In defence of those nurses who do attempt to improve patient care, the resources required to achieve even minimum care may not be available. So often nurses make the best of inadequate facilities and keep quiet, rather than publicising examples of poor standards of care. Nurses should be encouraged to exercise their professional responsibility and to record instances when they have to let patients down. They should voice their concerns loudly and publicly about failing the patients, rather than respond with a defensive silence.

A change to nurse managed units?

It is an anomaly that there are so few nursing homes for the elderly within the National Health Service (NHS). Frail elderly people who require continuing nursing care are faced with the choice of living in long-stay geriatric wards or finding the fees for a place in a nursing home in the private sector. Local authority residential homes also look after these old people but without the necessary nursing skills and resources (Wade *et al.*, 1983; Wilkin *et al.*, 1985). Scandalous conditions in some residential homes continue to be reported in the nursing press (Community Outlook, 1987) and the national press (Smith, 1986).

The case for nurse-managed NHS nursing homes has its advocates amongst nurses (Wade *et al.*, 1983) and some doctors (Batchelor, 1984), but there are medical and social work staff who are resistant to the idea (Dalley, 1983). Social workers fear that care will be run on sick-role lines removed from their control, and doctors perceive an erosion of medical control.

In England, although a few state nursing homes exist, initiatives by the Department of Health and Social Security (DHSS) have been taken only since its own sponsored study was completed (Wade *et al.*, 1983). This documented the provision of care of old people in long-stay geriatric wards, residential homes and private nursing homes. They concluded that the hospital environment is inappropriate for meeting the needs of old people requiring continuing care, and that local authority residential homes do not have the resources necessary to meet the nursing needs of their dependent residents. The authors recommended the phasing out of long-stay geriatric beds except for a few for 'holiday admissions' to give caring families a rest, and for short-stay admissions for medical and psychogeriatric assessment and treatment. Alternative provision should be provided in state nursing homes in which nursing care is organised along 'supportive model' lines, as distinct from 'protective', 'controlled' or 'restrained' models.

Evidence of each of these models was found in all kinds of setting in the Wade study; that is, in long-stay wards, residential homes and private nursing homes. The supportive model maximises residents' physical and psychological independence and favours individual choice, participation and self-determination. Barriers between the institution and the wider community do not exist. Relatives, volunteers and the children of staff are encouraged to be involved in everyday activities and to take the old people out shopping or on other trips. The residents contribute to the running of the home/ward by arranging outings and participating in decision making through their membership of residents' committees. The protective, controlled and restrained models are characterised by varying degrees of control, absence of choice and subordination to the care regime.

The highly acclaimed system of nursing home care in Denmark (Millard, 1983) took a lead in prompting the DHSS to continue to search for a 'best buy' by sponsoring a second major piece of research. This is being carried out by John Bond and his team at The Health Care Research Unit, University of Newcastle (Bond, 1984; Atkinson et al., 1986). Three NHS nursing homes have been set up in different parts of England, and they cater for the same kind of old person normally found in long-stay geriatric wards. The Bond research describes the dependency characteristics and provision and cost of care in the NHS nursing homes in comparison with conventional institutional settings for elderly people (acute medical and geriatric wards, residential homes and private nursing homes). The findings on the dependency characteristics confirm earlier research that all settings contain severely disabled old people (Wilkin et al., 1978; Wade et al., 1983), although the highest concentrations are found in geriatric wards and the NHS nursing homes (Atkinson et al., 1986).

We must wait for further publications from the Newcastle study to see, for example, whether the provision of care in the NHS nursing homes, which are headed by specially selected and trained nurses, follows more closely the supportive model of care advocated by the Wade study, or whether residents' dependency is related to the style of care. Miller (1985b) found that in a geriatric ward which changed from the traditional task-orientation to individualised care, patient dependency decreased even though factors such as medical policy, admissions and staffing levels remained much the same.

More work, however, is necessary in order to confirm a positive relationship between individualised care and residents' independence. Booth's (1985; 1986) study in residential homes for old people tests the 'induced dependency hypothesis', that homes run along institutionalised lines which deny residents control over their lives, tend to foster dependence amongst residents. A large number of homes (175) were categorised by cluster analysis according to their management style. Those with a *positive* style allowed residents freedom of choice and action and showed a positive approach to residents' abilities. Those homes with a *restrictive* style limited residents' freedom of choice and action, and took a restrictive view of their capabilities. Most of the homes fell between these two extremes and adopted a *mixed* style of management in that freedom of choice and action occurred in some daily living activities but restrictions and controls occurred in others.

No relationship was found between management style and level of dependency of the residents (measured by level of self-care, continence, social integration, orientation and mental state). This was the case even when the very positive homes were compared with the very restrictive. Booth had to conclude that there was no evidence to support the induced dependency hypothesis. Homes which prevented old people from having choice and control over their lives did not increase their levels of dependency. It may be that no support for the hypothesis emerged because the management regimes in all the homes were relatively similar. Even though the regimes were clearly distinguishable in a statistical sense, the differences between the homes in real terms might have been minimal in that, as Booth (1985) himself suggests, the differences may have been insufficient to affect the residents. It would be interesting to test the same hypothesis in nursing homes and long-stay geriatric wards.

Even if no reduction in dependency can be claimed in those homes which are organised along non-restricted lines, it is likely that the quality of residents' lives will be maximised in institutions with positive and individualised styles of care. In their review of the literature, Woods and Britton (1985) argue that, although an ideal institution may be unachievable because it is a contradiction in terms, there are identifiable features which will enhance quality of life. For example, essential staff attitudes are those which allow residents individuality as adults, dignity, self-respect, choice and independence (or dependence for those who wish it). The ideal institution would therefore allow residents privacy, would have the minimum of rules and regulations, would be rich in facilities and resources, and would have open access to the world outside. As in the Wade *et al.* (1983) 'supportive' model, the features characteristic of institutionalisation would be avoided, such as depersonalisation, block treatment, unvaried daily routine and social distance between staff and residents (King and Raynes, 1968).

Of course, residents may want some degree of social distance in that they may dislike intrusion by staff in their lives. It is important, as Woods and Britton (1985) make clear, that residents can manipulate their social distances and can interact closely with selected staff when they wish. Given the necessary status in a flexible and individual-centred environment, elderly residents will have the power to choose the kind of life they value. Staff will strive to achieve congruence between individual residents' needs and environmental constraints, and will aim for a variety of lifestyles which are close to those normally valued by society. Thus activities will be available but not imposed on residents, and they will be encouraged to continue those they enjoyed when younger.

Neither introducing nor maintaining change is easy to achieve, and so often activities newly introduced and apparently welcomed are abandoned when the initiator leaves (McCormack and Whitehead, 1981; Woods and Britton, 1985). In complex institutions such as hospitals, conflict and lack of communication between the numerous relevant groups may be common, as between nurses of different grade and shift, or between nurses and therapy staff (Woods and Britton, 1985). Georgiades and Phillimore (1975) predicted the likely failure of the 'hero-innovator' to achieve change. Their recipe for successful and enduring change consists of working with those forces in the institution which are most amenable to change, identifying a team of workers who can support and motivate each other, and concentrating on staff who have a certain amount of freedom and discretion in decision making. Having control over resources, obtaining permission to intervene from senior management, and instigating regular group meetings for mutual encouragement and support of those co-operating in the change, are also essential.

These factors contributed to the successful change made by Storrs and her colleagues when given the challenge of transferring 40 elderly women from two traditional long-stay wards to a renovated nursing home standing in its own grounds (Storrs, 1982). At the hospital the patients were extremely dependent, most were incontinent of urine and some were permanently confused. The care was organised along 'routine geriatric' lines; mealtimes were fixed, the food was dull and there was no choice. Daytime communal clothes were worn and most of the women did not wear knickers because of frequent incontinence. Although activities were encouraged, most of the patients spent their time sitting by their beds, passively watching activities or dozing. They went to bed before 7 p.m. and took night sedation in order to sleep well. Most could not sustain a conversation for more than a few minutes, and they could not summon the energy to take part in outings arranged by the staff.

The move to the nursing home gave these elderly women a very different environment. A homely atmosphere was developed with very few regulations. Residents were encouraged to bring their own furniture and possessions and to make their own decisions about mealtimes, bathing and dressing. Pensions were paid directly to them to be spent as they wished. Physical care was fitted in around their social activities, the reverse of the custom before. Storrs did not systematically evaluate the effects of the move, but she recorded some observations. Most of the residents showed a remarkable change in behaviour. They started to take part in activities and to go out; they became more alert and interested in conversation, more physically independent, and incontinence decreased markedly. The project showed that, given the commitment and motivation of enthusiastic staff, it is possible to change the behaviour of old people even after a long period of institutionalisation which enforces 'learned helplessness' (Seligman, 1975).

There is much support for the notion that old people who require continuing nursing care should not have to live out their lives in long-stay geriatric wards. Their quality of life is likely to be higher in homely nurse-managed units, as long as the nurse in charge has shed her or his medical cloak and is able to promote the psychosocial as well as the physical well-being of the residents.

PATIENT POPULARITY

The extensive research on nurses' attitudes towards different categories of patient has been comprehensively and critically reviewed by Kelly and May (1982). Their review demonstrates how often elderly patients are perceived by nurses as unpopular because of features related to certain clinical conditions, behaviours, social factors and attitudes of the patients. Nurses tend, for example, to show positive attitudes towards patients who make a dramatic recovery, or who have conditions requiring specific nursing skills or techniques. These skills are those closely related to acute medical specialties such as surgery and intensive care. The communication skills required in effective interpersonal interaction tend not to be recognised as belonging to this range of principally physical nursing skills.

Nurses' attitudes have been described as negative towards patients whose clinical condition is long-term and largely unresponsive to acute medical treatment, such as mutilation, incontinence, confusion, mental disturbance and terminal illness (Kelly and May, 1982; Ingham and Fielding, 1985). These problems are common among elderly patients, and may be present in combination. It is the 'acute-career' elderly patient who responds to the diagnosis-treatment-cure-discharge goals of acute medicine and who elicits favourable attitudes from medical and nursing staff (Evers, 1981b).

Some of the patient behaviours which are said to evoke negative attitudes in nurses are nonconformism, stubbornness, unpleasantness, anger, aggression, complaining, unco-operativeness, refusal to accept the dependent sick role or over-dependence (Kelly and May, 1982). It seems to be the case that nurses will have negative attitudes if the patient's demonstrated dependency is at odds with the level perceived by nurses. Those patients who convey positive attitudes are described in favourable terms by nurses. These patients are seen as understanding, amusing, optimistic, cheerful and grateful – attitudes which are more likely to exist in acute, short-term patients with curable disease. Patient attitudes which elicit negative attitudes among nurses are likely to be much more common for old people with multiple problems and communication difficulties.

Fielding's (1986) research on the attitudes of student nurses towards elderly patients confirms some of these findings. Although students showed favourable attitudes towards many of the elderly patients in geriatric and medical wards, a substantial number of patients were deemed unpopular by the students. Popularity depended on patients being pleasant, sociable, friendly, cheerful, conforming to the care regime and 'trying hard'. Unpopular patients were those who grumbled, who had communication difficulties, or who were regarded as unpleasant or inconsiderate. Often these were stroke patients in medical wards who were labelled by the nurses as 'geriatric' and untreatable, whereas similar problems in younger patients were deemed pathological and remediable. Fielding's research shows clearly a relationship between perceived patient popularity and student nurses' interpersonal communication difficulties. The students responded positively to patients who could communicate easily. They had difficulties with patients who were confused or who had a limited conversational repertoire. The students' objectives during conversations with patients were primarily concerned with completing nursing tasks. They tended not to use communication skills to achieve therapeutic goals, and when they tried to do this, their deficiency in these skills was apparent. The students themselves were aware of their inadequacies and became frustrated at their inability to meet the patients' needs.

Choosing to work with old people

Fielding (1986) also investigated student nurses' career choices with the explicit purpose of determining the proportion expressing an interest in working with old people. Students who had just started training were looking for excitement, interest and challenge from nursing, and they expected the perceived high-drama areas of maternity, paediatrics and accident and emergency to fulfil their expectations. The areas they expected to enjoy the least were the unknown and anxiety-provoking specialties of mental illness, geriatrics and operating theatres. Students who were at the end of their training endorsed as enjoyable and most rewarding those areas defined as exciting by the beginners: surgery, paediatrics and accident and emergency. The areas they enjoyed the least were also paediatrics, general medicine and geriatrics. The problem with the paediatric placement was unfortunate staff relationships, but the medical and geriatric wards were seen as heavy, tiring and dull. The tendency was for student nurses to regard geriatric nursing as requiring only 'basic' nursing care, i.e. little more than patience and understanding, in-sufficient for them to accept geriatric nursing as a specialty with unique skills. Few of Fielding's students contemplated a job in geriatric nursing and it was not seen as conducive to career progression. The view that specialising in the care of old people is professional suicide remains common today (Ingham and Fielding, 1985; Woods and Britton, 1985).

These results have serious implications for nursing training and practice. The taught course followed by Fielding's students was probably not untypical. It took a decremental view of ageing and placed the elderly person firmly in a medical context, with physicians doing a good deal of the teaching. No mention was made of nursing assessment and individualised care planning, and the information given on the process of ageing was often inaccurate. The students did not feel that they had a valuable educational experience, and regarded geriatric nursing as non-specialised care. These students saw no distinction between the care of old people in medical and geriatric wards and so their extensive experience in medical wards meant that they felt they would learn little on geriatric wards. These conclusions match closely those of Wells (1980), and suggest that very little progress has been made by nurse teachers in the field of elderly care. Undoubtedly many of the principles of nursing elderly people are common to nursing generally, but there is a large and growing body of knowledge about research into the process and effects of ageing and care of old people which many nurses specialising in this field do not know.

Fielding's study has shown that the routine geriatric style of nursing continues. The students regarded the psychogeriatric unit as more progressive, with its emphasis on reality orientation, drug therapy and electroconvulsive therapy. It is worth noting that all these treatments are the responsibility of professionals other than nurses, although nurses might take part in the therapy. Very little initiative was taken by nurses in the traditional geriatric wards to break the routine geriatric cycle. No emphasis was put on a person-orientated approach with individual assessment, rehabilitation and care designed to meet individual needs. Fielding endorses the suggestion made by Carlson and Wiseman (1981) that the approach taken in hospice care would be appropriate for old people. The emphasis in hospices is on total well-being and choice for the patient whenever possible, with full participation by the patient and family.

A change in the organisation of nursing care from a task-centred medical approach to primary individualised nursing might attract the energetic, innovative nurse as well as enhancing the well-being of frail old people. The rewards in caring for elderly people, and the emphasis on the importance of acquiring interpersonal communication skills, have been prominent topics in the nursing press in recent years. This may help to reduce the negative image of geriatric nursing. There is some evidence that the higher the attained level of nursing education, the more positive are nurses' attitudes towards old people (Ingham and Fielding, 1985; Fielding, 1986). This observation matches the impression that those who have graduated through degree courses in nursing often choose careers which involve the care of old people. These nurses have been through courses which give as much prominence to the psychosocial as to the physical needs of the patient, and they are therefore well equipped to promote the well-being of old people. These nurses are likely to reject the role of doctor's assistant, and may choose to work in nursing specialties which are not medically dominated. They are attracted to hospital or community nursing which allows them more autonomy than acute medicine.

INTERPERSONAL COMMUNICATION

The work on unpopular patients draws attention to the difficulties nurses have in communicating effectively with many elderly people. Interpersonal communication research in nursing has been carried out in different forms for some 20 years. Yet failure to communicate adequately features frequently in cases of complaint handled by the NHS ombudsman (Vousden, 1987). Patient satisfaction surveys have consistently found that the amount and content of information given to them by health care professionals constitute the single largest source of dissatisfaction for patients. The more recent intervention studies have pointed to the benefits of giving patients information (Macleod Clark, 1985). Structured information given to patients, before surgery or investigative procedures, has been shown to reduce patients' anxiety, stress and pain, and to promote their recovery in comparison to control patients who received usual care. These research studies confirm the common sense notion that giving patients information is a good thing. But the research may have inadvertently eclipsed the need to take individual differences into account. Most patients may indeed want detailed information, but some may not, or may want the details only when they feel ready for them. Nurses require a high level of skilled perception to assess the varying needs of each patient.

Observation of nurse–patient interaction started with workstudy projects in the 1950s and 1960s on patient dependency and nursing workload (Macilwaine, 1983; Macleod-Clark, 1983). These studies were designed to establish staffing requirements, but they inevitably recorded the time nurses spent with patients. They showed that nurses spent very little time in direct interaction with patients, and this was confirmed in later observation research by nurses, for example, with children in paediatric wards and with psychiatric patients (Altschul, 1972; Hawthorn, 1974; Cormack, 1976).

Recent research by nurses has increasingly used more sophsticated data collection and analysis techniques, using audio and video recordings, and has focused on the quality as well as the amount of communication between nurses and patients (Macleod Clark, 1983). The repeated findings from these studies are that nurses' interactions with patients are infrequent and brief, they are confined to physical care and treatment matters, and are almost invariably initiated by a nurse during the course of a physical task with a patient. In her study in surgical wards, Macleod Clark found that nurses use tactics which discourage prolonged conversation and which protect them from having to divulge information to patients (Macleod Clark, 1983).

In geriatric wards, although nurses spend most of their time in what they call 'basic' nursing, they spend very little time (less than four per cent) in personal contact and conversation with elderly patients (Macleod Clark, 1983). Wells (1980) found that more than half the verbal exchanges between nurses and elderly patients lasted less than 25 seconds. A Danish study revealed similar findings (Lorensen, 1983a). A large proportion of elderly patients wanted more information about their illness and treatment, and they complained that they had very little opportunity to discuss their concerns with health personnel.

The strategies nurses use to discourage prolonged conversation may be effective in reducing their anxiety if they feel unable to handle patients' questions (Menzies, 1959; Bond, 1983). Nurses may feel that lack of knowledge signifies incompetence, which they do not want to convey to the patient. Or they may regard it as the doctor's responsibility to give patients information. So often this is medical policy, yet the patient may choose to confide in the nurse rather than in the doctor. The resultant conflict may be difficult for the nurse to handle. Avoiding patients' signals for information may be a wise tactic for nurses to adopt, particularly if they know that they will not be able to follow up distressing information with adequate help. But nurses also discourage, or fail to notice, patients' requests for information which is neither particularly sensitive nor related to life-threatening problems.

This evidence highlights the importance of teaching interpersonal skills in nurse training. As with any technical skill, interpersonal skills must be learned, yet they have received little attention in conventional training. Most practising nurses have not been taught these skills, except for those who have been fortunate enough to find an effective role model whose communication skills they have recognised as important to good nursing. Others have not acquired these skills, and so have not become effective role models for the students who pass through their wards. The current emphasis in British nursing on individualised nursing care and the nursing process should be conducive to the teaching of interpersonal skills. Even so, few teachers feel comfortable with the experiential teaching methods which are appropriate: they and ward nurses need training themselves before they can effectively teach students, and before they can become good role models (Faulkner and Maguire, 1984).

Interpersonal communication through touch: a study in progress
Most of the research on interpersonal skills in nursing has focused on verbal communication. It is a reasonable assumption that, given the infrequent nurse–patient interactions and the inadequate conversation found in previous research, the range and frequency of non-verbal communication would also be low. This assumption prompted our team at King's College London to examine non-verbal communication with special reference to nurse–patient touch.

Non-verbal communication conveys important information about a person's emotional state, and a nurse's touch can be beneficial to patients in times of danger, incapacity or sickness (Barnett, 1972a). As we have seen, communication between nurses and patients, particularly verbal communication, has been the subject of recent research by nurses, but non-verbal communication in general, and touch in particular, have been relatively neglected in Britain. American research indicates that elderly patients are amongst those most deprived of caring, 'expressive' touch (Barnett, 1972b; Watson, 1975). The effectiveness of expressive nurse–patient touch has been demonstrated in several patient care settings: in reducing discomfort during labour (Lorensen, 1983b); in reducing pre-operative anxiety (Whitcher and Fisher, 1979) and the anxiety of patients in intensive care units (McCorkle, 1974); and for promoting the well-being of elderly frail and confused patients (Hollinger, 1980). Nurses are in a unique position to convey a caring attitude and to promote feelings of trust and self-esteem in patients. Yet many nurses find it difficult to give and to receive touch which is not directly related to a physical nursing task.

This background prompted our study which aimed to describe the amount and type of nurse–patient touch in hospital and nursing home settings for elderly people, and to establish any relationship between touch and the well-being of old people. We also proposed to identify those individual differences in nurses and patients which may affect their use and acceptance of touch (biographical details, nurses' attitudes to old people, reason for patient's admission, and preference for using and receiving touch); and to identify any association between patient dependency and well-being and nurse touch. Fieldwork for the study has been completed and data analysis is in progress. The samples consisted of 86 patients from acute and long-stay geriatric wards, a day hospital and a nursing home, and all the nurses (133) who cared for the patients during the observation periods.

Nurse–patient interaction and touch were observed using a schedule which involved observing individual patients at sample times throughout daytime hours (7.00–21.30) for each patient (Porter *et al.*, 1986; Le May and Redfern, 1987). Thorough training in the use of this schedule is necessary, and inter-observer reliability checks were made at regular intervals by a second observer. Patients' engagement and activity levels were observed using a technique developed by Felce *et al.* (1980); and patient well-being was assessed with Bradburn's (1969) Affect Balance Scale, and a short five-item well-being scale of our own. Patient dependency was assessed by the nurse in charge with the modified Crichton Royal Behavioural Rating Scale (Charlesworth and Wilkin, 1982).

The nurses and patients were interviewed in an attempt to elicit their preferences for using and receiving touch. We used a photographic exercise during the interview to encourage the interviewees to think about and discuss their feelings about touch without using direct questioning which might have introduced a social desirability bias. The photographs were presented in pairs. Each pair portrayed the same nurse and elderly patient communicating but in only one of the pairs was the nurse touching the patient. In addition to this, the nurses' attitudes towards elderly people were assessed with Kogan's (1961) Old People Scale.

The observation schedule emerged as a reliable research tool with consistently high inter-observer reliability coefficients on most of the components (test statistic Kappa ≥ 0.6, or ≥ 70 per cent agreement) (Cohen, 1960). These reliable components were the nature and duration of the interaction, when the touch occurred during the interaction, the patient's and the nurse's positions, the body area touched and the type of touch used. The components which failed consistently to reach our reliability criteria were the response of the recipient to each touch, verbal communication by the toucher, and the length of each touch episode. Extensive observer training did not succeed in raising the reliability of these three components. The length of each touch, which often is extremely short, with many touches following each other in rapid succession, was impossible to record accurately at the same time as recording the other components. The other two unreliable components required subjective interpretation by the observer which was difficult to standardise. These components were useful, however, in supporting a general comment about each nurse–patient interaction. This comment described the observer's impression of the content, the speed of touch and the communication patterns which occurred during the interaction in general, rather than focusing on each specific touch episode.

The results available so far show that most touch used by the nurses was task-defined and 'instrumental', and that there was much less spontaneous and 'expressive' touch. For the 86 patients observed, a total of 2590 touches were recorded during 830 interactions. Of these touches, 88 per cent were instrumental, 10 per cent were expressive, and 2 per cent were undefinable. The type of touch patients received varied between the settings, with significantly more (probability level <0.001) expressive touch occurring in the long-stay geriatric wards (16%) and the day hospital (12%) compared with the acute geriatric wards (6%) and the nursing home (7%). These findings support earlier research which demonstrated that nurses use relatively little touch with elderly patients.

Those patients who had been in the institutions for more than a month were touched more than those who had a shorter stay ($p < 0.05$); and those whose reason for admission was recorded as 'social' reasons received more expressive touch than those admitted for 'medical' reasons. Social reasons are often recorded by nurses and doctors when there is no definite medical diagnosis but the patient cannot continue to cope at home. These results suggest that the nurses may have recognised certain patients' needs for caring contact particularly when conventional medical treatment was not a priority.

Our results did not support earlier research (e.g., Barnett, 1972b) that the more dependent the patient the less the touch received. On the contrary, the reverse seemed more likely to be true, since we found that more dependent patients received more touch than less dependent patients, although the difference failed to reach significance ($p < 0.10$). The results also failed to reveal a significant relationship between the amount or type of touch patients received and their level of well-being. We had speculated that expressive touch might be positively related to patient well-being, but the findings suggested that if there was a relationship, it was more likely to be negative than positive. Those patients who rated themselves as relatively unhappy received more expressive touch than the happier patients, but this was not significant ($p < 0.10$).

The results so far have revealed important information about the amount and type of touch elderly people receive from nurses, and the differences among various settings and patients. Recommendations based on the findings will focus on the importance emphasised earlier of interpersonal skills for nurses working with these extremely frail and vulnerable elderly people.

CONCLUSIONS

Improving the quality of life of elderly people who require continuing nursing care is the principal theme of this chapter. The research on the organisation of nursing care in geriatric wards has shown that the individual needs of old people have been subordinated to the traditional care regime. We know that most patients want information about their illness, treatment and prognosis, yet research demonstrates consistently that they do not receive this information. Nurses have been shown to lack the interpersonal skills necessary to promote the well-being of elderly people. Elderly people who find themselves ending their days in long-stay geriatric wards can so quickly decline into an apathetic state of 'learned helplessness', in which any vestige of independence has long gone. Nurses see no challenge in this kind of work and choose instead to work in areas of excitment, drama and rapid change.

The research study summarised here on nurse–patient touch supports earlier work which has demonstrated the lack of interpersonal communication skills in nursing and the need for training in these skills. Happily, there is now recognition by the statutory bodies that communication skills training is necessary, and there are some nurses who choose the challenge of nursing old people. The superiority of individualised care, or the nursing process, in geriatric wards as compared with traditional task-orientated care, well demonstrated in Audrey Miller's work, points clearly to the importance of changing the organisation of nursing care. Changes are occurring, as in Alison Storrs' nursing home, Alan Pearson's Nursing Development Unit, and the experimental NHS nursing homes. But change is slow, and it will be a long time before the quality of care being achieved in these exceptional units reaches every old person in long-stay geriatric wards.

REFERENCES

Altschul, A. (1972). *Patient–Nurse Interaction.* Churchill Livingstone, Edinburgh.

Atkinson, D.A., Bond, J. and Gregson, B.A. (1986). The dependency characteristics of older people in long-term institutional care. In *Dependency and Interpendency in Old Age*, C. Phillipson, M. Bernard and P. Strang (Eds). Croom Helm, London.

Baker, D.E. (1983). 'Care' in the geriatric ward: an account of two styles of nursing. In *Nursing Research: Ten Studies in Patient Care*, J. Wilson-Barnett (Ed.). John Wiley & Sons, Chichester.

Barnett, K. (1972a). A theoretical construct of the concepts of touch as they relate to nursing. *Nursing Research*, **21**(2), 102–10.

Barnett, K. (1972b). A survey of the current utilization of touch by health team personnel with hospitalized patients. *International Journal of Nursing Studies*, **9**, 195–209.

Batchelor, I. (1984). *Policies for Crisis? Some Aspects of DHSS Policies for Care of the Elderly*. Occasional Paper No. 1, Nuffield Provincial Hospitals Trust, Oxford.

Bolt, D. (1983). Why we are worried about the process. *Nursing Times*, **79**(34), 11–12.

Bond, J. (1984). Evaluation of long-stay accommodation for elderly people. In *Gerontology: Social and Behavioural Perspectives*, D.B. Bromley (Ed.). Croom Helm, London.

Bond, S. (1983). Nurses' communication with cancer patients. In *Nursing Research: Ten Studies in Patient Care*, J. Wilson-Barnett (Ed.). John Wiley & Sons, Chichester.

Booth, T. (1985). *Home Truths: Old People's Homes and the Outcome of Care*. Gower, Aldershot.

Booth, T. (1986). Institutional regimes and resident outcomes in homes for the elderly. In *Dependency and Interdependency in Old Age*, C. Phillipson, M. Bernard and P. Strang (Eds). Croom Helm, London.

Bradburn, N. (1969). *The Structure of Psychological Wellbeing*. Aldine, Chicago.

Carlson D. and Wiseman G. (1981). Hospice concepts applied to the aging. In *Care of the Ageing*, L.A. Copp (Ed.). Churchill Livingstone, Edinburgh.

Charlesworth, A. and Wilkin, D. (1982). *Dependency Among Old People in Geriatric Wards, Psychogeriatric Wards and Residential Homes, 1977–1981*. Research Report No. 6. University of Manchester Psychogeriatric Unit, Manchester.

Clarke, M. (1978). Getting through the work. In *Readings in the Sociology of Nursing*, R. Dingwall and J. McIntosh (Eds). Churchill Livingstone, Edinburgh.

Cohen, J. (1960). A coefficient of agreement for nominal scales. *Educational and Psychological Measurement*, **20**(1), 37–48.

Community Outlook (1987). An old age scandal. *Community Outlook*, Editorial, March.

Cormack, D.F.S. (1976). *Psychiatric Nursing Observed*. Royal College of Nursing, London.

Dalley, G. (1983). The nursing home: professional attitudes to the introduction of new forms of care provision for the elderly. In *Ageing in a Modern Society*, D. Jerrome (Ed.). Croom Helm, London.

Evers, H. (1981a). Tender loving care. In *Care of the Aging*, L.A. Copp (Ed.). Churchill Livingstone, Edinburgh.

Evers, H. (1981b). The creation of patient careers in geriatric wards: aspects of policy and practice. *Social Science and Medicine*, **15A**, 581–8.

Faulkner, A. and Maguire, P. (1984). Teaching assessment skills. In *Recent*

Advances in Nursing, 7: Communication. A. Faulkner (Ed.). Churchill Livingstone, Edinburgh.

Felce, D., Powell, L., Lunt, B., Jenkins, J. and Mansell, J. (1980). Measuring activity of old people in residential care. *Evaluation Review,* **4**(3), 371–87.

Fielding, P. (1986). *Attitudes Revisited: An Examination of Student Nurses' Attitudes Towards Old People in Hospital.* Royal College of Nursing, London.

Georgiades, N.J. and Phillimore, L. (1975). The myth of the hero-innovator and alternative strategies for organisational change. In *Behavioural Modification and the Severely Retarded,* C.C. Kiernan and F.P. Woodford (Eds). Associated Scientific Publications, New York.

Hawthorn, P. (1974). *Nurse – I Want My Mummy!* Royal College of Nursing, London.

Hollinger, L. (1980). Perception of touch in the elderly. *Journal of Gerontological Nursing,* **6**(12), 741–6.

Ingham, R. and Fielding, P. (1985). A review of the nursing literature on attitudes towards old people. *International Journal of Nursing Studies,* **22**(3), 171–81.

Kelly, M.P. and May, D. (1982). Good and bad patients: a review of the literature and a theoretical critique. *Journal of Advanced Nursing,* **7**(2) 147–56.

King, R.D. and Raynes, N.V. (1968). An operational measure of inmate management in residential institutions. *Social Science and Medicine,* **2**, 41–53.

Kogan, M. (1961). Attitudes towards old people: the development of a scale and an examination of its correlates. *Journal of Abnormal and Social Psychology,* **62**, 44–54.

Le May, A.C. and Redfern, S.J. (1987). The nature and frequency of nurse–patient touch and its relationship to the wellbeing of elderly patients. In *Collaborative Research and its Implementation in Nursing,* M. Sorvettula (Ed.). Proceedings of the Workgroup of European Nurse Researchers' Conference, Helsinki, 1986. Finnish Federation of Nurses and Nursing Research Institute, Helsinki.

Lorensen, M. (1983a). Evaluation of the elderly person's need for nursing care to maintain optimum self-care capability. In *Research – A Challenge for Nursing Practice,* E. Hamrin (Ed.). Proceedings of the Workgroup of European Nurse Researchers' Conference, Uppsala, 1982. Swedish Nurses' Association, Stockholm.

Lorensen, M. (1983b). Effects of touch in patients during a crisis situation in hospital. In *Nursing Research: Ten Studies in Patient Care,* J. Wilson-Barnett (Ed.). John Wiley & Sons, Chichester.

Macilwaine, H. (1983). The communication patterns of female neurotic patients with nursing staff in psychiatric units of general hospitals. In *Nursing Research: Ten Studies in Patient Care,* J. Wilson-Barnett (Ed.). John Wiley & Sons, Chichester.

Macleod Clark, J. (1983). Nurse–patient communication: an analysis of conversations from surgical wards. In *Nursing Research: Ten Studies in Patient Care,* J. Wilson-Barnett (Ed.). John Wiley & Sons, Chichester.

Macleod Clark, J. (1985). The development of research in interpersonal skills in nursing. In *Interpersonal Skills in Nursing: Research and Applications,* C.M. Kagan (Ed.). Croom Helm, London.

McCorkle, R. (1974). Effects of touch on seriously ill patients. *Nursing Research,* **23**(2), 125–32.

McCormack, D. and Whitehead, A. (1981). The effect of providing recreational activities on the engagement level of long-stay geriatric patients. *Age and Ageing*, **10**, 287–91.

Menzies, I. (1959). A case study of the functioning of social systems as a defence against anxiety. *Human Relations*, **13**(2), 95–121.

Millard, P.H. (1983). Long-term care in Europe: a review. In *Care of the Long-Stay Elderly Patient*, M.J. Denham (Ed.). Croom Helm, London.

Miller, A.F. (1984). Nursing process and patient care. *Nursing Times Occasional Paper*, **80**(13), 56–8.

Miller, A.F. (1985a). Does the process help the patient? *Nursing Times*, **81**(26), 24–7.

Miller, A.F. (1985b). A study of the dependency of elderly patients in wards using different methods of nursing care. *Age and Ageing*, **14**, 132–8.

Mitchell, J.R.A. (1984). Is nursing any business of doctors? A simple guide to the 'nursing process'. *British Medical Journal*, **288**, 216–19.

Pearson, A. (1983). *The Clinical Nursing Unit*. Heinemann, London.

Porter, L., Redfern, S.J., Wilson-Barnett, J. and Le May, A.C. (1986). The development of an observation schedule for measuring nurse–patient touch, using an ergonomic approach. *International Journal of Nursing Studies*, **23**(1), 11–20.

Seligman, M.E.P. (1975). *Helplessness: On Depression, Development and Death*. Freeman, San Francisco.

Smith, A. (1986). The old folk at home. *Guardian*, November 12; Four chips and a bucketful of spite. *Guardian*, November 19.

Storrs, A. (1982). What is care? *British Journal of Geriatric Nursing*, **1**(4), 12–14.

Vousden, M. (1987). When the care collapses. *Nursing Times*, February 25, 16–17.

Wade, B., Sawyer, L. and Bell, J. (1983). *Dependency With Dignity*. Occasional Papers on Social Administration No. 68. National Council of Voluntary Organisations. Bedford Square Press, London.

Watson, W. (1975). The meanings of touch: geriatric nursing. *Journal of Communication*, **25**(3), 104–12.

Wells, T. (1980). *Problems in Geriatric Nursing Care*. Churchill Livingstone, Edinburgh.

Whitcher, S. and Fisher, J. (1979). Multidimensional reaction to therapeutic touch in a hospital setting. *Journal of Personality and Social Psychology*, **37**(1), 87–96.

Wilkin, D., Mashia, T. and Jolley, D.J. (1978). Changes in behavioural characteristics of elderly populations of local authority homes and long stay hospital wards, 1976. *British Medical Journal*, **2**, 1274–6.

Wilkin, D., Hughes, B. and Jolley, D.J. (1985). Quality of care in institutions. In *Recent Advances in Psychogeriatrics: No. 1*, T. Arie (Ed.). Churchill Livingstone, Edinburgh.

Woods, R.T. and Britton, P.G. (1985). *Clinical Psychology with the Elderly*. Croom Helm, London.

Part Three

PROSPECTS: THIRD AGE LIVES IN THE NEXT GENERATION

Mark Abrams

Age Concern Institute of Gerontology
King's College
University of London

13 THIRD AGE LIVES IN THE NEXT GENERATION: CHANGING ATTITUDES AND EXPECTATIONS

INTRODUCTION

It is widely recognised that the eight and a half million people aged 65 years or more in Britain in 1986 cannot for most purposes be regarded as a homogeneous group. Some were born when Queen Victoria was Empress of India, while others were born long after her grandson had ascended the throne. The government's statistical accounts of the elderly population have increasingly subdivided elderly people into two age bands: the younger (aged 65–74 years) and the older (aged 75 years or more). The people in these two groups differ in their economic circumstances, household conditions, health, and also in the age at which they experienced such events as the First World War, the Great Depression, the launching of the Welfare State, the election of the first majority Labour Government, the widespread use of antibiotics and the successful launching of interplanetary satellites. Such differences have contributed to the shifts in attitudes and expectations between the younger and the older elderly of the 1980s, and may also lead to differences in the attitudes and expectations of the younger and older elderly of the year 2001.

This chapter will attempt to anticipate some of the differences in the younger and the older elderly's attitudes and expectations at the end of the century. A helpful starting point is to set out some of the main facts about both the economic and social conditions of the elderly of the early 1980s and their attitudes and expectations. The first information to be considered (Table 13.1) is a secondary analysis of data from the *1982 Family Expenditure Survey* (Department of Employment, 1983). The sample was drawn from the United Kingdom population and did not include the three per cent of elderly people living in 'communal establishments', i.e. not in private households. The sample consisted of 7428 households, and of these 1842 (25.1 per cent) were households whose head was aged 65 years or more. These households did not include all persons aged 65 years or more in private households, since a small number would have been living as non-heads in the households of younger people. Figures are given for the two age bands of elderly heads of households and for men and women. Among households headed by persons aged 75 years or more, not only were female heads predominant, but they were also better off in terms of average weekly expenditure per person. Among households where the head was aged 65–74 years, average weekly expenditure per person was similar irrespective of the sex of the head of the household.

Among the younger elderly heads of households (aged 65–74 years), women constituted 35 per cent of all heads; in households where the head was aged 75 or more the proportion headed by a woman rose to nearly 60 per cent (Table 13.1). Any comparison between younger and older elderly groups must

Table 13.1 Some demographic characteristics of elderly households, by age and sex of head: United Kingdom, 1982. Data from *1982 Family Expenditure Survey* (Department of Employment, 1983).

	Age of head of household			
	65–74		75 or more	
	Male	Female	Male	Female
Average number of males	1.1	0.1	1.1	0.1
Average number of females	0.9	1.1	0.7	1.1
Total persons	2.0	1.2	1.8	1.2
Per cent of total aged 65 or more	75	85	91	87
Average age of head (years)	69	70	79	80
Year of birth of head	1913	1912	1903	1902
Life expectation of head (years)	10	13	6	8
Per cent of heads living alone	13	35	23	48
Sample size	740	406	308	390

Table 13.2 Average weekly household income: United Kingdom, 1982. Data from *1982 Family Expenditure Survey* (Department of Employment, 1983).

	Men		Women	
	65–74 £	75+ £	65–74 £	75+ £
Normal total *gross* income	116	86	70	67
Sources				
Wages and salaries	21	9	10	8
Self-employment	4	1	1	1
Investments	13	6	6	6
Annuities, private pensions	19	13	7	7
Social security benefits	51	50	40	41
Imputed from owner occupation	8	6	5	5
Other	1	1	1	0
Disposable income: total	104	80	64	62
Disposable income: per head	50	40	51	47

consider this difference in the sex composition of the two age bands. In both of the elderly age groups the average household headed by women was much smaller than that headed by a man. This was largely because a greater proportion of women lived alone, and, at least until recently, women have married men older than themselves and tended to outlive them.

The bulk of the *1982 Family Expenditure Survey* deals with household monetary incomes and it ignores social incomes, for example, in the form of free transport. The sources and amount of these monetary incomes and expenditures on goods and services are reported. In male-headed households in 1982, those with younger elderly heads were better off; gross household incomes were 35 per cent higher and expenditure per person was 25 per cent higher (Table 13.2). Of their additional £30 a week, £15 came from gainful employment and £7 from private pensions. Among female-headed elderly households the differences between the two age groups were much smaller. In terms of gross income the younger elderly were only slightly better off, and in

Table 13.3 Average weekly household expenditure: United Kingdom, 1982. Data from *1982 Family Expenditure Survey* (Department of Employment, 1983).

	Age group (years)	
	65–74 £	75+ £
Housing	18.3	15.9
Fuel, light, power	7.5	7.4
Food	9.9	5.0
Alcoholic drink	3.4	2.0
Tobacco	2.3	1.3
Clothing and footwear	5.2	3.3
Durable household goods	4.8	2.6
Other goods	6.1	4.3
Transport and vehicles	9.0	3.7
Services	10.6	7.5
Miscellaneous	0.2	0.1
Total	87.2	63.1
Per person	50.0	43.0

Table 13.4 The elderly's possessions: Great Britain, 1985.

	Men (%)		Women (%)	
	65–74	75+	65–74	75+
Car	59	34	40	19
Washing machine	76	58	72	50
Deep freezer	55	39	50	28
Telephone	80	66	81	67
Personal cheque book	61	49	47	35
Personal credit card	27	16	12	6
Taken holiday, past year	54	37	57	42
House/flat, five rooms or more	62	51	55	43
Colour television set	85	77	83	71

the amounts they received from various sources the two groups of female-headed households were almost identical. If sex is ignored, much of the difference in income between the two age groups is due to the relative poverty of older men (as compared with younger elderly men) and to the large proportion of female heads of households that are aged 75 years or more.

The average younger elderly household had a weekly household expenditure per person that was 16 per cent higher than that of the average older elderly household (Table 13.3). The differential was substantially larger for expenditure on alcohol and tobacco, clothing and footwear, transport and vehicles and durable household goods. Some of the lower expenditures by the older elderly, for example, on alcohol and tobacco, reflect differences in the sex composition of the two age groups; in part they reflect the fact that fewer of the older elderly travel to and from work, fewer have driving licences, and most have already acquired all the necessary durable household goods.

The annual *National Readership Survey* for the media industry uses a sample sufficient to provide substantial numbers of interviews with both younger elderly people (3370 in 1985) and older elderly people (2037). Both heads of households and other individuals are sampled and the survey deals not only with media consumption but also with the durable goods possessed by either the respondent or by the household of which he or she is a member.

Neither men nor women aged 75 years or more, in the light of these figures, were recognisable in 1985 as full members of the 'acquisitive society' (Table 13.4). Only small minorities had taken a holiday, defined as at least four nights away from home, during the 12 months before the interview. Even fewer possessed a credit card, a deep freezer, or a car; and levels of ownership among the older elderly were consistently lower among women than men. For both sexes the outstanding form of participation in the consumer world is the high proportion who have a colour television set. Irrespective of sex or age, the average elderly person spends over three hours of each day watching television.

Three other characteristics of the respondents' circumstances demonstrate the importance of distinguishing older elderly from younger elderly: the age at which they finished their full-time schooling, their marital status, and their household type. Four in five of the older elderly of both sexes had a terminal education age of 14 years or less; for younger elderly the proportion was slightly under 70 per cent. Of the older elderly women, only 21 per cent were married, in contrast to 50 per cent of younger elderly women. Of the older elderly women, 63 per cent lived alone, but among younger elderly women the corresponding figure was no more than 39 per cent.

Members of the two age groups naturally differ in the age at which they experienced various historical events. In 1981 the median age of the younger elderly was 68 years, while that of the older elderly was 78 years. The latter were born in 1903 when the United Kingdom, having won the Boer War and consolidated its world-wide imperial power, could afford to dispense with the extra twopence in the pound income tax necessitated by the costs of the war. In 1903 one alternative to such a reduction was to follow the long-established examples of New Zealand and Germany and to introduce a modest old age pension. This latter option was rejected by a Parliament in which the majority of members took the view that the 'deserving' elderly in need would be taken care of by private philanthropy, while the 'undeserving' could, and should, reap the fruits of their self-inflicted shortcomings in the workhouse.

SHARED LIFE EVENTS OF THE OLDER COHORT

The median older elderly person of 1981 had finished full-time schooling half way through the First World War and although then only 13 years of age, had probably spent a year or two (whether boy or girl) working in a war-related factory. On becoming a legal adult at the age of 21 years in 1924, the future elderly of 1981 could celebrate or deplore the formation of Britain's first minority Labour Government under Ramsay MacDonald. After a few months in office, another General Election restored Stanley Baldwin to office as leader of a Conservative government for a period marked by the General Strike in 1926 and a steady rise in unemployment. By the time of the Great Depression in 1932, when 23 per cent of all insured workers were unemployed, our median future older elderly person was aged 29 years. More than a third of all coal miners and nearly half of all iron and steel workers were unemployed. When the unemployed workers of the Jarrow shipyards completed their march to London, they were able to witness a sight that had become familiar in the towns of south-east England: small groups of unemployed miners from South Wales singing forlornly and holding out their caps for pennies.

Presumably not many of those aged 29 years in the depression years could afford such a gesture. Rowntree's second survey of York in 1935 found that of all unemployed heads of households, nearly one-third were aged 30–39 years (Rowntree, 1941). The *New Survey of London Life and Labour*, directed by Lewellyn Smith with the assistance of William Beveridge, found that in Greater London in 1931, nearly half (46 per cent) of all insured unemployed persons were aged 20–34 years (Smith and Beveridge, 1932). Moreover, by 1932 most of those born around 1903, whether employed or unemployed, were married; the Census taken in 1931 found that two-thirds of all males in Britain aged 25–34 years were married. And those who were married were also the parents of young children and infants.

The typical wife who had been born in 1903 had married at the age of 24, and half had produced a second child by 1930 (Abrams, 1946). By 1933, however, the economic depression had taught those born in 1903 that children were an extravagent indulgence; in 1933 births per 1000 women aged 15–44 years reached an unprecedented low and were half the figure recorded in 1903 (Mitchell and Deane, 1962). When a sample of the survivors of those born at the beginning of the century was interviewed in 1977, over one-third of the women said they had never had any children and only 20 per cent had had three or more children. The older elderly people of 1981 were the first generation to produce children who grew up in families where siblings and cousins were few or nonexistent.

During the remainder of the 1930s, levels of unemployment fell below 12 per cent in only one year and the real earnings of those in full-time employment only reached their pre-depression level in 1938 (Mitchell and Deane, 1962). By then the older elderly of 1981 were aged 35 and had witnessed the violent establishment of fascist governments throughout much of Europe. The would-be British version, formed and led by Sir Oswald Mosley, fell short of success. In the 1930s the British preferred a different type of folk hero – or rather father-figure – King Georve V. According to one historian writing of the 1930s, 'the old King was loved and respected by all . . . he remained the symbol of the British family – a symbol of a generation that looked back beyond . . . the Lloyd George era of the adventurer with the sharp swords and the glittering prizes, the Churchills and Birkenheads, to the world of Victoria and the draped gun carriages at Windsor and the old certainties and the tears of imperial things' (Raymond, 1960). There was an occasional dissident such as Victor Gollancz with his 'Left Book Club' or the unknown trouble-maker, 'who (in 1935) unfurled a banner reading "Thirty Years of Hunger and War" in Fleet Street during the Jubilee procession' (Raymond, 1960).

In 1939 when World War Two began, the infant of 1903 was aged 36 years. This time there was no talk (as in 1914) of 'it will all be over by Christmas'. This time it was a matter of gas masks, air raids and blackouts, evacuation of the young and the old to 'safe' areas, conscription of men and women and the rationing of almost all foods and clothes. One major social consequence of the war was that it enabled the government to force upon the general population a diet that was vastly more healthy than half the population had had, or had preferred, to consume. National sample surveys carried out before the war had shown that, 'the diet of as much as half the population, and that the poorer half, was deficient in varying degrees in those nutrients that are essential, not indeed to life, but to vigorous health . . . many people were going seriously short of calcium, iron and the vitamins A, B, and C' (Hammond, 1951). During the war, synthesized vitamin B_1 was added to flour, vitamins A and D added to margarine, calcium deficiency was made good by encouraging milk and potato production, 'standard' bread offered in place of white bread and the production of green vegetables encouraged. Among imported goods, high priorities were given to cheese and dried egg powder and at the same time food subsidies held down the prices of bread, oatmeal, eggs and fresh milk.

It is probable that the food policy adopted in World War Two and maintained for the early post-war years played an appreciable part in increasing slightly the life expectation of both men and women. In 1953–55 (when those born in 1903 were aged 50–52 years), the average woman aged 50 years had a life expectation of a further 27 years; while in 1930–32 the average life expectation of a woman of 50 had been 24 years. For men the comparable increase had been from $21\frac{1}{2}$ to $22\frac{1}{2}$ years. In contrast, during the preceding 20 years from 1911 to 1931 there had been absolutely no increase in the life expectation of either men or women aged 50 years.

There is little evidence that the nutritional benefits of food rationing generated enthusiasm among the general public. On the other hand, the steps taken by the wartime coalition government toward the foundation of a welfare benefit system and a free health service were welcomed by most people of all classes and all age groups. In June 1941, when most of Britain's allies had either surrendered to Hitler's armies or else been occupied by them, the government formed an Interdepartmental Committee, under the chairmanship of Sir William Beveridge, 'to undertake . . . a survey of the existing national schemes of social insurance and allied services . . . and to make recommendations'. In arriving at his recommendations, Beveridge assumed that there would be three central and essential elements of post-war social policy: children's allowances for all parents, a comprehensive health and rehabilitation service for all citizens, and the maintenance of full employment (Beveridge, 1942).

The Labour Government elected in 1945 implemented all three, and in 1948 established what the electorate considered to be its greatest achievement, the National Health Service. In 1949 the annual cost of *all* social services was £1800 million – four times the average annual figure of £450 million of central government expenditure during 1935–39. However, the amount voted by Parliament toward contributory old age pensions had increased by little more than 50 per cent. This discrepancy should not have come as a surprise to those who had read the chapter in the Beveridge Report, entitled 'The problem of age'. It warned that, 'it is dangerous to be in any way lavish to old age until adequate provision has been assured for all other vital needs such as the prevention of disease and the adequate provision of the young. . . . The problem for the future is how persons who are past work can be given a guarantee against want (without) throwing an intolerable financial burden on the community' (Beveridge, 1942). Apparently few of those for whom the prospect of soon being 'past work' found much that was either new or objectionable in Beveridge's values, since many of them had learned in childhood to accept 'want'. Indeed, acceptance was identified by the first generation of social gerontologists as an important means of adjustment to ageing.

The older elderly of 1981 (with a median birth year of 1903) reached retirement age in 1963 if female and in 1968 if male. In 1968 the standard rate of retirement pension for a man was £4.50 a week plus £2.80 for a wife, a total of £7.30. In the same year the median weekly income of households where the head was aged 64 years or less was £31.00. By 1978 those still living who had been born in 1903 or earlier were aged 75 years or more and qualified as members of the older elderly age group. For a majority of these people adjustment to later life necessitated not only acceptance but also disengagement; that is, withdrawal from almost all the active roles available to the rest of the adult population. This had already been made clear by the *1977 General*

Table 13.5 Participation in sports and activities, 1977. Data from *1977 General Household Survey*.

Sports and activities	Age group (years)					
	30–59		60–69		70+	
	Male (%)	Female (%)	Male (%)	Female (%)	Male (%)	Female (%)
Outdoor						
Bowls	1	nd	2	nd	2	nd
Athletics/jogging	x	x	x	0	x	0
Golf	5	1	3	1	2	x
Football	3	nd	x	nd	x	nd
Rugby	x	nd	0	nd	0	nd
Cricket	1	nd	x	nd	0	nd
Tennis	2	1	x	x	x	0
Swimming	3	2	1	1	x	x
Fishing	5	1	2	x	1	0
Walking two miles or more	19	18	20	16	13	7
Any outdoor sport[a]	34	23	26	18	17	7
Indoor						
Badminton	2	2	x	x	0	0
Squash/fives	3	1	0	0	0	0
Swimming	6	4	1	1	x	x
Table tennis	3	1	x	x	0	0
Bowls	2	1	2	x	1	x
Billiards/snooker	9	1	4	x	2	0
Darts	13	4	4	1	2	x
Keep fit/yoga	1	2	x	1	x	x
Any indoor sport[a]	29	12	9	3	5	1

[a]   including activities not separately listed
x   less than 0.5%
nd   no data

Household Survey in Great Britain. The total sample of over 23 000 people aged 16 or more included 1015 men and 1801 women aged 70 years or more. Respondents were asked if they had engaged in various activities at any time in the four weeks before the interview.

They were first questioned about active participation in ten outdoor sports and activities and eight indoor sports and games. Among men aged 30–59 years, one-third had taken part during an average four-week period in at least one active outdoor sport or game (Table 13.5). Among men aged 70 or more, however, five in every six had failed to take part in any outdoor activity, and of those who had, only 20 per cent had done anything except take a walk of at least two miles. One would have thought that the differential participation in indoor games and activities between the two age groups would have been less substantial; but in fact it was greater, perhaps because all these indoor activities took place away from home. Of eight indoor activities, only two, snooker and darts, attracted the active participation over a four-week period of as many as two per cent of those aged 70 or more years. Apart from the seven per cent who had taken a walk of two miles or more in the four weeks before the interview, older elderly women had almost entirely ceased to participate in either indoor or outdoor sports and games (Table 13.5). The same survey enquired about outings, sightseeing and visits to places of entertainment. A similar picture

Table 13.6 Participation in outings in previous four weeks: Great Britain, 1977. Data from *1977 General Household Survey.*

	Men (%)			Women (%)		
	30–59	60–69	70+	30–59	60–69	70+
Open-air outing	16	14	10	17	14	9
Visiting historic buildings, museums, etc.	14	12	6	15	11	5
Visiting theatre, ballet, cinema, etc.	17	10	6	15	12	9
Out for meal or drink	75	56	41	62	41	26
Going to clubs/societies	10	9	9	11	15	16
Social and voluntary work	9	9	6	12	12	6

emerged of disengagement on the part of the older male and female elderly.

Possibly the high level of disengagement on the part of the older elderly arises from the fact that the surveyed activities call for physical fitness. The lower levels of disengagement recorded for other activities (Table 13.6) may be because they provide companionship and because the older elderly like to spend their time and resources maintaining lifelong cultural interests. Another factor is that the proportion of middle class people was higher among those aged 70 years or more than among those aged 30–59 years; life expectancy among middle-aged working class men and women has been and is appreciably lower than among middle class people.

SHARED LIFE EVENTS OF THE YOUNGER COHORT

The median aged at 68 years of the younger elderly person in 1981 was ten years younger than that of the median older elderly person. Consequently the events that played a large part in shaping people's expectations and attitudes occurred when they were ten years younger. Someone born in 1913 missed the Boer War, and was almost certainly still at school at the time of the General Strike in 1926. 'Almost certainly', because in the school year ending in March 1927, of all the children attending elementary schools, 90 per cent left school at the age of 14.

The educational experience of a minority of those born in 1913 had been affected by the war-time activities of H.A.L. Fisher. In December 1916, Fisher, then Vice-Chancellor of Sheffield University, had been invited by the Prime Minister, Lloyd George, to join his government as President of the Board of Education. He accepted and began to visit the schools of the country. After inspecting London's elementary schools he expressed the view that there was a greater difference between the worst and the best, than there was between the best of them and either Eton or Winchester. He set about bringing good education to a larger proportion of the nation's children. Between 1919 and 1927 government expenditure on education in England and Wales more than doubled from £19.4 to £44.3 million. Over the same period the retail price index fell by over one-fifth so that real expenditure on education trebled. For some pupils at elementary schools there were scholarships to secondary schools, and for some at secondary schools there were State Scholarships to enable them to go to universities and other institutions of higher and further education. Between 1920 and 1927 the number of pupils in England and Wales aged 16 or more years attending secondary schools increased from 13 500 to

38 200. This was hardly a revolution, but by 1927 for the first time in Britain a handful of working class children were receiving the broader secondary education that had hitherto been monopolised by middle class children.

In the early 1930s, the worst years of the Great Depression, those born around the year 1913 were in their late teens: almost all had completed their formal education, for in 1931 only 14 000 full-time new students were admitted to all British universities. A few had found employment either as apprentices or else in dead-end jobs such as messenger-boys or domestic servants; very few had married and many of those who had were living with their parents. It was altogether a wretched start to adult life. When war broke out in 1939 and they were in their mid-twenties, the military conscription of young men solved the employment problem for many. Between mid-1938 and mid-1941, the strength of the armed forces increased by nearly three million and the complement of the women's auxiliary services grew from virtually nothing to over 100 000. The number of women in civilian employment increased by 1.3 million. By June 1941 the total of registered insured unemployed men and women had fallen to less than 200 000, including very few of those born around the year 1913.

By 1948, when the National Health Scheme was launched, the survivors of the infants born in 1913 were aged 35 years. Most men and women had been demobilised from military or quasi-military service; approximately three-quarters of both sexes were married and both they and their very young children were enjoying the benefits of the welfare state. In the fiscal year 1949–50, current expenditure on social services by all public authorities reached £1470 million and provided maternity grants, school meals and mid-morning milk, child allowances, housing subsidies and free health services for all. In 1954 commercial television broadcasting started and the following year saw the end of all food rationing. By June 1955 the total number of registered unemployed men and women was no more than 200 000, little more than one per cent of the total civilian working population: not only had full employment been achieved but there seemed to be no good reason for it ever to diminish.

Of course, not everyone benefited at all times. At the end of the 1950s the wholly-unemployed total doubled, but this was a brief set-back and by 1965 the total was down to 300 000. It increased slightly each year thereafter, but not until 1975 did the unemployed total start to move firmly towards one million. At this date the median younger elderly person was aged 62 years, only three years short of the male retirement age.

In summary, by 1975 the median survivor of the younger elderly could look back on a life which had started with four years of war and then experienced sequentially 20 years characterised by widespread unemployment and poverty, another six years of war, and, in startling contrast, almost 30 years of full employment, steadily rising real incomes, and a bureaucracy whose allotted task was to ensure their well-being in old age. By 1975 the population aged 65–74 years was enjoying living conditions which an earlier generation, and indeed they themselves when young, would have called luxury. This had occurred despite the fact that four-fifths of them had left school at the age of 14 years or less.

Some of their main achievements as consumers are shown in Table 13.7. A majority were equipped not only with vacuum cleaners, gas or electric cookers, washing machines, refrigerators, and much increased room space, but also with enough leisure to spend at least three hours a day watching television; and a majority of these addicts had a colour television set (Joint Industry Committee

Table 13.7 Possessions and characteristics of people aged 65–74 years: Great Britain, 1974. Data from *1974 National Readership Survey* (JICNRS, 1984).

	Men (%)	Women (%)
Car	42	29
Electric or gas cooker	97	98
Vacuum cleaner	89	89
Washing machine	64	57
Refrigerator	78	77
Central heating	33	32
Telephone	42	42
Own house/flat outright	47	44
Dwelling with five or more rooms	62	56
Spouse still living	78	47
Watching television at least three hours daily	66	70

for the National Readership Survey, 1974). And judging by the content of the daily newspapers which they mostly read – *The Daily Express*, *The Daily Mirror* and *The Sun* – they were not worried by Carnaby Street, 'swinging London' or rebellious students.

By 1977 the survivors of those born in 1913 were aged 64 years and about to join the ranks of the younger elderly. The *1977 General Household Survey* (GHS) suggests that in comparison with those aged 30–59 years, their levels of participation in outdoor and indoor sports and activities were low but only substantially so with regard to indoor activities (see Table 13.5). Among men this may have been because some indoor sports and games, such as darts or snooker, were then dominated by men in their thirties and forties. Among women of both age groups in 1977, rates of participation in indoor and outdoor sports and activities were negligible. One exception was 'walking two miles or more', but even for this activity the proportion of participating women fell with age, whereas among the eldest men the proportion slightly increased. In terms of their participation in outdoor and indoor sports and games, women, unlike men, had almost completely disengaged by the time they were in their sixties.

The GHS also provides information on people's participation in outings and cultural pursuits. In comparison with those aged 30–59 years, the younger elderly had either the same rates of participation, as in undertaking voluntary social work, or else only slightly lower rates, as with open-air outings, going to clubs and attending society meetings. The only activities with substantially lower rates of participation were those involving fairly large spending, such as going out for meals (see Table 13.6).

VARIATIONS IN ATTITUDES AND EXPECTATIONS

By 1981 some significant differences had emerged in the attitudes and values of the two groups of elderly people. In that year the European Values Systems Study Group undertook a sample survey of the values, social attitudes and expectations of the adult population in several European countries and the results for Great Britain have been published (Abrams *et al.*, 1985). Some of the striking differences between the younger and older elderly of 1981 are shown in Table 13.8. This shows that, compared with the older elderly of 1981, the younger elderly were much less involved in religious activities and beliefs, much less antagonistic to non-white and non-Anglo-Saxon minority groups, left-wing extremists and unmarried mothers; they were more interested in

Table 13.8 Variations in attitudes and values by age in 1981. Data from Abrams *et al.* (1985).

	1981 age group (years)			
	45–54 (%)	55–64 (%)	65–74 (%)	75+ (%)
Belong to a religious organisation	25	27	29	46
Do voluntary work for a religious organisation	10	13	1	13
Attend church, chapel, etc. at least once a week	14	24	11	23
Would not like as neighbours:				
People of different race	12	12	11	32
Left wing extremists	32	29	35	50
Unmarried mothers	3	3	9	16
Politics:				
No interest at all	23	26	20	34
Right wing in politics	13	22	19	38
Have great deal of confidence in:				
The Church	18	36	29	40
The Police	39	57	54	72
Parliament	11	15	21	28

party politics, less right-wing in their own political attachments, and less likely to express confidence in the activities and achievements of the Church, the Police and Parliament.

When asked to use an eleven-point scale to express satisfaction with their lives (0 = completely dissatisfied, 10 = completely satisfied), the younger elderly were consistently less satisfied with their circumstances in 1981 and with their conditions five years previously, and more pessimistic about their level of life satisfaction in 1986. Their early experience may have been less effective in conditioning them to 'adjust through acceptance' and to find satisfaction in their current circumstances. The younger elderly were less satisfied with their current financial situation and less likely to anticipate improvement. They also gave less support to the statement that, 'Parents' duty is to do their best for their children even at the expense of their own well-being'. When asked to assess the acceptability of various forms of deviant behaviour, the younger elderly gave a significantly higher justification score to five of the 19 types: claiming State benefits to which you are not entitled; keeping money that you have found; having an affair although married; abortions; and divorce. Clearly more of the younger elderly of 1981 than their predecessors had accepted the 'liberation' attitudes adopted by intellectuals during the 1930s and which became commonplace during the third quarter of the century.

ELDERLY PEOPLE IN 2001

The older elderly in 2001 will be the survivors of those aged 55 to 64 years in 1981 plus the few survivors of those aged 65 or more years in 1981. Among the former group, the average life expectancy was 16 years for men and 20 years for women. Women will therefore constitute at least three-quarters of all those aged 75 or more years at the beginning of the next century. The younger elderly in 2001 will be the survivors of those aged 45–54 years in 1981; they were born in the years 1926 to 1936. Their knowledge of the First World War would have been either from books or from the reminiscences of their elders, and the oldest was still a schoolchild when the Second World War broke out. The Great Depression in one way benefited them: between the early 1920s and the early 1930s the average annual total of live births fell by a quarter, helping to raise earnings and job opportunities during the late 1940s and early 1950s when this generation entered the labour market. When they married during the 1950s and early 1960s, they were the first generation to enjoy the full benefits of the welfare state: maternity grants; child allowances; free medical care; school meals; and housing subsidies. Between 1951/1 and 1961/2 public expenditure on social security benefits in the United Kingdom increased from £703 million to £1675 million, almost doubling real expenditure per head.

In 1975, when the survivors of this cohort were aged 40–49 years, four-fifths of all employees were covered by their employer's sick pay arrangements and 65 per cent of male employees and 50 per cent of female employees were covered by employers' private pension schemes. By 1981–82, when they were aged 45–54 years, the demographic and social conditions of the representative member resembled someone in a stereotypical, middle-age, middle income household. He or she was living with a spouse and one child; over 80 per cent were in full-time or part-time employment, less than one in ten were living alone and even fewer were widowed (Table 13.9). Nearly one-third had a terminal education age of 16 years or more, and only a minority had finished their schooling before reaching the age of 15 years. In these respects they were 'better off' than those aged 55–64 years. The latter were living in smaller households, and more were living alone. Less than half were in either full-time or part-time employment, while one in eight was already widowed and almost three-quarters had finished their schooling by the age of 14 years (Table 13.9).

At the beginning of the 1980s the gross weekly income of households whose heads were aged 45–54 years was considerably larger that that of the average UK household. It was probably equally ahead of the median gross income of the households where the head was aged 55–64 years (Table 13.10). Not surprisingly, when in the 1981 European Value Systems Study respondents answered the question. 'How satisfied are you with the financial situation of your household?', the average score of those aged 45–54 years was 7.4 as compared to 6.8 for those aged 55–64 years. Among both older and younger groups, only small proportions reported much involvement with religious organisations. At the same time, their objections to such minority groups as 'people of a different race' and 'unmarried mothers' as neighbours were negligible. Levels of confidence in such basic social institutions as the Church, the Police and Parliament were very low, particularly among the younger group of whom only 11 per cent expressed great confidence in Parliament. Is there a possibility that even when this cohort reaches retirement age, they will favour non-parliamentary methods for expressing their opinions and achieving their ends? They were in their late twenties and early thirties during the 1960s and watched, even if few participated in, the then unconventional but often successful methods of making political, social and economic demands.

The 1983 General Household Survey covered the respondents' participation in leisure activities in the previous four weeks. The figures for those aged 45–59 years suggest that those who will be the younger elderly in 2001, compared with those aged 30–44 years, had substantially withdrawn from most outdoor and indoor leisure activities apart from taking a two mile walk (Table 13.9). Their participation in outdoor outings, for example, visits to the countryside, sightseeing, visits to museums and to places of entertainment, was slightly less than those of younger people, but for all age groups participation rates were

Table 13.9 Some demographic and social conditions in 1981 of the 'younger' and 'older' elderly of 2001. Data from Abrams *et al.* (1985).

	1981 age group	
	45–54	55–64
Persons in average household	3.0	2.4
Per cent living alone	9	13
Per cent in full-time employment	58	35
Per cent in part-time employment	23	11
Per cent married	84	75
Per cent divorced, separated	3	4
Per cent widowed	5	13
Per cent single	7	8
Number of children born	2.7	2.5
Terminal education age:		
14 or less	42	72
15	20	7
16–17	23	13
18+	8	8

Table 13.10 Median gross weekly household income, by age of head of household 1982. Data from *1982 Family Expenditure Survey* (Department of Employment, 1983).

	£	Index
All UK householders	154	100
Age:		
40–49	227	147
50–59	192	125
60–64	130	84

low. Judging by their replies to various attitude and behaviour questions, the following contrasts between the elderly of given ages in the year 2001 as compared with the same age group in the early 1980s can be forecast.

The older elderly
This age group in 2001 is likely to be:

(a) much less intolerant of people of a different race, of left-wing extremists and of unmarried mothers;
(b) less interested in politics;
(c) less ready to describe themselves as right-wing politically;
(d) less confident in the Church and a great deal less confident in the Police and in Parliament;
(e) less likely to belong to any religious organisation, but those who do belong will be just as active as today's members and just as likely to attend services regularly.

The younger elderly
This age group in 2001 is likely:

(a) to show no reduction in their dislike of people of a different race, left-wing extremists and unmarried mothers as neighbours;

(b) to include a slight increase in the minority with no interest at all in politics;

(c) to include fewer people who describe themselves as right-wing politically;

(d) to have even less confidence in the Church, the Police and Parliament;

(e) to include an even smaller minority who belong to a religious organisation;

(f) to have a larger number involved in voluntary work for a a religious organisation. The present extent of regular church attendances by a small minority will probably be maintained.

AFFLUENCE AND EXPECTATIONS: THE ELDERLY IN 2001

Since 1970 there has been considerable improvement in the real incomes of elderly people: it is difficult to assess the impact that this has had on the attitudes and expectations of the present and future elderly. The real income of pensioners increased during 1970–85 at an average annual rate of 2.2 per cent (Dawson and Evans, 1987). The annual rate of increase in real income was 3.1 per cent from social security benefits and 3.8 per cent from occupational pensions: these increases more than offset the decline in employment earnings. The real incomes of recently retired married couples (with the husband aged 65–69 years) increased by almost 40 per cent and the proportion receiving an occupational pension rose from 57 to 70 per cent.

By the year 2001, the most common type of multi-income household is likely to be that of the pensioner receiving a state pension, an occupational pension and income from investment. Their main political demands are likely to be for zero inflation and for state pensions to be linked to the earnings of the working population. Pensioners will number at least 10 million and will form a fourth of the electorate: they will be healthier than today's elderly, better educated, less conditioned by early years of accepted poverty, and more courted by the producers of goods and services. They will be organised and led by a generation of younger elderly who as young adults witnessed the launching of Beveridge's Welfare State, and participated, if only as voters and television viewers, in the political battles to reshape it for a more affluent and acquisitive society than Beveridge ever anticipated.

By 2001 it is unlikely that successful retirement will be viewed as disengagement from the adult world but rather as a re-engagement on equal terms. More and more people will appreciate Freud's assessment when aged 57 years of the choices which faced him in retirement: 'The readiest safeguard (against unhappiness) is voluntary isolation, keeping oneself aloof from other people.... There is another and better path: that of becoming a member of the human community ... (and) one gains the most (from this) if one can heighten the yield of pleasures from sources of intellectual activity' (Freud, 1930).

There are two routes by which the elderly of the twenty-first century could achieve this participation: either by forming numerically substantial communities of their own along the lines of similar developments in the United States, or by breaking down the barriers set up by the non-elderly to exclude them as full members from adult society. Whichever course is taken, by the beginning of the next century there will be a generation of younger elderly people fitted by education, material resources and good health to play a full part in either or both of these alternatives. The present circumstances of the elderly, pushed into a post-adult sector of society in which they increasingly tend to live alone, will certainly not be feasible even with a growing army of paid and voluntary carers. Our society, or at least many of its most powerful representatives, has become vociferous about 'the burden' of an ageing population and seems likely to encourage more self-reliance and mutual support among elderly people themselves.

REFERENCES

Abrams, M. (1946). *Condition of the British People, 1911–1945*. Gollancz, London.

Abrams, M. (1984). Supplementary analysis and commentary on the 1982 Family Expenditure Survey. Unpublished.

Abrams, M., Gerard, D. and Timms, N. (Eds) (1985). *Values and Social Change in Britain*. Macmillan, London.

Beveridge, W. (1942). *Social Insurance and Allied Services*. HMSO, London.

Dawson, A. and Evans, G. (1987). Pensioners' incomes and expenditure, 1970–1985. *Employment Gazette*, **95**(5), 243–52.

Department of Employment (1983). *1982 Family Expenditure Survey*. HMSO, London.

Freud, S. (1930). *Civilisation and its Discontents*. Jonathan Cape, New York.

Hammond, R.J. (1951). *History of the Second World War: Food*, Vol. 1. HMSO, London.

Joint Industry Committee for the National Readership Survey (JICNRS) (1974). *The National Readership Survey 1974*. JICNRS, London.

Mitchell, B.R. and Deane, P. (1962). *British Historical Statistics*. Cambridge University Press, Cambridge.

Raymond, J. (Ed.) (1960). *The Baldwin Age*. Eyre & Spottiswoode, London.

Rowntree, B.S. (1941). *Poverty and Progress*. Longman Group, London.

Smith, L. and Beveridge, W. (1932). *New Survey of London Life and Labour*, Vol. 3. P.S. King & Son, London.

Brian Groombridge

Institute of Education
University of London

14 EDUCATION AND LATER LIFE

THE RIGHT TO EDUCATION THROUGHOUT LIFE

> What has surprised me is that the numbers of retired and elderly people coming to classes has been so very large. One class in community history that I am taking at the moment in a small village near Bradford has about 50 people in it. It took my breath away, because I'd just put out 12 chairs. I had to get 24, then 36, and then the headmaster had to come in to help me shift them all as everybody came streaming in!
>
> (Tutor-organiser quoted in Groombridge, 1987)

Educational gerontology has been defined by the pioneering American authority, Professor David A. Peterson, as:

> a field of study and practice that has recently developed at the interface of adult education and social gerontology ... (it) is the study and practice of instructional endeavours for and about aged and aging individuals. It can be viewed as having three distinct though related aspects: (1) educational endeavours for persons who are middle-aged and over; (2) educational endeavours for a general or specific public about aging and older people; and (3) educational preparation of persons who are working or intend to be employed in serving older people in professional or paraprofessional capacities.
>
> (Peterson, 1976)

In this article I am mainly concerned with the first of Peterson's categories, while accepting as he does in his several reworkings of this definition, that the three cannot be rigidly kept apart.

The *Declaration of Human Rights*, adopted by the United Nations in 1948, mentions 'teaching and education' in its very first sentence; as a chief means whereby respect for rights and freedoms shall be promoted. The actual right *to* education appears in Article 26:

> (1) Everyone has the right to education. Education shall be free, at least in the elementary and fundamental stages. Elementary education shall be compulsory. Technical and professional education shall be made generally available and higher education shall be equally accessible to all on the basis of merit.
>
> (2) Education shall be directed to the full development of the human personality and to the strengthening of respect for human rights and fundamental freedoms. It shall promote understanding, tolerance and friendship among all nations, racial or religious groups, and shall further the activities of the United Nations.

Rights, as the Declaration asserts, provide 'a standard of achievement for all peoples and all nations', to be secured by 'progressive measures, national and international, to secure their universal and effective recognition and observance . . .' (United Nations Organization, 1948).

Proclaiming rights is one thing: getting them implemented is notoriously quite another. The gap between international law and reality is not always a consequence of political failure or ill will. The interpretation of rights takes time, and indeed may vary over time, as in this case. When rights to education were promulgated, those who formulated them could not have had in mind all the possible applications and consequences of that declaration. It would not necessarily occur to them that these rights might one day be expressly invoked in favour of the oldest members of society.

In 1982, the connection between these rights and this constituency was made explicitly and categorically by the World Assembly on Ageing in Vienna. The Assembly, convened by the United Nations Centre for Social Development and Humanitarian Affairs, adopted the *Vienna International Plan of Action on Ageing* (United Nations Organization, 1983). As well as making recommendations under such customary and expected heads as 'Health and nutrition', 'Housing and environment', 'Social welfare', 'Income security and employment', the Plan less predictably included eight recommendations about education (Nos. 44–51). These recommendations were grounded in education 'as a basic human right'.

> As a basic human right, education must be made available without discrimination against the elderly. Educational policies should reflect the principle of the right to education of the ageing, through the appropriate allocation of resources and in suitable education programmes.
>
> (Recommendation 45, United Nations Organization, 1983)

Education features in the Plan because when addressing the problems caused by the near-universal ageing of the world's populations, the World Assembly did not construe older people as in themselves constituting the problem. Instead of treating them as burdensome dependants, the Assembly was expected 'to provide a forum "to launch an international action programme aimed at guaranteeing economic and social security to older persons, as well as *opportunities to contribute to national development*" ' (United Nations Organization, 1983: my italics).

As its full name implies, the British organisation, Forum on the Rights of Elderly People to Education (FREE), also bases its advocacy on human rights. Formed in 1981 to be both a clearing house for the developing movement for education and the elderly and a lobby pressing for improvements in education for older people, FREE launched its Manifesto at the end of 1983 at a meeting in the House of Commons (Glendenning, 1985). The preamble includes these statements:

> Justice between age groups requires us . . . to ensure that older people in Britain should benefit as far as they possibly can from the educational system which has been so greatly expanded by their own economic efforts. Worse educated as children and young persons than any of their successors . . . , they should now have access, as of right, to all the intellectual, cultural and aesthetic facilities and practical skills, which in their own judgement, they need and desire.
>
> (Glendenning, 1985)

One of the signatories to the FREE Manifesto was Dr Peter Laslett, the distinguished historical demographer, a leading figure in British gerontology, and founder chairman of the University of the Third Age in Cambridge. The Manifesto shows the influence of a statement which Glendenning (1985) calls his *cri de guerre: An Educational Charter for the Elderly*, first published in *New Society* on 13th March 1980. This Charter was the introduction to a report full of challenging proposals, entitled *The Education of the Elderly in Britain* (Laslett 1980; revised in Midwinter, 1984). It also polemically expressed a rights-based approach:

> This charter . . . is intended as a charter for all British persons, as they are now, or as they will finally be. It consists of five educational *rights*. The right to a fair share of the educational budget of the nation: the right to the abandonment of the identification of education with youth: the right of access to all educational institutions on their own terms: the right to a 'distance teaching' organisation, to bring education for the elderly into the home: and the right to recognition of their unique intellectual and cultural value.
>
> (Midwinter, 1984)

The concept of 'right' may not fit all of these proposals equally well, but Laslett's recommendations, coupled with those of the *International Plan of Action*, provide a starting point for an appraisal of the developments in this field.

To begin the discussion of recent developments in Britain and elsewhere, one definition should be offered and some general points made. By education, I shall not mean anything reducible to 'school' or 'college' but for any systematic opportunities for learning which are socially organised. It will be evident that these developments are indeed international; that they already display great variety; and that they are provided under a wide range of organisations. This is the more impressive in that it is not so long since the very juxtaposition of 'education' and 'elders' would have caused puzzlement or disbelief. Their conjunction with health, welfare and pensions was more familiar and is indeed still the underlying source of anxiety among politicians about the costs of ageing populations.

Laslett has argued that, 'the elderly have never previously been thought to have specifically educational needs at all, let alone rights. . . . The exercise of these educational rights might reduce the demands of the aged for care. . . . It is reasonable to suppose that the better informed, active and interested the elderly become, the less help of this kind they will need' (Laslett, 1984).

As recently as 1985, James regretted that 'the juxtaposition of the concepts of education and ageing is unfamiliar and open to misunderstanding', since the 'traditional and established view in much of the Western world is that education is principally for the young', and that creating 'learning opportunities for adults or taking an interest in the needs and contributions of older people is seen as much less important and worthwhile' (James, 1985). The Finnish gerontologist, Sihvola (1983), welds the two concepts together within the context of international studies of well-being and the quality and mode of life:

> Fresh research from the field of gerontology shows that the individual's probable life-expectancy is lengthened as the quality of life is raised by enriching and diversifying his or her educational, professional and recreational opportunities. . . . Education is a resource which can help

people to augment the material and social conditions of their well-being. But education is also a means by which individuals can become aware of needs and interests and relate them to their abilities and qualifications. With the aid of education, the individual can further expand his or her range of activities and see more clearly than before the significance of earlier choices and actions, and thus direct future activities along lines that best serve both interests and needs.

Sihvola is among those in many countries who now assert the need for a new literalness in the philosophy and relation of 'lifelong' education, finding meaning in a tautology:

> Lifelong education thus assumes new significance when seen from the standpoint of the totality of life. From this viewpoint the main emphasis is on developmental possibilities and personal achievements as continuing through the entire lifespan and into the later stages of old age.
>
> (Sihvola, 1983)

DIVERSITY OF INTERNATIONAL INITIATIVES

The juxtaposition, education for elders, is becoming familiar in Britain, largely thanks to publicity surrounding universities of the third age, the educational aspects of the Age Well campaign and other manifestations. The international reach of this phenomenon needs, however, to be emphasised. In preparing its submission on education to the World Assembly on Ageing, Unesco used statements and case studies from eighteen member states in Africa, Latin America and the Caribbean, North American and Europe. 'Education and later life' may mean *t'ai chi* for elders in the parks of Shanghai; training for their 'residual economic role' in the Soviet Union; participating in liberal adult education study circles in Sweden; providing (with difficulty in the face of urbanisation) for the maintenance of cultural continuity in some developing countries; role-playing in intergenerational workshops about three-tier family living in Singapore; as well as, more familiarly, being on a study tour in or from the United States with Elderhostel, or following a course with a *université du temps libre* (*troisième âge*) in any of the francophone countries (Unesco, 1982).

The emergence of a new wave of elderly, purposive learners and students, is changing the whole aspect of education itself. These 'endeavours', as Peterson would call them, may originate in at least four ways.

1. They may be undertaken by quite new organisations, brought into being for the purpose, as in the Retirement Education Centre in Bedford or in all the universities of the third age in Britain.
2. They may arise as new activities started by established educational institutions, as when colleges of further education, traditionally concentrating on vocational courses for the young, arrange programmes for retired men and women; when the folk high school movement in Denmark, historically associated with the social education of young people, successfully launched courses for pensioners; when the Inner London Education Authority's adult education service extended its Special Needs policies to provide earmarked resources for older students; or when the Polytechnic of North London branched out with a new programme entitled 'Learning in Later Life'.
3. They may be new educational activities provided by bodies and organisations that are not primarily educational, as exemplified by: pre-retirement

courses, run by private industrial concerns; educational activities (intended as something more than occupational therapy) in residential homes and geriatric wards; educational television series for older viewers such as *The 60–70–80 Show* (BBC), *Getting On* (Central) and *Years Ahead* (Skyline Productions/Channel Four); oral history, creative writing and craft workshops provided by Age Concern, Help the Aged and other welfare agencies; social research (with elderly people doing the research) or health fairs arranged by Pensioners' Link; or, as in Leicestershire, library clubs for senior citzens.

4. They may be created through some kind of collaboration or partnership between agencies in the different categories already mentioned. For example, French universities of the third age are voluntary organisations independent of but co-operating with their parent, statutory, universities; or local education authorities may provide classes in centres run by social services departments.

The foregoing selection of developments in different countries distinguished four ways in which educational endeavours for elders may originate. These distinctions correspond to an internationally accepted convention for analysing education systems: in this usage, such systems can be formal, non-formal or informal. Formal systems comprise education conducted by statutory or chartered institutions set up expressly for that purpose (schools, colleges, universities). Non-formal systems refer to organisations which provide education but which mainly exist for other social purposes (such as churches, trade unions, public service broadcasting, single issue political lobbies). Informal systems comprise voluntary movements, grass roots organisations or the relatively spontaneous, lightly structured activities of friends, neighbours, fellow hobbyists and other enthusiasts.

When Laslett and others say that older people should have unconditional access to education because its advance was enabled by their work, they seem to have the formal system in mind. When Midwinter and others proclaim 'age' as 'opportunity', it is often the informal sector that is being invoked and celebrated. These distinctions are not merely theoretical: they are directly relevant to questions of responsibility for policy and resource allocation, and hence for ensuring that rights are implemented. Do current initiatives stem from formal sector adult education, in particular as an extension of opportunities for mature people in general to the oldest generations in particular? Or are they coming from older people themselves, out of British traditions of mutual aid and an associative culture? Other significant questions could relate to the interaction between one sector and another. For example, are self-help organisations of older learners (informal sector) also able to act as lobbies to promote access to schools, colleges and universities (formal sector)? Conversely, do voluntary educative clubs and societies derive support from or even owe their existence to formally established educational bodies? Such questions are important in practice for promoters and planners; they are also important in theory for research and formative evaluation.

Issues arising from these distinctions as to auspices overlap with 'curricular' matters (recognising that the concept of 'curriculum' has itself connotations from the formal sector). Who decides what is to be learned and how? Older people themselves, as individuals, or collectively as in universities of the third age in Britain? Professional educators or professionals who are not educators, for example, in caring agencies? Or are decisions about what is to be learned in some way shared between learners and professionals, either through overt negotiation of the curriculum or through the operation of market forces (Groombridge, 1983)?

BRITISH DEVELOPMENTS: A MOVEMENT?

Developments such as these have not yet been comprehensively researched in Britain, where they are still comparatively recent, but they have been described (Glendenning, 1980; 1985; Johnston and Phillipson, 1983; Midwinter, 1982; 1984; Norton, 1984; 1986). Pre-retirement education has been evaluated by Coleman and Groombridge (1982) and Phillipson and Strang (1983). Glendenning (1985) describes education for older adults in Britain as a developing movement. It certainly feels like a movement to those involved: one finds older learners themselves or professionals acting as animators, trail blazers and flagwavers, together with several organisations of the different kinds already indicated. The anecdote at the head of this article captures the atmosphere. The scale of these developments is not known, but there has been a conspicuous quickening of the pace in recent years. When a survey for *Education and Retirement* (Groombridge, 1960) was undertaken there was little education for older adults to be discovered in Britain. Subsequently there have been pioneering endeavours in different parts of the country owing much to the persistence of visionaries. The change, when these isolated ventures became the beginnings of the movement, occurred around 1978 (Glendenning, 1985). In July 1986, FREE published the first *Directory of Educational Initiatives Involving Older Adults*, in which Dianne Norton, co-ordinator of FREE since its foundation, listed over 230 such initiatives. The first universities of the third age in Britain (Cambridge and London) were started in 1981 and 1982 and there are now 120 (Norton, 1986). Through FREE and more recently through the creation of the Association of Educational Gerontology, the activists in this movement have had some sense of solidarity and achievement.

Developments in Britain challenge stereotypes of old age at both ends of a spectrum. One stereotype often prompts the view, held even by some enthusiasts for education in later life, that because older people value education as an end itself, they are not interested in studying for degrees or other qualifications. At the other extreme, another stereotype current among the elderly themselves as well as professional carers, is that at their feeblest and frailest, in geriatric hospital wards or even in residential homes, elderly people are incapable of learning and not the slightest interested in education.

As to the former: in 1982 nearly 3000 of the 64 500 Open University undergraduate students were aged over 60. The Open University Older Students' Research Group discovered that these students, who were making up for missed opportunities or lack of opportunities in the past, half of whom left school at 16 years or earlier, did as well as younger students. They tended to get better marks than the under-60s for their continuous assessment work but poorer marks on examination, especially the over-70s (Open University, Older Students Research Group, 1984). As to older people in hospitals or homes, the research of Jones (1982) and the practice of Newman (1986), Poulden (1980) and others, indicates that where there is life, there remains a capacity for learning in art, poetry, movement, French and current affairs. Moreover, given that the label 'education' need not be on display, even the most disadvantaged and demoralised older people may respond to what is an undisguised invitation to take part in an organised occasion for learning.

The main features of the middle ground, which in effect make up the education in later life movement in Britain are these:

1. A lively informal sector involving something like 10 000 people in universities of the third age and other self-programming groups.
2. A few local education authorities with articulate policies and a probably larger number of specific institutions in different branches of the formal sector (usually inspired by individual members of staff) involving some tens of thousands of older adults as students.
3. A growing number of endeavours in the non-formal sector; as medical or welfare organisations add educational work to their repertoire of strategies, as the media and leisure industries become aware of the potential audiences and markets being created by the changing population structure, and as employing bodies accept the need for new forms of pre-retirement education.

The informal sector

The voluntary part of the movement can be exemplified by FIRCONE, a long-established group in Birmingham, and by the University of the Third Age in Cambridge, usually reckoned to be the first U3A in Britain. FIRCONE was a precursor of the movement and flourishes still. It was set up in the mid-1960s (different sources give different foundation dates) under the umbrella of the Birmingham Retirement Council. FIR stands for Friends in Retirement and the fircone which is its logo is said to be of a species which crops twice a year instead of only once. Between 2500 and 3000 people take part in a programme of art, craft, music, practical subjects, history and languages, all the groups being run by volunteer instructors. Each group has a leader and these leaders make up the committee in charge of activities (Norton, 1986).

Most U3As have about 25–30 members. Cambridge is one of the largest with some 500 members, but its ethos and programme, as described by Futerman (1984) are typical. The U3A in Cambridge, founded in June 1981, started by arranging three streams of activity: weekly foundation lectures, drawing on the wealth of local intellectual talent, and often serving as tasters for related series of seminars; weekly seminars on such subjects as art history, political science, music, English literature, and practical classes in sculpture, painting and drawing; language workshops at different levels, including Mandarin Chinese, Latin, Ancient Greek, Modern Greek, Russian and Serbo-Croat as well as modern European languages at all levels of fluency. These streams have evolved (for example, classes in English literature have become a structured Modern English Literature course lasting three years), and to them have been added research activities, a newsletter, a community services group (involving housebound members in study), study travel abroad and a variety of social activities.

The formal sector

The commitment to adult education of London's metropolitan administration, successively the London County Council and the Inner London Education Authority (ILEA) has always been exceptional (Devereux, 1982). Its reputation in this field is worldwide and its contribution to education for the elderly extends the traditions on which this reputation is based. At the time of writing the future of ILEA is in doubt but, in view of its significance to this paper's theme, its role in this field needs to be given particular attention. In recent years, ILEA has been strongly motivated by the pursuit of equal opportunities. Its policies have led to various forms of affirmative action in favour of unemployed men and women, ethnic minorities, single parents, disabled people and other disadvantaged or, as they came to be termed, 'special needs' groups. Measures to secure the right to education did not at first include older adults, but in 1981 ILEA asked an experienced adult educator, Dorothy Underwood, to collaborate with Age Concern (Greater London) in a survey of adult education with the elderly. The project was in effect more than a survey: it raised consciousness among adult educators, people in the older age groups and their representatives of an area of opportunity and of an unfamiliar but positive aspect of social policy. ILEA backed the recommendations of the Underwood Report (1983) and adopted policies leading to: increased provision at generously reduced fees and at convenient times of the day; extra provision and promotion, stimulating demand; and a shift in the composition of ILEA's adult student population.

One Principal of an adult education institute in south-west London reported, for example, that whereas in 1981–82 there were 1536 older students, two years later there were 2123 out of about 13 000: a sixth of his students were of pensionable age. ILEA provides for elders, the robust and the frail, in homes, hospitals and hospices as well as through its network of adult education institutes, sometimes in classes for all ages, sometimes in specially designated ones (Underwood, 1983; Groombridge, 1985). To maintain the momentum of its work with older adults, especially at the level of policy formation and curriculum development, ILEA has set up EdROP (Educational Resource Unit for Older People), which has, among other activities, begun to probe the problematic nature of 'special needs' as a basis for securing equal opportunities founded on a concept of human rights.

In other parts of the formal sector, a reputation for interest in education in later life has been acquired by several establishments: for example, Braintree College of Further Education, Hatfield Polytechnic, North Hertfordshire College, Middlesex Polytechnic, the Polytechnic of North London, Manchester College of Adult Education, Newark Technical College, Birkbeck College and King's College (University of London), Debden House Residential College, and the Department of Adult Education at the University of Leeds (Johnston and Phillipson, 1983; Groombridge, 1985; Glendenning, 1985; Norton, 1984; 1986). It may be significant that some of the best known of these centres are in further and advanced further education, not in the adult education branch of the formal sector. This may be because adult education cherishes a tradition of open access, is wary of making provision expressly for any particular segment of the public, and hence many of its practitioners are opposed to anything which suggests to them that education is endorsing the separateness or reinforcing the segregation of the elderly. On the other hand, most of FREE's individual members are adult educators who have extended their institutions into this field of work. Interesting questions arise: which branch of the formal sector is most apt to develop this work? What are the comparative advantages and disadvantages of development through the different branches?

The non-formal sector

A mass of activity in the non-formal sector could be represented by two contrasting endeavours; broadcasters addressing a national audience of around half a million older people at a time, and a field agency working with small groups of elderly adults in a particular locality. Broadcasters in Britain have been the vehicle promoting interest in education about ageing and for the elderly. As long ago as 1965, the BBC produced *Forward to Retirement* and in 1967 ABC Television Ltd commissioned a series and an accompanying paperback, *The Middle Years*, a subject at that time of little interest to social scientists (but see Fogarty, 1975). There have been several such series on all channels since. When Channel 4 was created, with a remit to cater for minority groups, it decided to include older viewers as one of these groups. *Years Ahead* began transmission in November 1982, a magazine programme seeking to entertain, inform, advise and educate older viewers and those interested in the well-being of older people. One evaluation of the series concludes with these words:

> The great attraction and the great strength of *Years Ahead* lie in its responsiveness and its capacity for change. It has sometimes been patronising to its viewers and it has often lacked humour.... It has produced items which have been breathtakingly beautiful to look at and profoundly moving in their content; and others which have so painfully missed their mark that one has viewed them with mounting disbelief. Getting lost is the price it occasionally pays for breaking new ground; yet ... there is ample evidence ... that in the daily lives of a considerable number of elderly people it plays an important and valued role.
>
> (Willcocks, 1984)

Pensioners Link started neighbourhood-based health education courses for older people in the outer London Borough of Barnet in 1981. These courses were planned in co-operation with pensioners themselves, as well as health visitors, community workers from the local authority, the Community Health Council and voluntary organisations. They were motivated by the knowledge that being and staying healthy is of crucial concern to pensioners. On the one hand, they are probably the largest 'consumer' group of both hospital and community based health provision, yet on the other they are generally less informed than other age groups about their health, less aware of their rights and more intimidated by the health service. As part of Age Well, a joint campaign by the Health Education Council and Age Concern, these courses were evaluated by participants (elders, co-ordinators and speakers). They reached some hundreds of pensioners, nearly 200 of whom took part in the evaluation survey. It concluded, 'A snapshot portrait of a regular participant would show a woman, over 70 years of age, who lives alone in rented accommodation. She would have left school at 14 and would probably describe herself as working class.' (Meade, n.d.).

THE BRITISH SCENE ASSESSED

What has been called, by Jones (1986) and others, 'the liberation of the elders', could have immense value throughout the world for older people, and for educational systems and societies. The movement in Britain has achieved enough during ten years to give a sense of this potential and a sense of its values, even though the scale and impact has so far been modest. Adult education is an amorphous and variously defined field, but evidence from the early 1980s of low late-age participation rates has only been confirmed by recent enquiries (Abrams, 1980; Midwinter, 1982). A survey of attendances at courses during 1977–80 showed that 27 per cent of the enrolment were aged under 25 years, 44 per cent were aged 25–44 years, 23 per cent 45–64 years and only seven per cent aged 65 years or more (Advisory Council for Adult and Continuing Education, 1982). The reasons for this massive non-participation by older people have been closely examined (Glendenning, 1980; Midwinter, 1982).

The experience of the past ten years in Britain indicates that older people gain from the recognition that: growth is still possible, at any age, and that the delights, rewards and satisfactions, as well as the pains and frustrations, of learning can be available to everyone; being a mature student or a purposive learner is a role with dignity and status; and the creation of voluntary organisations provides a range of worthwhile occupations. Nearly one in ten of the 1000 members of the University of the Third Age in London, for example, find outlets for their creative and administrative talents in leading the study groups, running the office, and staffing the numerous committees.

Education can be valuable in the reconstruction of old age, and in enabling older people to play their full part in the humane development of society. Education itself stands to gain in the process through the intervention of mature people, whose motives are usually less instrumental than those of younger students. They have resources of knowledge and experience to share with younger people, and bring many educational communities into better balance by creating settings in which different generations may meet on common ground.

Society at large stands to gain by rooting out the ageism which construes old people as essentially dependants, patients, or clients and a burden; by recognising older adults as a neglected resource, with time, energy, ideas, knowledge and experience which could be deployed for the common good; through education itself, new programmes of research and new forms of informed citizenship. Something like this vision has inspired much of the work of educational gerontologists in Britain, as with the vision of elders as pioneers of the post-industrial society (Jones, 1986).

All that can soberly be claimed to date is that a start has been made. The movement started relatively late in Britain compared with, say, Denmark, which in 1960 began to adapt its Folk High Schools with elders in mind. In France, a fast-moving trend began with the first Université du Troisième Age in 1972, and the United States has been developing programmes for older adults since the 1950s. Britain does not compare in terms of participation by the eligible population or the numbers of agencies involved. All too correct is the observation that, 'education for older people in Britain has ... hardly begun. Like cricket in Philadelphia, its existence is exotic rather than ubiquitous' (Norton, 1982).

The rights having been asserted and promulgated, they must now be claimed and implemented. This calls for policies and lively inaugural practice in all sectors.

> Suddenly the education of elderly people in the United Kingdom has become an important issue. A matter of months ago it scarcely seemed, in the public mind, a crucial question despite the steadfast efforts of a few selfless pioneers and activists. Now, quite abruptly in the time-scale of social policy, it is a matter of moment.
>
> (Midwinter, 1982)

The most pressing need at present is that there should be more opportunity for education in later life, but there should also be good, argued, tested, negotiated answers to the question: What is it for? It is surely right to advocate that, 'there will be a need to move beyond vagueness and imprecision in discussion about the aims and purposes of education for older adults' (Battersby, 1984). But Battersby is on weaker ground when he implies that this is a task for educators. It is too important to be left exclusively to the professionals among them. Pierre Vellas, the originator of the first Université du Troisieme Age at the University of Toulouse, set a standard for curricular innovation when he included sports and swimming in the programme as well as more conventional academic pursuits (Reeves, 1980). Education in later life, as at other stages, should relate to physical and mental well-being and health and to emotional, aesthetic, intellectual and creative growth. According to some experienced commentators, reality falls way below these noble aspirations. Midwinter writes:

> As for subject matter, a glance at the schedules of those authorities which do offer specialist courses to the elderly is not always rewarding or inspiring either in choice of theme or its treatment. At one extreme, there is a condescendingly therapeutic note about some of the crafts and physical exercise lessons on offer, and much too conscious and strained a jollity about making people healthier in mind and body. At the other extreme are those military-sounding survival courses which suggest that retirement is some kind of siege to be negotiated with fortitude ... 'cooking for one' or 'living on a reduced budget' ... One perhaps should not caricature those who are at least making an effort to fulfil what they genuinely see as an actual need, and, like so much in education, it is a matter of style. Manchester's 'car maintenance for widows' and 'cookery for widowers' were reported as being carried off with some *elan*. What is necessary is to pull off the paradoxical trick of considering the educational needs of older people without being ageist.... It has all that daunting and unpalatable flavour to which, sadly, elderly people have grown accustomed, of crumbs from the table.
>
> (Midwinter, 1982)

Among the hindrances to the development of a more positive and appropriate curriculum are the attitudes which pervade education and society. Negative and pathological stereotypes prevail: we tend to imagine that cerebral dexterity ceases at 60 or 65. Some courses in music appreciation and general studies recognise great capability but many are confined to a variety of crafts (Evans, 1985). Norton (1982) goes further: 'There is a certain ageist characteristic about these forms of provision.... Rights, technical and moral, must be recognised, clarified and publicised.' Even the enlightened ILEA has been caught in the dilemma of the extent to which elderly people should be regarded as a special needs group. In many cases, retired adults are the backbone of the normal classes in art, languages, music appreciation and crafts: they take their place on equal terms with their neighbours and, apart from reduced fees, are not treated in any special way by the Adult Education Institutes (Underwood, 1983).

> The ILEA operates Equal Opportunities and Special Needs statements, both of which relate to age. In practice, older learners have come to be seen as having special education needs. (It argues) that older learners are better served, in relation to curriculum, access and educational development, by an Equal Opportunities policy which is mediated by special needs, rather than by a strong Special Needs approach with its emphasis on losses and deficits of old age.
>
> (Cooper and Bornat, 1987)

Even this statement is marked by a degree of political caution. Cooper and Bornat go on to argue that, 'a strong Special Needs policy ... encourages a narrow perspective on what it is to grow old, which is at odds with experience and research', whereas 'a strong Equal Opportunities policy which includes disability and special needs alongside gender, race and class should help to ensure that development matches the needs and experience of individual learners'.

DIRECTIONS FOR DEVELOPMENT

To progress beyond the inadequate quantity and to improve the quality of the educational opportunities and activities in later life that have been described, at least four broad areas of reform must be achieved in Britain.

Formal agencies

Formal education authorities and institutions must be encouraged to adopt explicit and positive policies for the age group, grounded in a much fuller and informed understanding of the preferences, interests and potential of an immensely diverse and changing section of the population. Some practical steps have already been taken to facilitate this change, such as funding by the Department of Education and Science to enable the Unit for the Development of Adult and Continuing Education to prepare a handbook of guidance for local education authorities.

Informal and non-formal agencies

Their multiplication, innovation and growth in the field deserves far more support and encouragement from central and local government, the private sector and voluntary agencies. At present, the few bodies which are attempting to provide opportunities for participation are existing from hand to mouth and examples of good practice are in imminent danger of being overwhelmed by the gathering pace of the social movement.

The content and objectives of education activity

Even informal and self-help initiatives are still too heavily influenced in their activities by an inappropriate adherence to educational models derived from schooling. This stricture applies most strongly to the formal sector, in which the remaining traces of condescension towards elderly people must be challenged. As recommended by the Vienna Action Plan (United Nations Organization, 1983), the emphasis must move towards education for the development of individuals and of society. If professional educators can free themselves from simplistic views of elderly people's educational interests and capabilities, and join together with people in middle and later life for new forms of collaboration and curriculum development, the ingredients for substantial progress will be in place.

Challenging images of ageing and later life

These reforms will depend to some extent on deeper changes in society. Since ageing and its management are everyone's business, we all have to disengage from the images of ageing imbibed from stories in childhood, from our literary heritage and pervasively from our culture. The novelist Alison Lurie (through the reflections of the 54-year old scholarly heroine of *Foreign Affairs*) has expressed the conceptual deception and cultural prejudice that many of us have acquired.

> In the world of classic British fiction ... almost the entire population is under fifty, or even forty, as was true when the novel was invented. ... In most novels it is taken for granted that people over fifty are as set in their ways as elderly apple trees, and as permanently shaped and scarred by the years they have weathered. The literary convention is that nothing major can happen to them except through subtraction. They may be struck by lightning or pruned by the hand of man; they may grow weak or hollow; their sparse fruit may become misshapen, spotted or sourly

crabbed. They may endure these changes nobly or meanly. But they cannot, even under the best conditions, put out new growth or burst into lush and unexpected bloom.

(Lurie, 1985)

The development of education in later life will require in part a cultural revaluation of old age, but education will itself also make a dynamic contribution to that transformation.

REFERENCES

Abrams, M. (1980). *Education and the Elderly*, Research Perspectives on Ageing. Age Concern Research Unit, Mitcham, Surrey.

Advisory Council for Adult and Continuing Education (1982). *Adults: their Educational Experience and Needs*. Advisory Council for Adult and Continuing Education, Leicester.

Battersby, D. (1984). Education in later life: what does it mean? *Convergence: International Journal of Adult Education*, **18**, 1–2.

Benjamin, S. and Allen, I. (1967). *The Middle Years*. TV Publications Ltd, London.

Coleman, A. and Groombridge, J. (1982). *Preparation for Retirement in England and Wales*. National Institute of Adult Continuing Education, Leicester.

Cooper, M. and Bornat, J. (1987). *Combatting the Woolly Bunny: Equal Opportunity or Special Need*. Education Resource Unit for Older People, Inner London Education Authority, London.

Devereux, W.A. (1982). *Adult Education in Inner London 1870–1980*. Shepheard-Walwyn, London.

Fogarty, M. (1975). *40 to 60: How We Waste the Middle Aged*. Bedford Square Press, London.

Futerman, V. (1984). The University of the Third Age in Cambridge. In *Mutual Aid Universities*, E. Midwinter (Ed.). Croom Helm, London.

Glendenning, F. (Ed.) (1980). *Outreach Education and the Elders: Theory and Practice*. Beth Johnson Foundation and Department of Adult Education, University of Keele, Stoke-on-Trent.

Glendenning, F. (Ed.) (1985). *Educational Gerontology: International Perspectives*. Croom Helm, London.

Groombridge, B. (1960). *Education and Retirement*. National Institute of Adult Education, London.

Groombridge, B. (1983). Adult education and the education of adults. In *Education for Adults: Adult Learning and Education*, M. Tight (Ed.). Croom Helm and The Open University Press, London.

Groombridge, B. (1985). The impact of older learners in traditional systems of education: a British survey. Paper delivered at Thirteenth International Congress of Gerontology, New York.

Groombridge, B. (1987). Older students: the perceptions of educational providers in Great Britain. *Journal of Educational Gerontology*, **2**(1), 19–30.

James, D. (1985). Foreword. In *Educational Gerontology: Inernational Perspectives*, F. Glendenning (Ed.), pp. 1–3. Croom Helm, London.

Johnston, S. and Phillipson, C. (Eds) (1983) *Older Learners: The Challenge to Adult Education*. Bedford Square Press, London.

Jones, S. (Ed.) (1976). *Liberation of the Elders*. Beth Johnson Foundation and Department of Adult Education, University of Keele, Stoke-on-Trent.

Jones, S. (1982). Learning and meta-learning with special reference to education for the elders. Unpublished PhD thesis, University of London.

Jones, S. (1986). The elders, a new generation. *Ageing and Society*, **6**, 313–32.

Laslett, P. (1980). Educating our elders. *New Society*, 13 March.

Laslett, P. (1984). The education of the elderly in Britain. In *Mutual Aid Universities*, E. Midwinter (Ed.). Croom Helm, London.

Lurie, A. (1985). *Foreign Affairs.* Michael Joseph, London.

Meade, K. (n.d.). *Challenging the Myths: a Review of Pensioners' Health Courses and Talks.* Health Education Council, London.

Midwinter, E. (1982). *Age is Opportunity: Education and Older People.* Centre for Policy on Ageing, London.

Midwinter, E. (Ed.) (1984). *Mutual Aid Universities.* Croom Helm, London.

Newman, C. (1986). *Potential for Activity in Residential Homes.* Age Concern Greater London, London.

Norton, D. (1984). The University of the Third Age nationwide. In *Mutual Aid Universities*, E. Midwinter (Ed.). Croom Helm, London.

Norton, D. (1986). *FREE Directory of Educational Initiatives Involving Older Adults.* Age Concern England, Mitcham, Surrey.

Open University, Older Students Research Group (1984). Older students in The Open University. Open University, Milton Keynes.

Peterson, D.A. (1976). Educational gerontology: the state of the art. *Educational Gerontology*, **1**(1), 62.

Phillipson, C. and Strang, P. (1983). *The Impact of Pre-retirement Education: A Longitudinal Evaluation.* Department of Adult Education, University of Keele, Stoke-on-Trent.

Poulden, S. (1980). Art for the elderly in hospitals and residential care: some examples. In *Outreach Education and the Elders: Theory and Practice*, F. Glendenning (Ed.). Beth Johnson Foundation and Department of Adult Education, University of Keele, Stoke-on-Trent.

Reeves, J. (1980). The Universities of the Third Age. Unpublished Diploma in Adult Education, University of London.

Sihvola, T. (1983). Education, ageing and the quality of life. *Convergence: International Journal of Adult Education*, **18**(1–2), 58–62.

Underwood, D. (Ed.) (1983). *Joint Project Report.* Inner London Education Authority and Age Concern Greater London, London.

Unesco (1982). *Education et Personnes Agées, Contribution de l'Unesco*, Paper to the World Assembly on Ageing. Unesco, Paris.

United Nations Organization (1948). *Declaration of Human Rights.* Document A/811, United Nations Organization, New York.

United Nations Organization (1983). *Vienna International Plan of Action on Ageing.* World Assembly on Ageing, Vienna.

Willcocks, J. (1984). *Years Ahead: Broadcasting and the Educational Needs of the Elderly.* Independent Broadcasting Authority and Department of Extra-Mural Studies, University of London, London.

Anthony Warnes

Department of Geography and
Age Concern Institute of Gerontology
King's College
University of London

15 RESPONDING TO THE CHALLENGE OF AGEING

Viewed historically, it is difficult to understand why the gradual emergence in Britain of a more balanced age structure should be regarded as a 'problem of ageing'. What we have to our credit as humanists and good husbanders is a great reduction in premature death since the nineteenth century. . . . This should be a matter for satisfaction. Paradoxically, however, we are alarmed by our success. Perversely, we speak about the 'crippling' burden of old age, forgetting that the extraordinarily youthful structure of Victorian society entailed a phenomenal rate of growth in numbers and was accompanied by great losses from morbidity and mortality among children and young people. I believe that the present alarm is unjustified . . . and that unless saner views prevail, great harm may be done to the public welfare.

(Titmuss, 1955)

INTRODUCTION

The title of this chapter was adopted for the final of the public lectures with which Age Concern England and King's College, University of London, marked the inauguration early in 1986 of the Age Concern Institute of Gerontology (ACIOG). Those lectures provided the initial stimulation for this volume. Now as then, the intention is not to summarise the preceding contributions, but rather to take up some of the recurring and common themes, particularly those which have a bearing on the agenda for academic gerontology and the relationships between its priorities and social policy and practice. Gerontology is a young field of study in Britain, just at the stage of seeking both more independence from its parent disciplines in biology, medicine and sociology* and more intimate liaisons between attractive and stimulating individuals and ideas. The prospective marriage partners are seeking permanent homes, means of support and are actively debating to which goals their time and energy should be devoted and how they can be most useful within their society.

The terms 'sociology' and the 'social sciences' are commonly misrepresented and derided, particularly among those who are suspicious of critical approaches to existing social forms but also among practitioners of the natural and medical sciences. Both terms are properly given an epistemological definition, as in this chapter, which refers to 'the science or study of the origin, history and constitution of human society' (Shorter Oxford English Dictionary). In this sense, sociology studies all social forms and conditions including those which feature today in the academic disciplines of economics, political science, anthropology, human geography, demography and social psychology. For a spirited and full exposition see Runciman (1983).

The foundation of ACIOG as a multidisciplinary research institute and the gradual drawing together of a community of gerontologists within the College and from the Age Concern movement has many novel features for all the participants. The prizes of collaboration, of greater effectiveness and productivity in research or advocacy, and of mutual instruction among us, are to be reaped only after a preliminary period of learning. Different disciplinary approaches, problems and preoccupations have to be appreciated, new skills of communication learnt, and a common agenda between academics and the articulators of applied gerontology agreed. The conception and first years of ACIOG have been fascinating and instructive: this chapter will try to make good use of the perspectives that have been gained in its review of the achievements of this field of study and the tasks that it must pursue.

'Responding to the challenge of ageing' self-consciously adopts the problematic terminology which colours so much discussion of the implications of a growing elderly population with rising expectations. This is done not to support the view that accomplished or prospective ageing represents a crisis or even exceptional problems for our societies, but rather to put such interpretations under a critical and sceptical spotlight. It was argued in Chapter 5 that, in the United Kingdom and several European countries, neither the evidence from our demographic history nor a dispassionate interpretation of population projections provides much support for premonitions of crisis. The affluent western nations have already accommodated the major transition in our age structures brought about by the decline in fertility to near-replacement levels: in Europe several of the countries which have the greatest relative elderly populations, such as Sweden, Switzerland or the Federal Republic of Germany, appear to have been among the most successful in developing arrangements for their income support, effective health and social services, and in the exploration of new activities and social roles in retirement and the 'third age'. It is the less developed countries just beginning to undergo the transition that must learn how to adapt their societies to support a greater representation of elderly people and to direct towards them a reasonable share of the material, health and quality of life improvements that they experience.

Far sighted epidemiologists, demographers and biomedical researchers do see, however, the possibility of a further impetus to demographic ageing, stemming from reductions in the lethality of the most common diseases and disorders of later life rather than a further fall in fertility. These can occur whether or not there are major breakthroughs in our understanding of the biochemical and physiological bases of senescence: they are projections of the improvements in diagnosis, treatment, management and preventive practices that are already evident. Further contributions to the increase of life expectancy at the ages of 60, 70 or 80 years do seem likely from cohort effects, whereby successive birth groups, having experienced better nutrition, housing and working conditions than their predecessors, as well as a host of socioeconomic improvements, as in education and leisure, reach later life with lower susceptibilities to certain common incapacitating and lethal conditions. On the other hand, there are trends in many countries, such as the increase of drug abuse, alcoholism, or complacency concerning the virility of infectious diseases, which make real the possibility of a retrogression in mortality.

Many features of our individual futures are unpredictable and unknown: our usual response is not to worry about what we cannot know. With the future size of the elderly population, however, there is a firm basis for forecasts of numbers up to six or seven decades ahead. Our ignorance of other facets of the future leads us to believe, often against our better judgement, that it will be just like now but with greater numbers. Maybe this is the underlying explanation of the tendency to see growth as a problem and the reason why the phrase 'the challenge of ageing' strikes a chord. Political debate and action concentrates on the problems of today: it tends to leave successes alone. Its view of the elderly population is therefore dominated by the problems of the least healthy and the least advantaged: its view of the future of the elderly simplistically multiplies these problems. It is more probable that gerontologists, welfare organisations and politicians will be most concerned in 2040 with problems that we cannot now conceive. The challenge we face from ageing is hardly at all a matter of uncomfortable financial adjustments, but more to develop the social formations and institutions which promote the welfare and quality of later life. We need not to begrudge but to capitalise on the success in achieving increased life expectancy and the immense reduction in premature sickness and death that it implies.

THE GROWTH OF GERONTOLOGY

Organised observations and thought concerning senescence and the nature of old age have been evident in most literate societies (Beauvoir, 1970; Freeman, 1979). According to one modern view, among the most perceptive early contributions was that of the Admirable Doctor, Roger Bacon (c. 1214–1294), in recognising that an interaction of heredity with physical health produced increasing vulnerability over time (Hendricks and Hendricks, 1986). Three centuries later, Francis Bacon (1561–1626), in founding a new system of scientific investigation based on observation and inductive reasoning, turned his attention in The History of Life and Death to the possible causes of ageing. Concerted academic investigation of these topics perhaps began with the biometric work of the Belgian astronomer-mathematician Adolphe Quetelet (1796–1874) and of Sir Francis Galton (1822–1911). Two closely related areas of academic enquiry have emerged: firstly, gerontology has developed as a recognisable field of study within physiology, biochemistry, psychology and the social sciences, with a focus on the processes of ageing and the circumstances and needs of elderly people. Secondly, geriatric medicine has emerged as a hospital-based speciality concerned with the diagnosis and treatment of the mental and physical disorders which have a high incidence among elderly people (Barker, 1987; Andrews and Brocklehurst, 1987).

While it is mainly since the Second World War that social gerontology has developed, and to a far greater extent in the United States than elsewhere until recently, its antecedent roots extend to a diversity of social enquiries during the nineteenth century. In Britain, for example, Charles Booth and Seebohm Rowntree, pioneers of the country's tradition of empirical and applied social study, were both acutely conscious of the concentration of poverty and social isolation among elderly people. After his monumental survey of poverty in London, Booth is indeed remembered for his tireless and eventually successful campaign to establish a State weekly-paid old age benefit (Booth, 1894).

Social gerontology concentrates upon the social, economic and demographic conditions of elderly people. Like geriatric medicine, it has a strong applied bent which leads it to focus on the casualties of old age, in this case, those who are most disadvantaged or incapacitated. Clearly there is common ground: thoughtful geriatricians are keenly interested in the continuing care and support of their discharged patients and in the intricacies of the management of multidisciplinary care teams, while practical social gerontologists are often preoccupied with the financing, organisation, management and regulation of institutional accommodation for a similar group of sick or dependent elderly people.

The contemporary vanguard: gerontology in the United States
The expansion and achievement of gerontology in the United States are attested by the high standards of two long-established journals (*The Gerontologist* and the *Journal of Gerontology*), its prominent position within their universities and the quality of the research conducted in a number of Institutes of Gerontology, and the publication of the second editions of a remarkable trilogy of reflective research digests and an encyclopaedia (Binstock and Shanas, 1985; Birren and Schaie, 1985; Finch and Schneider, 1985; Maddox, 1987). The longevity and scale of gerontological research surprises tiro social gerontologists: using a liberal definition of the field, Shock (1951) listed 18 000 published items for the period 1900–1948, and his supplementary bibliography six years later added another 16 000 titles and noted that the number of journals in gerontology had increased from four in 1948 to 17 in 1957 (Anderson, 1960; Shock, 1957). So extensive has the bibliography become that a listing for the period 1954–1974 produced 50 000 entries (Birren and Clayton, 1975).

Gerontology teaching and research in the United States has recently been reviewed by Peterson (1987). Doctoral dissertations in ageing have increased from about 53 per year during 1956–1968 to around 360 per year during 1976–1982. A 1976 review found that 631 colleges and universities offered at least one credit course in gerontology, and by the early 1980s as many as 800 of the accredited institutions of higher education in the United States had ageing-related courses, at least half of which led to a gerontology credential. Peterson points out that a tabulation of this kind masks the nature of university gerontology. Many large institutions now have several relevant courses on the same campus, for example, in a gerontology centre, and in schools of social work, public administration, medicine, nursing, allied health, psychology, sociology and the humanities. The centres of teaching and research which have grown to national stature includes those at the Universities of Southern California, Duke, Michigan, Chicago, Brandeis, Washington, Wisconsin, Utah, South Florida, North Texas State, and California at San Francisco.

Only scattered and superficial information is received on this side of the Atlantic about current developments in these centres, but one interesting trend appears to be the gaining strength of the representatives of the natural sciences over those attached to social policy and welfare practice in determining their priorities. The levers assisting this shift include: the growing interest of biomedical scientists and the National Institute on Aging and other funding agencies in fundamental problems of senescence in humans; the funding which is available for research on the aetiology and management of senile dementia; the larger grants which biomedical research wins when compared to social research; and the reduced enthusiasm during the Reagan administration for public sector social programmes. Altered directions of development appear to be adding to rather than retarding the growth of institutional gerontology, and 'all indicators support the conclusion that gerontology instruction is growing very rapidly and in the near future can be expected to become a part of most liberal arts curricula as well as a scientific and professional specialisation at the graduate level in at least 30 per cent of higher educational institutions' (Peterson, 1987).

The establishment of gerontology has proceeded unevenly among other affluent nations. 'If the recognition of aging as a social problem is recent, then the recognition that it is a problem for social science is more recent still.'

Maddox and Campbell (1985) made this observation for the United States, but it is apposite for European countries. In a review and celebration of 40 years of gerontological research in The Netherlands, which began within psychology and medicine, it is stated that research started to develop during the 1950s and has undergone rapid expansion in the last ten years (Heuvel and Santvoort, 1987). Of the 52 listed centres pursuing gerontological research, 20 have primary interests in the behavioural and social sciences or social care practice. Social gerontology has become established as a component of the institutional social science research capacity of universities or of public administration in Scandinavia, West Germany, Austria and Israel in Europe. Vigorous growth has also been evident in Australia, Canada and Japan.

The recent growth of gerontology in Great Britain

Only in the last decade has Britain seen comparable increasing interest in the development and pursuit of gerontological scholarship. For many decades exceptionally able individuals, such as Alex Comfort and Peter Medawar in biology, and Peter Townsend in applied social studies, contributed books and studies that achieved remarkable scientific, scholarly and policy influence. British social gerontology's protracted infancy was most nurtured by those directly or indirectly involved in the elaboration of social policy and the improvement of social welfare practice. Its roots, in the nationally distinctive collaboration between the collectivistic State approach to social welfare which came to full fruition at the end of the Second World War, and the tradition of critical social commentaries grounded in empirical studies, are evident in Richard Titmuss' 1955 essay on 'Pensions systems and population change'. The introduction to his essay, from which the header quotation is taken, is not only a splendid lambasteing of attitudes which we still have not buried, but reveals in his stated objective, 'to discuss certain aspects of social provision for old age', the strengths and also the bounds of most social gerontology in Britain until the 1970s.

During the last decade, gerontology courses within social studies degrees have been successfully established at The Open University and at several universities and polytechnics. Extra-mural certificates and diplomas now are taught in London and Birmingham. The first Masters in Science courses in gerontology will begin in 1988 at King's College London and the University of Keele and others are planned at the Universities of Manchester and Liverpool and at The Open University. There have been comparable developments in postgraduate training opportunities in geriatric medicine, the broadening scope of which is indicated by the spreading adoption of the phrase 'Health Care of the Elderly' to describe the medical departments responsible for these courses.

There have also been institutional developments in research, with the early specialised centres growing first from the voluntary bodies concerned with the welfare of elderly people. One great impetus came during the Second World War with the disruption to elderly people's lives from the dispersal of families, and with their vulnerability to accidents during blackouts and in disorganised, blitzed urban areas. Local old people's welfare committees in 1941 spawned the National Committee on Old People's Welfare, which has subsequently evolved into more than a thousand local Age Concern groups under the co-ordinating body Age Concern England (Coleman, 1975). A parallel development in 1943 was the creation of The Nuffield Foundation with a budget of £10 million, much of which was devoted to the care of old people. The National Corporation for the Care of Old People (NCCOP) grew out of the Foundation in 1947 and over the next 30 years it evolved important roles in information gathering, research, publications and the development of the only specialised library in social gerontology in the country. In 1980 NCCOP changed its name to the Centre for Policy on Ageing, and subsequently it has developed its contributions to policy-related research and publication.

During the late 1970s Age Concern England (ACE) established a research unit with Mark Abrams as the first Director. This rapidly established a reputation for publishing valuable thematic reviews of the circumstances of elderly people in Britain and innovative social research (Abrams, 1978; 1980; Age Concern England, 1977–; Barker, 1984). Chapter 9 of this volume gives a good account of the productive alignment within ACE of motivations to encourage more vigorous and effective social policies, improved professional training and practice, and more incisive applied research. The involvement of the Age Concern Research Unit with psychogeriatricians and local authority social service departments in service development for mentally frail elderly people living in the community has been particularly productive. It is from this substantial base, and from complementary gerontological interests within King's College in the life sciences, medicine, nursing studies, law, education, demography, geography and social policy, that in January 1986 was formed the Age Concern Institute of Gerontology as a research and teaching unit within the College.

Other research units have been developed by enthusiastic individuals and groups. One of the earliest and most distinctive is the Centre for Environmental and Social Studies in Ageing, formed within the Polytechnic of North London by Leonie Kellaher, Sheila Peace, and Diane Willcocks. Another active group is found at the University of Keele, where long-standing interests in adult education have combined productively with critical and structuralist research in the field of social policy. In 1988, the University created a Centre for Social Gerontology under the direction of Chris Phillipson who has been appointed to the first chair ascribed to social gerontology. Among several attempts to establish disciplinary-based gerontology centres within British universities, pioneers included a biological unit at Hull, the Rank-Xerox Unit on Ageing created by Peter Laslett within the Economic and Social Research Council group on the History of Ageing at Cambridge, and a social policy group at Exeter, but the most eclectic has been the Institute of Human Ageing at Liverpool. Founded around the expertise of Denis Bromley in social psychology and in psychogeriatrics of John Copeland, and after a lengthy period of consolidation, the Institute is now broadening its disciplinary interests and research. During the 1980s, new university units with gerontological objectives include the Centre for Applied Gerontology at Birmingham, a Research Unit for the Care of the Elderly at Bath, and a nascent social and anthropological grouping at Bangor, North Wales.

There have been significant concentrations of gerontological expertise in other universities. It is likely that the new centres are encouraging at least some further groupings of previously autonomous but proximate interests. One of the most substantial concentrations of gerontological research capacity, for example, has grown up in the University of Manchester. It possesses a Giegy Unit in Geriatric Medicine, an Age and Cognitive Performance Unit directed by Patrick Rabbitt, and gerontological interests in academic nursing, primary health care and the Hester Adrian Research Centre (which has specialised in disability). The first British academic journal in social gerontology, *Ageing and Society*, is now in its eighth volume and has established a high scholarly standard and a noted role in widening the subject's debates.

THE AGENDA FOR GERONTOLOGY

Tasks in understanding

A theme common to many branches of gerontology is the extent to which it is logically and concretely possible to differentiate the pathological effects and correlates of long life from the manifestations of normal ageing. As Richard Adelman, Director of the Institute of Gerontology in the University of Michigan, concisely expressed the difficulty during the inaugural lectures, 'much that is ascribed to ageing is in fact the manifestation of disease, inappropriate life style or incompetent social policy'. All contributors to the public lectures and to this book probably agree that there is a significant avoidable fraction in today's levels of incidence, severity, discomfort and incapacity which arise from diseases and ill-health in later life.

Some commentators emphasise the weaknesses in contemporary medical and social care practice, such as the low priority which has been given to health education and preventive measures, or the similarly neglected problems on hospital discharge of liaison with community physicians, nursing and social welfare services in the long-term management of treatment. Others stress the proportions of ill-health and mortality which they attribute to damaging behaviours, from alcohol abuse and smoking to physical inactivity and non-optimal nutrition. A related view, expressed in Chapter 4, is that too many elderly people are prematurely resigned to sensory declines or ill-health, in contrast to the health educator's maxim that health is improvable at any age. A third line of argument points to the material disadvantage of large fractions of the elderly population, even among the richest nations. Late-age mortality rates correlate inversely and strongly with income and social class, and there are differentials by marital status and among the regions of Britain (Townsend and Davidson, 1982; Whitehead, 1987). A specific hypothesis of this topic is that the excess mortality in Britain during exceptionally cold weather is produced by a lethal interaction between economic disadvantage, the passive acceptance of privation and discomfort, and an ignorance of physiology. This problem, illustrative of many others, can only be ameliorated or removed by a consortium of scientific, educational, and policy reform efforts (Wicks, 1978).

A consensus belief in the avoidability of some proportion of the disorders and discomforts of later life is not matched by a consensus agenda for their removal. Two interrelated tasks face gerontologists before this could be agreed. Firstly, there are problems of understanding which require concerted and systematic investigation. Until we understand the molecular and genetic basis of ageing, how can we assess the extent to which age-related decrements in organ function result from these processes or from misuse, abuse or neglect? What are the risk factors for senile dementia; how can it be diagnosed at an early stage; and can the conditions be managed more effectively? What kinds of exercise, if any, improve morbidity and mortality? What kinds of preventive health measures are operational, affordable and effective? What are the causal connections between a person's socioeconomic position and his or her susceptibilities to disease and disorders?

Improved or changed understanding should lead to better policies, professional practice and everyday habits. The second category of problems for gerontology therefore begin with the implementation of knowledge; in this, the experience of a body like Age Concern, and its network of interested organisations and individuals throughout the country, are of exceptional value. The task includes discovering how today's elderly population, and that of future decades, can most benefit from existing but unapplied knowledge and from further advances. How does new knowledge translate to changed medical and care practice? How do we best educate and train professionals to adopt changed practices? What form and content of health education programmes are most likely to influence the behaviour of people?

The biomedical, epidemiological and actuarial problems involved in predicting the future course of late age mortality and average life expectancy are clearly relevant to the prevalence of ill-health at different ages. A key issue for public policy and medical and social care practice is the ratio between unhealthy and healthy years in any increment of life expectancy. These matters raise a problem fundamental to any positivist investigation: how do we observe and measure our subject? At the present time, data on the health status of the population is extremely sparse in most western countries, and we are particularly deprived in Britain. A recent study of health changes among the oldest old in the United States was able to draw on: (a) national cause-specific mortality data; (b) morbidity and disability data from the Duke University longitudinal study on ageing (although this refers to only 267 persons with a mean age of entry of 71.3 years); (c) data from a 1982 National Long-Term Care Survey on functional disabilities in the elderly (65+ years) non-institutionalised population; and (d) repeated National Nursing Home Surveys which included the health characteristics of the residents (Manton and Soldo, 1985). In this and other studies, great ingenuity is deployed to bring together informative statistics on health variations in populations, but our efforts in understanding will be hampered as long as we have to rely on such partial and indirect records and as long as the skill of the researcher is so consumed with data assembly and transformation.

It is a sad paradox that the best information on the health of the population in most western countries comes from statistics on deaths, with lesser contributions from morbidity data on the prevalence of diagnosed diseases. Cross-sectional surveys through the entire, healthy and unhealthy, population are normally either local and unrepresentative or superficial, relying often on self-rated and unstable indicators. Only a few longitudinal studies have been established at several centres in the United States and Europe. While most of these are local, small scale, based on unrepresentative populations, and concerned principally with physiological and cognitive measures, the productivity of the findings and insights from the best enquiries, as in Baltimore, Duke, Bonn and Göteborg, demonstrates their enormous potential (Table 15.1). Only shorter-term longitudinal studies have yet been reported in Britain. Mark Abrams' (1980) survey of elderly people aged 70 years or more living in four towns of England remains the only example with strong socioeconomic content: most of the pioneers repeat the preoccupations of the USA and European studies and are particularly favoured by cognitive psychologists for their studies of changes in mental functioning with age (Davidson et al., 1987; Rabbitt, 1982).

No country has a standing, nationally representative longitudinal study. The reason is that both clinical surveys and the management of nationwide, repeated, follow-up social surveys are extremely expensive, and despite vigorous advocacy for them, the required scale of funding implies substantial government or foundation support and has nowhere been forthcoming. In Britain there is, however, the possibility of converting a survey of the health, educational histories, employment, marriage and reproduction of a national random sample of children born in a few weeks of 1947 into a study of human development and change throughout the life course (Wadsworth, 1986).

There have been several recent developments in British health data.

Table 15.1 The principal longitudinal studies on ageing in the United States and continental Europe. This table has been constructed from several entries in Maddox (1987), viz. Baltimore Longitudinal Study (N. W. Shock), Duke Longitudinal Studies (E. B. Palmore), Longitudinal Studies Europe (U. M. Lehr), National Institute of Mental Health Human Aging Study (R. N. Butler), and Normative Aging Study (D. J. Ekerdt). Specific studies are referenced.

Name	Duration	Characteristics of sample	Sample size	Sampling method	Principal topics
Baltimore (Shock et al., 1984)	1958–	Men Women living alone	598 335	Referral	Biomedical, clinical, physiological, psychosocial
Duke I	1955–76	Aged 60–90 in 1955 Eleven examinations	271	Selected volunteers	''
Duke II	1968–76	Aged 46–70 in 1968 Four examinations	502	Probability from health insured group	''
Duke III (Busse and Maddox, 1985)	1972–	Aged 65+ in 1972 Survivors in 1980	1 000 300	Representative community survey	Complete physical, mental and social examination
Seattle (Schaie, 1983)	?1962–83	Local people			Psychometrics
Retirement History Survey (Institute on Aging, 1984)	1969–79	Aged 58–63 in 1969 Men Women living alone	11 153 8 132 3 021	Representative of USA, recent retirees	Living arrangements Employment history Widowhood
National Institute of Mental Health (Birren et al., 1963)	1955–66	Aged 65–92 in 1955			Physiological, mental health, personality

Study	Period	Birth/age	N	Sample	Measures
Normative Aging (Bossé et al., 1984)	1963–	Men born 1884–1945 Healthy on entry Bias to high status	2 280	Boston, live in community	Biomedical, clinical, ophthalmological, audiological, social network
Basle (Gsell, 1968)	1955–65	In age groups 13–22, 31–39, 45–59 in 1955	100	Employees of company	Biomedical, physiological
Netherlands (Van Zonnenfeld, 1981)	1954–74	Age 65–100 in 1954	3 174	Nationally representative	Psychosocial, cognitive
Göteborg I	1969–	Age 70 in 1969 Repeats in 76, 79, 81		Göteborg, live in community	Clinical, psychological
Göteborg II (Svanborg, 1988)	1976/7–	Women aged 70 in 1976/77		"	"
Budapest (Lengyel, 1979)	1965–80	Age 60–75 in 1965	215	Budapest	Health status
Kiev (Mankowsky and Mints, 1979)	1973–				Physiological, clinical
Bonn (Thomae, 1984)	1965–	Age 65–70 in 1965 Age 55–60 in 1965		Bonn	Physiological, social, psychological
Jerusalem (Shanan, 1985)	1973–83	Age 48–73 in 1973?	134	Urban	Coping behaviour

Collations and analyses of data from general practitioners have been tried (Royal College of General Practitioners, 1982). Successive General Household Surveys have included since 1976 questions on self-rated measures of health. These have showed a rising trend of the percentage of the population reporting illness, but there must be a strong possibility that this is an artefactual effect. The large sample size and national representativeness of the GHS does permit, however, valuable cross-sectional analyses (Arber, 1987). One of the most innovative developments in British official statistics in recent years has been the linking of a one per cent sample of records from the 1971 national census with information for the survivors at the time of the 1981 census and with any intervening registered vital events. The Office of Population Censuses and Surveys (OPCS) Longitudinal Study (LS) enables mortality to be analysed in relation to the full range of census variates (Fox and Goldblatt, 1982). The limitations of mortality as a surrogate for health remain for the LS but it provides many other analytical opportunities, as Chapter 8 in this book demonstrates.

Local statutory and voluntary health advisory groups are now producing a spate of health surveys for local areas. Examples of such sources and the uses to which they can be put are explored by Whitehead (1987), who comments, 'the development of ways of measuring health has not kept pace with theory'. While traditional mortality and morbidity statistics still predominate, there have been concerted attempts to develop and use quality of life measures like the Nottingham Health Profile, which provides a subjective indicator of the experience of illness in the community (Hunt and McEwen, 1980; Macintyre, 1986).

The weakness of the subject's observational base reveals the youth of gerontology. It may be that the colour of the debate and concern with the implications of ageing can be attributed to our dependence on cross-sectional studies and understanding. If we could document more fully the differences between people of a given senior age in 1920, 1950 and 1980, then there would be fewer worthless speculations about the circumstances and service demands of people at the same age in 2010 or 2040. Directions of change, positive and some negative, would be documented, and a better founded debate could proceed on their trajectories. Academic gerontologists and those who seek to promote the welfare and interests of older people therefore recognise a common interest in stimulating longitudinal studies: it is not fanciful to say that if we are to respond to the challenge of ageing, this is where we must start.

Understanding and improving the daily lives of elderly people

There are equally formidable problems, and data deficiencies, in the study of the sociology of the life course and of later life. Modern societies are characterised by change. Neither the shared experiences, nor the variations among those born in any one decade, will be a complete guide to the life courses of those born in succeeding years (Hagestad and Neugarten, 1985). Social scientists have recently decried the lack of attention to 'normal ageing'. It is probably true that social gerontology's early focus on the deficiencies of residential, hospital and domiciliary services for frail and disadvantaged elderly people, however justifiable in humanitarian or policy terms, fostered an image among politicians and bureaucrats of later life (among the masses, if not prospectively for themselves) as problematic and distressful. Studies of non-pathological ageing would produce a deeper understanding of the lives, attitudes, contributions to society, and aspirations of healthy, independent and socially integrated elderly people; antecedent factors would be explicated, perhaps enabling their diffusion (Bossé *et al.*, 1984). But given the hetero-geneity of human populations, and the strong changes in successive cohorts' experiences and opportunities, statistical normality is difficult to recognise in logic or in practice.

Social studies of the circumstances of elderly people, and particularly those which have applied intent, have also to accommodate to the epistemological phenomenon that their enquiries alter their subjects. This is a particularly acute difficulty in panel research, for the members can hardly avoid detecting the investigators' approved models of behaviour. The formal effect, that no representation is independent of the observer, is part of the Einsteinian paradigm of the natural sciences, and is partly found in biomedical research as the placebo response. In social research, however, the effect is less often a nicety and its presence is more variable and unpredictable.

Another and similar difficulty in social investigations, blurring the distinc-tion between neutral study and the promotion of change, is that most novel but well-grounded critical expositions upon existing social forms or institutions, lead to changes in policy, practice and present trends. A simple domestic example is that the discovery of an association between the high consumption of milk products and heart disease stimulates a decline in consumption. An indecently hasty political response arose in Britain during an unusually cold spell in February 1987: wide publicity of the association between low room temperatures and the country's excess winter deaths, together with dramatic newspaper accounts of individual elderly people unable for financial reasons to heat adequately their homes, stimulated an overnight relaxation of the criteria for paying exceptional heating benefits. This issue illustrates well a feature common to many in applied gerontology: the attendant problems will only be ameliorated or removed through a consortium of efforts by clinicians, researchers in the life sciences, critical studies of social policy, and well-informed and skilful advocacy. It is therefore particularly apposite that, in the formalisation of a substantial multidisciplinary research and teaching group in a British university, the Age Concern Institute of Gerontology will have access to the complementary and practice-orientated experience of our titular volun-tary body.

To list the aspects of later life about which we have little more than rudimentary knowledge would be a lengthy exercise, despite the vast growth of social gerontological research and writing during the last two decades. The strengths of British social gerontology have been, firstly, in critical appraisals of social welfare policy and practice, as exemplified a quarter of a century ago by Peter Townsend's influential attack in *The Last Refuge* (1962) on the unneces-sarily insensitive and inhumane practices within residential homes, now categorised throughout the English-speaking world by the term 'institutional-isation'. Another strength is in constructive and imaginative approaches to aspects of social administration, as with the multiple studies in progress of the implementation of domiciliary support services for mentally or physically frail elderly people. Among the most substantial of these endeavours has been that conducted at the University of Kent with the co-operation of that county's Social Services Department (Davies and Challis, 1987).

Following Townsend's own shift from concrete and specific forms of social administrative practice, leading spirits in a younger generation have developed a distinctive contribution to social gerontology in the form of structuralist or politico-economic analyses and theory concerning the goals and forms of current social policies towards older people (Phillipson, 1982; Phillipson and Walker, 1986; Townsend, 1981; Walker, 1981). Cognitive psychologists and psychogeriatricians have contributed one further corpus of excellent and innovative work in British gerontology, incidentally doing more than other disciplinary groups to establish bridges between both social and biological researchers and the path-breaking field of geriatric medicine. More specialised strengths are in adult and third-age educational theory and practice, the social and humane dimensions of geriatric nursing, the social history of old age, environmental and geographical studies of elderly people's situations, and in epidemiology and historical demography.

On the other hand, there are substantial areas of relative neglect, which can be identified by comparing British social and behavioural work with the range of chapter topics in the second edition of Binstock and Shanas' (1985) state-of-the-art handbook. Perhaps the broadest relative weakness is in the attention given to the micro- and meso-scale social forms of friendship, interpersonal relations, family and household structures, social differentials in later life, voluntary associations and ethnic, religious and cultural variations. In recent decades, British sociology has looked to European theorists more than American positivists for its inspiration: a consequence appears to be the dearth of studies in the sociology of non-pathological (rather than normal) old age. A conspicuous gap is in the economics of ageing. Apart from commentaries on pensions funding, largely from the perspective of macroeconomic management, few British economists have taken any interest in the subject. Other gaps in Britain are in the more specialised studies of the spiritual response to human senescence and mortality, thanatology, and, somewhat in contrast, electoral behaviour.

Some aspects of old age lives are changing so rapidly that it is difficult to envisage that the quest for better understanding will ever be satiated. Among the topics which are attracting research but with insufficient resources are: the dynamics of household formation and trends among elderly people; the changing nature of familial, intergenerational and friendship relationships and of people's largely unexpressed reciprocal expectations; the implications of the rapid increase of per capita assets (and of inherited wealth) among those reaching old age on their expectations, activities and expenditure patterns; and the consequences of the higher rates of divorce, remarriage and of less durable sexual unions since 1950 on the prospective social networks, relationships and integration of elderly people. All these involve factors which are likely to transform the circumstances of elderly people in the affluent nations of the world in the next years and decades (Warnes, 1988).

The impossibility of a clear distinction between academic study and a programme for change within the social sciences is most evident in the field of social administration. This subject faces another daunting agenda in Britain at the end of the 1980s. From 1945, if not the late 1930s, a universal eligibility model was adopted, with the State taking the dominant role in administration, for the development of enhanced pensions, income supplements to raise every elderly person above a minimum subsistence level, and to create access to health, residential and domiciliary social services without income barriers. It appeared to be reinforced during the mid-1970s by a cross-party consensus for a national uprated, earnings related retirement pensions scheme (SERPS), still under the management of central government, but even then the stresses involved in the expansion, financing and effective management of the burgeoning health and social services were evident. Successive Conservative administrations have made plain their antipathy to state, socialist, and universalist approaches. They have weakened SERPS, encouraged private sector provision in residential, nursing and health care, and, most recently, provoked a radical re-examination of the principles and financing of the National Health Service.

The principal elements of the Conservatives' preferred arrangements are vociferously expressed; that individuals should take more responsibility for their own and their families' welfare throughout the life course, that those who have greater income should be encouraged to purchase services of superior quality, and that there should be a reallocation of responsibilities from the statutory to the voluntary and, particularly, the private sectors. However, it is not clear to what extent, or in which fields of policy, the present administration believes that its duty is to provide no more than a safety net for the most disadvantaged casualties of society; or to what extent it accepts the evidence from our neighbouring European nations, that it is efficient, consistent with the views and aspirations of the majority of the population, and promotes social cohesion for the state to retain a much larger role.

Whether one focuses on the implementation of 'community care' policies as a preferred alternative to long-term institutional care, or on the financing of acute medical treatments and chronic illness care, or again on how to encourage individuals to do more to invest for their last decades; the suspicion insistently recurs that the government is acting not from a well grounded view of the circumstances and conditions of old age that it wishes to promote, but more from quite separate motives, to reduce public expenditure and the compass of the government's role. They cannot, however, be entirely condemned as mere ideologues or as duplicitous: neither the political parties of the centre and the left, nor even many gerontologists, have elaborated their positive views. Speculations concerning the evolution of life in old age are rare and no more than exploratory (Gutmann, 1987; Hobman, 1978; Laslett, 1987; Silverman, 1988). Few have given detailed consideration to the ideal bases and extent of social differentials that we should seek for the later, economically-inactive ages, a serious omission when our societies give prime position to work as a source of income and status (Midwinter, 1985; Streib, 1985).

Truly the scientific, scholarly, advocacy and governmental agendas are large. The 'challenge of ageing' is not, however, how to cope with increasing numbers – it is much more to do with the management of the population's changing preferences, expectations and needs. If the 'challenge' is daunting, that is mainly because of our present ignorance. A collaborative effort is now being constructed, to increase our understanding of ageing and the changing nature of elderly people's lives, to translate this understanding into more rigorous descriptions of both present trends and forecasts, and to debate and to determine the changes in public policy and the conduct of our economic and social affairs that are most likely to bring advantage. Inequalities arising from the haphazard incidence of illness (during working ages or in old age), of parent and caring roles, of bereavement in old age, or of exceptionally long life, need to be better described and subject to the critical attention of social philosophy and political manifestos. None of this is in any way exceptional for either the academic or the political enterprises, nor is there any reason for believing that our ability to sustain improvements in the health and welfare of elderly people has lessened. It is to be hoped that the alarmist opinions and the vocabularies fit for intractable problems have had their day. They will at least have served one useful function, if, as seems likely, they have had some part in the recent expansions and innovations in the field of gerontology in Britain.

REFERENCES

Abrams, M. (1978). *Beyond Three Score and Ten: A First Report on a Survey of the Elderly.* Age Concern England, Mitcham, Surrey.

Abrams, M. (1980). *Beyond Three Score and Ten: A Second Report on a Survey of the Elderly.* Age Concern England, Mitcham, Surrey.

Age Concern England (1977–). *Profiles of the Elderly.* Age Concern England, Mitcham, Surrey.

Anderson, J.E. (1960). Research on aging. In *Aging in Western Societies,* E.W. Burgess (Ed.), pp. 354–76. University of Chicago Press, Chicago.

Andrews, K. and Brocklehurst, J.C. (1987). *British Geriatric Medicine in the 1980s.* King Edward VII's Hospital Fund, London.

Arber, S. (1987). Gender and class inequalities in health: understanding the differentials. In *Inequalities in Health Within Europe,* A.J. Fox (Ed.). Gower, Aldershot, Hampshire.

Barker, J. (1984). *Black and Asian Old People in England,* Research Perspectives on the Elderly. Age Concern England, Mitcham, Surrey.

Barker, W.H. (1987). *Adding Life to Years.* Johns Hopkins University Press, Baltimore.

Beauvoir, S. de (1970). *La Vieillesse.* Gallimard, Paris. Translated as *Old Age,* Deutsch, London, 1972.

Binstock, R.H. and Shanas, E. (Eds) (1985). *Handbook of Aging and the Social Sciences,* 2nd edition. Van Nostrand Reinhold, New York.

Birren, J.E. and Clayton, V. (1975). History of gerontology. In *Aging: Scientific Perspectives and Social Issues,* D.S. Woodruff and J.E. Birren (Eds), pp. 15–27. Van Nostrand Reinhold, New York.

Birren, J.E. and Schaie, K.W. (Eds) (1985). *Handbook of the Psychology of Aging,* 2nd edition. Van Nostrand Reinhold, New York.

Birren, J.E., Butler, R.N., Greenhouse, S.W., Sokoloff, L. and Yarrow, M.R. (1963). *Human Aging: A Biological and Behavioral Study,* PHS 986. United States Government Printing Office, Washington D.C.

Booth, C. (1894). *The Aged Poor in England and Wales.* Macmillan, London.

Bossé, R., Ekerdt, D.J. and Silbert, J.E. (1984). The Veterans Administration Normative Aging Study. In *Handbook of Longitudinal Research,* S.A. Mednick, M. Harway and K.M. Finello (Eds), pp. 273–89. Praeger, New York.

Busse, E.W. and Maddox, G. (1985). *The Duke Longitudinal Studies of Normal Ageing: 1955–1980.* Springer Publishing Co., New York; E. Palmore (Ed.) (1981). *Social Patterns in Normal Aging: Findings From the Duke Longitudinal Study.* Duke University Press, Durham, North Carolina.

Coleman, P.G. (1975). Social gerontology in England, Scotland and Wales: a review of recent research. *The Gerontologist,* **15,** 219–29.

Davidson, I.A., Copeland, J.R.M., Dewey, M.E. *et al.* (1987). The Liverpool study of continuing health in the community: progress with the year three survey. In *Social Gerontology: New Directions,* S. di Gregorio (Ed.), pp. 224–31. Croom Helm, London.

Davies, B.P. and Challis, D. (1987). *Matching Resources to Needs in Community Care.* Gower, Aldershot, Hampshire.

Finch, C.E. and Schneider, E.L. (Eds) (1985). *Handbook of the Biology of Aging,* 2nd edition. Van Nostrand Reinhold, New York.

Fox, A.J. and Goldblatt, P.O. (1982). *Socio-Demographic Mortality Differentials: Longitudinal Study 1971–75,* Longitudinal Study Series No. 1. HMSO, London.

Freeman, J.T. (1979). *Aging: Its History and Literature.* Human Sciences Press, New York.

Gsell, O. (1968). Die Basler Studie über longitudinale Alternsforschung. In *Herzund Atmungsorgane im Alter*, R. Schubert (Ed.), pp. 16–28. Steinkopff, Darmstadt.

Gutmann, D. (1987). *Reclaimed Powers: Towards a New Psychology of Men and Women in Later Life.* Basic Books, New York.

Hagestad, G.O. and Neugarten, B.L. (1985). Age and the life course. In *Handbook of Aging and the Social Sciences*, 2nd edition, R.H. Binstock and E. Shanas (Eds), pp. 35–61. Van Nostrand Reinhold, New York.

Hendricks, J. and Hendricks, C.D. (1986). *Aging in Mass Society: Myths and Realities*, 3rd edition. Little, Brown and Co., Boston.

Heuvel, W.J.A. van den and Santvoort, M.M. van (1987). Gerontological research and science management and policy in The Netherlands. In *Forty Years of Gerontological Research in The Netherlands*, special issue, *Tijdschrift voor Gerontologie en Geriatrie*, **18**(2a), 158–64.

Hobman, D. (1978). *The Social Challenge of Ageing.* Croom Helm, London.

Hunt, S. and McEwen, J. (1980). The development of a subjective health indicator. *Sociology of Health and Illness*, **2**, 231–46.

Institute on Aging/Pacific North West Long-Term Care Center (1984). *The Social Security Administration's Retirement History Study* (compiler L.R. Hatch). University of Washington Press, Seattle.

Laslett, P. (1987). The emergence of the third age. *Ageing and Society*, **7**, 133–60.

Lengyel, E. (1979). A longitudinal study on aged people in Budapest. In *Recent Advances in Gerontology*, H. Orimo, K. Shimada, M. Iriki and D. Maeda (Eds). Excerpta Medica, Amsterdam.

Macintyre, S. (1986). Health and Illness. In *Key Variables in Social Investigation*, R. Burgess (Ed.). Routledge & Kegan Paul, London.

Maddox, G.L. (Ed.) (1987). *Encyclopedia of Aging.* Springer Publishing Co., New York.

Maddox, G.L. and Campbell, R.T. (1985). Scope, concepts and methods in the study of aging. In *Handbook of Aging and the Social Sciences*, 2nd edition, Binstock and Shanas (Eds), pp. 3–31. Van Nostrand Reinhold, New York.

Mankowsky, N.B. and Mints, A.Y. (1979). A longitudinal study of human ageing conducted at the Kiev Institute of Gerontology. In *Recent Advances in Gerontology*, H. Orimo, K. Shimada, M. Iriki and D. Maeda (Eds). Excerpta Medica, Amsterdam.

Manton, K.G. and Soldo, B.J. (1985). Dynamics of health changes in the oldest old: new perspectives and evidence. *Milbank Memorial Fund Quarterly*, **63**(2), 206–85.

Midwinter, E. (1985). *The Wage of Retirement.* Centre for Policy on Ageing, London.

Peterson, D.A. (1987). University centers and programs. In *Encyclopedia of Aging*, G.L. Maddox (Ed.), pp. 676–9. Springer Publishing Co., New York.

Phillipson, C.R. (1982). *Capitalism and the Construction of Old Age.* Macmillan, London.

Phillipson, C.R. and Walker, A. (Eds) (1986). *Ageing and Social Policy: A Critical Assessment.* Gower, Aldershot, Hampshire.

Rabbitt, P. (1982). How do old people know what to do next? In *Aging and Cognitive Processes*, F.I.M. Craik and S. Trehub (Eds), pp. 79–98. Plenum, New York.

Royal College of General Practitioners (1982). *Morbidity Statistics from General Practice 1970–71: Socio-Economic Analysis.* Office of Population Censuses and Surveys, Studies in Medical and Population Subjects 46. HMSO, London.

Runciman, W.G. (1983). *A Treatise on Social Theory.* Cambridge University Press, Cambridge.

Schaie, K.W. (Ed.) (1983). *Longitudinal Studies of Adult Psychological Development.* Guilford Press, New York.

Shanan, J. (1985). *Personality Types and Culture in Later Adulthood*, Contributions to Human Development, Vol. 12. Karger, Basel.

Shock, N.W. (1951). *A Classified Bibliography of Gerontology and Geriatrics.* Stanford University Press, Stanford, California.

Shock, N.W. (1957). *A Classified Bibliography of Gerontology and Geriatrics: Supplement 1, 1949–55.* Stanford University Press, Stanford, California.

Shock, N.W. *et al.* (1984). *Normal Human Aging: The Baltimore Longitudinal Study of Aging.* United States Government Printing Office, Washington D.C.

Silverman, P. (Ed.) (1988). *The Elderly as Modern Pioneers.* Indiana University Press, Bloomington, Indiana.

Streib, G. (1985). Social stratification and ageing. In *Handbook of Aging and the Social Sciences*, 2nd edition, R.H. Binstock and E. Shanas (Eds), pp. 339–68. Van Nostrand Reinhold, New York.

Svanborg, A. (1988). The health of the elderly population: results from longitudinal studies with age–cohort comparisons. In CIBA Foundation Symposium, *Research and the Ageing Population*, pp. 3–12. Wiley, Chichester.

Thomae, H. (1984). The Bonn longitudinal study of ageing: an approach to differential gerontology. In *Prospective Longitudinal Research*, S.A. Mednick and A.E. Baert (Eds), Oxford University Press, Oxford.

Titmuss, R.M. (1955). Pensions systems and population change. *Political Quarterly* **26**(2). Reprinted in *idem, Essays on the Welfare State*, 3rd edition (1976). Allen & Unwin, London.

Townsend, P. (1962). *The Last Refuge.* Routledge & Kegan Paul, London.

Townsend, P. (1981). The structured dependency of the elderly: the creation of social policy in the twentieth century. *Ageing and Society*, **1**(1), 5–28.

Townsend, P. and Davidson, N. (1982). *Inequalities in Health: The Black Report.* Penguin, Harmondsworth, Middlesex.

Van Zonnenfeld, R.I. (1981). Health in progressive old age. In *Prospective Longitudinal Research*, S.A. Mednick and A.E. Baert (Eds). Oxford University Press, Oxford.

Walker, A. (1981). Towards a political economy of old age. *Ageing and Society*, **1**(1), 73–94.

Wadsworth, M.E.J. (1986). Serious illness in childhood and its association with later life achievement. In *Class and Health: Research and Longitudinal Data*, R.G. Wilkinson (Ed.). Tavistock, London.

Warnes, A.M. (1988). The demography of ageing. In *Anaesthesia and the Aged Patient*, A.T. Davenport (Ed.), pp. 9–26. Blackwell Scientific Publications, Oxford.

Whitehead, M. (1987). *The Health Divide: Inequalities in Health in the 1980s.* Health Education Authority, London.

Wicks, M. (1978). *Old and Cold.* Heinemann, London.

GLOSSARY

The glossary is designed to assist the reader with terms and concepts employed in the chapters of this book. Emphasis is placed on the terms which are most pertinent to ageing and old age. Terms which have been fully explained in the text do not appear here, so the index should also be consulted. No attempt has been made to provide a comprehensive guide to chemical, biological, medical, psychological or sociological terms, for which subject dictionaries should be consulted. The following sources have been drawn upon in developing this glossary:

M. Coe (Ed.) (1985). *Oxford Illustrated Encyclopaedia: The Natural World.* Oxford University Press, Oxford.

J. Hendricks and C.D. Hendricks (1986). *Aging in Mass Society: Myths and Realities.* Little, Brown & Co., Toronto.

G.L. Maddox (Ed.) (1987). *Encyclopedia of Aging.* Springer Publishing Co., New York. Distributed in Great Britain by Edward Arnold.

E.A. Martin (Ed.) (1980). *Concise Medical Dictionary.* Transworld, London.

C.T. Onions (Ed.) (1973). *The Shorter Oxford English Dictionary.* Clarendon, Oxford.

achieved status   an achieved social position attained as a result of a person's efforts or talents. *Compare* ascription.

ageing, aging   the former is the spelling in Great Britain, the latter the spelling in the United States of America. *See* ageing effect and normal ageing.

ageing effect   a change in a characteristic such as sensory acuity or vulnerability which is either correlated with or has a causal association with increasing age. *Compare* cohort effect and period effect.

ageism   false or questionable generalisations, usually expressing negative or derogative attitudes or inferences, about elderly people or individuals with little or no basis in evidence.

Alzheimer's disease   a progressive form of dementia associated with irreversible brain syndromes, first recognised among young and middle aged adults and associated with a global impairment of cerebral function (presenile dementia), but which in recent decades has been increasingly recognised as a disorder with a high incidence in the latest years of life, hence senile dementia of Alzheimer's type (SDAT).

angioplasty   surgery to reconstruct blood vessels.

ascription   in sociology: privileges, roles and characteristics bestowed upon individuals by virtue of either their identity, for example, as grandparents, or by their membership of an identifiable group such as 'the old', for example, the age-defined entitlement to state pensions leads to the status of pensioner. False ascriptions, such as the view that elderly people have severely attenuated sexuality, are a manifestation of ageism (q.v.).

atheroma, atherosclerosis   disease of the walls of the arteries in which fatty plaques develop on their inner surfaces and predispose the development of blood clots (thrombi) with eventual obstruction of the blood flow.

avascular   bloodless.

burden   a synonym with emotive or ideological connotations for cost or expenditure, now commonly applied to the cost of income support of health care of the elderly population, and evincing a conscious or unconscious agenda to marginalise (q.v.) the age group. *See* structuralism.

centenarian   a person who has attained 100 years of age.

cerebral tumour   an abnormal growth or neoplasm in the brain.

cholinergic system   system in which transmission of nerve impulses is mediated by the neurotransmitter acetylcholine.

cohort   a group of people born in the same year or longer period who experience events at the same age and thereby share social, economic or attitudinal characteristics, for example, those born in the 1910s experienced high rates of unemployment and economic hardship in their early adult years. The distinction between cohort and period effects (q.v.) is not accepted by all investigators. Different cohorts born in successive periods, however, may all experience an historical event, the basis of the period effect, but at different ages, the basis of the cohort effect. *Compare* ageing effect and period effect.

cohort-survival projections   *See* life table.

community care   describes forms of care for the physically or mentally frail elderly (or others) which lie between hospital care and support by co-resident family at home. Its precise meaning in social and health administrative circles has changed several times during the last 50 years: at one time it referred to care and support provided in residential institutions, but it now refers to the complex of self-consciously organised voluntary, statutory and private sector support provided to frail or dependent (q.v.) elderly people living in their own homes. *See* deinstitutionalisation.

comparative statics (study)   an investigation which compares cross-sectional (q.v.) data from two or more dates or specific times. Some insights into change over time result but the method is an indirect approach to the study of growth and development and may give a misleading impression. This form of study is much less costly and demanding than a longitudinal study (q.v.).

cross-sectional study   an investigation which consists of observations made at one particular time. When used to compare individuals of different ages, it may give rise to incorrect inferences about change through time or ageing effects (q.v.) partly as a result of the existence of cohort effects (q.v.) that cannot be identified using this methodology. *Compare* longitudinal study.

cytogerontology   the study of ageing at the cellular level. *See in vitro.*

deinstitutionalisation   refers to a complex of policies in social and health administration which seek for both financial and humanitarian reasons to minimise the role of institutions in providing long-term care for the chronically ill, frail or dependent populations. *See* community care.

dementia   a chronic or persistent disorder of the mental processes due to organic brain disease. Implies predominantly irreversible conditions such as Alzheimer's disease (q.v.) but is sometimes applied to other, treatable conditions.

demographic ageing normally refers to the changing rates of fertility and mortality (q.v.) in a population which bring about a rising proportion of elderly people: rarely refers to a rise in the average age of a population.

demographic transition a summary term for the sequences of demographic changes which have lead from high mortality and fertility rates in pre-industrial societies to low mortality and fertility in late- or post-industrial societies. Characteristically the fall in mortality rates precedes the fall in fertility rates, and there are lagged adjustments to the age structure.

denaturation changes in the physiological and physical properties of proteins brought about by extremes of temperature, X-rays or chemicals.

deoxyribonucleic acid (DNA) a nucleic acid occurring principally in the nucleus of cells and forming the hereditary material of living organisms. DNA molecules comprise four nucleotides; each contains a sugar, a phosphate group and a nitrogenous base. The nucleotides form into two parallel strands held together in a double helix by chemical bonds. Replication of the DNA molecule precedes cell division so that copies occurring in the chromosomes are passed to each of the daughter cells. The sequence of nitrogenous bases acts as a code for making proteins. The code is copied on to a molecule of ribonucleic acid (RNA) and transferred from the nucleus to the cytoplasm of the cell, where the assembly of protein takes place.

dependency the condition of being more than normally dependent upon others. For individuals this may be for practical or instrumental help by relatives, informal and paid carers or for material and monetary support. For an age group such as the elderly, dependency may be in terms of a net positive transfer of money to the age group to finance health care or pensions, principally from the working age group. Dependency ratios are crudely indicated by age group ratios, for example, 60+ years/18–59 years, and more refined measures examine (a) the numbers actually in work and receiving retirement benefits, and (b) the value of transfers from one group to another. *Compare* reciprocity.

dermis the layer of 'true' skin below the epidermis or outermost layer.

digoxin a substance obtained usually from the leaves of foxglove (*Digitalis purpurea*) plants, used medicinally for its beneficial effect on the heart.

diploid describing cells, nuclei or organisms in which normally there are two sets of chromosomes. *See* genome.

disposable soma theories theories which speculate on the evolutionary mechanisms or functions of the differential between the duration of an individual's reproductive life and the somatic (whole organism) life. A recent version postulates that a higher organism which reproduces repeatedly thereby invests more energy into the creation and effectiveness of its germ cells at the expense of somatic maintenance. This makes impossible the high quality repair of somatic cells and is the basis of a finite life span (q.v.) through the progressive accumulation of damaged cells.

Down's syndrome an hereditary disorder due to a chromosome defect and characterised by a variety of physical characteristics, mental subnormality and a reduced life expectancy. The neuropathology of this condition has some features in common with those of Alzheimer's disease (q.v.) among elderly people. *See* progeroid syndromes.

elderly somewhat old; verging on old age; of or pertaining to old age. These grammatically precise adjectival usages, taken from the Oxford English Dictionary, are rarely respected in commentary on older people. The adjective has become a euphemistic synonym for old, and it is now commonly used as a noun, implying elderly or old people. The term has also acquired inconsistent and ageist (q.v.) taxonomic usages among different professionals and scholars, which confuses administrators, politicians, journalists and the general public. Geriatricians and nurses tend to apply the term to old people who are frail, sick and their patients; politicians to the age group which is eligible for state pensions and other old-age benefits; and entrepreneurs to people in the age groups susceptible to the purchases of commodities designed for retired or old people (including some aged less than 60 years). Attempts to develop a differentiating terminology have been crude and insufficiently precise, for example, very old people, those aged more than 75, 80 or 85 years, have been given the solecism 'very elderly' and the inelegant 'old-old'. A worse grammatical blunder, which uses 'the ageing' for old people, is current in North America and Australia although rare in Britain.

electroencephalology   the study of electrical impulses in the brain. Includes electroencephalography (EEG) in which impulses are detected by placing electrodes on the scalp.

endocrine   originally ductless as applied to glands of the body, now virtually synonymous with hormone. Endocrine glands include the thyroid, pituitary, ovary and testis.

endoscope   an instrument for examining the inside of a body organ.

enzyme   a protein that acts as a catalyst in a biochemical reaction by binding with the substrate (q.v.) and converting it into a product. Ribonucleic acid (RNA) (q.v.) is now considered to act as an enzyme.

epidemiology   the study of the incidence (q.v.) and prevalence (q.v.) of diseases, formerly associated particularly with infectious epidemics, but now including non-infectious conditions of which the prevalence may be related to the environment or to ways of life.

fibroblast   cells in connective tissues, those which support, bind or separate specialised tissue or organs, which are responsible for the production of many of the materials of such tissues.

free radical   unstable oxygen molecules which can attack polyunsaturated fatty acids and cross link with other molecules including proteins and DNA (q.v.). They therefore possess the potential for creating biologically abnormal molecules: this mechanism is the basis of a free radical theory of biological ageing.

gangliosides   glycolipids (q.v.) found in nerve cell membranes.

genome   the genetic component of a cell.

geriatrics, geriatric medicine, nursing or dentistry   the study and practice of medical and nursing care for elderly people. *Compare* gerontology and thanatology.

geront   Greek: old man, hence gerontocracy, government by elderly men.

gerontology   the study of old age and ageing processes. *Compare* geriatrics and thanatology.

glaucoma   a group of diseases in which pressure inside the eye increases and causes progressive damage.

glomerulus   the network of blood capillaries within the cuplike end (Bowman's capsule) of the nephron, the region of blood filtration in the kidney.

glycogenesis   the conversion of glucose into glycogen, occurring chiefly in the liver and the muscle. *See* phosphorylation.

glycolipid   a lipid (q.v.) containing a sugar molecule.

glycolysis   the conversion of glucose in the cytoplasm of cells to pyruvic acid.

household   a co-resident group normally in private dwellings. Problems of defining households arise in subdivided dwellings or in groups containing more than one sexual union or married couple. One possible index is the group that regularly shares meals or meal preparation. *Compare* living arrangement.

household head   the person who is the principal earner or decision taker in a household. Rapidly becoming obsolete with the growing symmetry of husband's and wife's economic roles and influence.

hypothalamus   a region of the third ventricle of the brain, linked with the thalamus (q.v.) and the pituitary gland.

iatrogenic   resulting from treatment by medical personnel, often used of disease or disability.

incidence rate   rate of inception or onset of a disease or disorder, often expressed in terms of sick persons or episodes per 1000 of those at risk. *Compare* prevalence rate.

infarction   the death of part or all of an organ as a result of a lack of blood.

institutions   1. In sociology, any group with a recognised or definable membership formed for a particular purpose, ranging from a card-playing circle to a multinational corporation or political organisation.   2. In gerontology and social administration, the term frequently refers to those institutions which specialise in the care and support of physically and mentally frail or socially dependent elderly people. *See* deinstitutionalisation.

in vitro   Latin: literally 'in glass', i.e. in an artificial setting. Refers to the cultivation of cells in the laboratory, as practised in cytogerontology (q.v.).

in vivo   Latin: in a living host environment. Refers to the study of cells in living tissues. *Compare in vitro* (q.v.).

levodopa (L-dopa)   drug used in the treatment of Parkinson's disease, a precursor of the deficient neurotransmitter, dopamine.

life course   used in social studies to denote the study of an individual's or a group's development and change throughout life; in gerontology with a view to enriching the understanding of a person's psychology or social situation in old age. Increasingly preferred to life span (q.v.) which is reserved for its biological and demographic meaning.

life expectancy   in demography and epidemiology, the expected duration of life of an individual, estimated by the mean age of death in a population given stated age-specific mortality rates. Life expectancy may be measured from birth (and is conventionally represented as E_0) or from any other age, for example, 65 years (E_{65}). In most contemporary societies female life expectancy exceeds that of males, particularly at older ages.

life potential   *See* life span.

life span   for an individual, the maximum or potential duration of life if entirely free of disease or accident. Because genetic variations produce considerable variations in individual life potentials, the average life span of a species or a population is the arithmetic mean of the individuals' potentials. It can rarely be estimated with great confidence. Most authors give a range of 110 to 115 years for maximum individual human life potential.

life table   a device in mathematical demography for representing fertility and mortality conditions by one- or five-year age groups in a population at a particular date. It is the basis of cohort-survival methods of projecting the size, age and sex structure of future populations.

lipids   chemical compounds in organic solvents which have nutritional importance, for example, fats and steroids.

lipofuscin   a normally brownish, autofluorescent pigment staining for fat and polysaccharides associated with ageing, most common in the cells of heart muscle, nerves and the liver.

lithium   a drug used in the treatment of manic depression, schizophrenia and similar psychiatric disorders.

living arrangement   used in social statistics and demography to refer to the dwelling type and co-resident group of a person, for example, to distinguish private households (q.v.) from groups or individuals living in institutions (q.v.).

longitudinal study   an investigation which observes phenomena through time and therefore has direct information about growth and development. *Compare* cross-sectional study and comparative statics.

lysosome   organelles or structures in the cytoplasm of every mammalian cell containing hydrolytic enzymes (q.v.) which are responsible for the controlled breaking down of substances which are either of value to the cell or unwanted.

marginalisation   the exclusion of an age or a social group from a society's normal privileges or roles. This may arise as a by-product of cultural norms or social policies with other aims or functions but is often seen as systematic and purposeful.

metabolism   collective term for all chemical reactions taking place in an organism. Includes catabolism, whereby complex substances are broken down, and anabolism, whereby new compounds are built up.

metabolite   a substance involved in metabolism (q.v.).

mentation   mental action; a state of mind.

microsomes   minute fragments of cellular material produced from heterogenous material, for example, membranes and ribosomes (q.v.), by homogenisation in a blender or centrifuge.

micturition   urination.

mitochondrion (*pl.* **mitochondria**)   organelles or structures in the cytoplasm of cells which are the principal sites of their energy production and fatty acid synthesis, and which may show significant ageing effects (q.v.) such as increased fragility, modified functional properties and changes in the physical state of their inner membranes.

morbidity   the state of being diseased, normally applied to populations rather than individuals. *See* prevalence rate.

myocardium   heart muscle.

necrosis   mortification; the death of some or all cells in an organ or tissue, caused by disease, physical or chemical insult or interference with the blood/oxygen supply.

natural (population) change or increase   the change in the size of a population brought about by the net balance of births and deaths in a defined period. Distinguished from actual change, which includes also net migration change.

need   a complex concept which expresses a level of requirement for a resource (e.g., income, care, housing, social support) which is regarded as a minimum or a right. If the level is defined by individuals or groups for themselves, the term 'perceived need' is used; if the level is defined by actual usage, the term 'expressed need' is used and is approximately equivalent to the economic concept of effective demand; and if the level of need is defined by an elite or professional group, the term 'normative need' is used.

normal ageing a concept much debated in the biology, medicine and sociology of ageing which refers less to statistical normality (the average condition) than to the absence of pathological factors such as disease. The attempt is to describe the course of a human life in the absence of severe environmental insults, so isolating either (in sociology) the characteristics and development of ageing in healthy and socially-adjusted individuals or (in biology and medicine) the physiological decrements which arise from intrinsic ageing processes. A problem with the concept is that among individuals who attain very great age, the absence of pathologies is statistically abnormal.

oestradiol the major female sex hormone produced by the ovary.

oöcyte a cell of the ovary that undergoes a distinctive form of division to form an ovum.

paradigm a set of assumptions and theoretical interpretations about phenomena which are shared by the great majority of scholars or scientists in a field; hence paradigm-shift, when there is a wholesale change in such assumptions, as occurred with the acceptance of the theory of relativity. The term has been degraded in social studies in recent decades through its application to minor concurrent differences in aims, attitudes and theoretical positions of investigators.

Parkinson's disease a disease affecting predominantly the extrapyramidal (movement co-ordinating) part of the nervous system, most commonly contracted in middle or late life, characterised by difficulty with voluntary movement, muscle rigidity and involuntary tremors.

pensionable age, pensionable population common terms to refer to the population eligible for state retirement benefits or pensions (whether they receive them or not), viz., in the United Kingdom, males aged at least 65 years and females aged at least 60 years are eligible. A confusing term, particularly useless for international comparisons.

peptide a molecule consisting of two or more amino acids linked by peptide bonds (q.v.) between the amino group and the carboxyl group.

period effect in demography and social studies, a characteristic distinctive to a cohort (q.v.) or a population born or living at a certain time, for example, the shared experience of a war or economic depression, or the memory of the death of a statesman or king. *Compare* ageing effect and cohort effect.

period (or point) prevalence *see* prevalence rate.

phosphorylation the combination of an organic molecule with a phosphate group, as in the liver and kidney where it is involved in the breakdown of the carbohydrate glycogen, or in the mitochondria where it is associated with energy retention.

pituitary gland the master endocrine gland, attached beneath the hypothalamus (q.v.) at the base of the skull.

polypeptide a molecule of three or more amino acids (e.g., proteins) linked by peptide (q.v.) bonds.

population pyramid a diagram which represents the age structure of a population, normally by representing the size of successive one- or five-year age groups with horizontal bars arranged around a vertical scale of ages, with males to one side and females to the other.

presbys   Greek: old man or elder; hence presbyopia, the decreasing power of the eye lens to change its shape and therefore to focus at or accommodate different distances (gave Latin *presbyter*, elder of the church).

prevalence rate   rate of current sickness in a population, often expressed in terms of sick persons or episodes per 1000 of those at risk, measured either at a particular time (point prevalence) or over a stated period (period prevalence). *Compare* incidence rate.

progeria, progeroid syndromes   premature ageing; rare conditions with a genetic basis that produce premature ageing, the best described being Werner's syndrome (q.v.) or progeria of the adult and Hutchinson Gilford syndrome or juvenile progeria. *Compare* Down's syndrome.

protease   proteolytic enzyme (q.v.): a digestive enzyme associated with the breakdown of protein.

psychotropic   affecting psychological function, usually applied to drugs.

racemization   change of a molecule from an optically active to an inactive form due to heat, light or chemical reagents, without changing its structure.

reciprocity   in social psychology, an approximate balance between an individual's 'giving' to another and their receipts from that person. The evaluation may in the case of strangers be for the dyad alone, over a short time and consciously material (exchange reciprocity), while among close relatives the evaluation may extend over a person's lifetime, involve several people or be seen in an intergenerational calculus (communal reciprocity).

retirement   the withdrawal from paid employment, which in western nations during this century has become virtually mandatory at a stated age for all except the self-employed. It is comparatively rare in most less developed countries. *See* pensionable age and third age.

ribonucleic acid (RNA)   nucleic acid, closely similar in structure to deoxyribonucleic acid (DNA) (q.v.) and involved in acting as the gene messenger; the structural basis of ribosomes (q.v.) and the carrier of amino acids to the ribosomes for synthesis of proteins designated by mRNA.

ribosome   a particle, consisting of RNA and protein, that occurs in cells and is the site of protein synthesis. *See* deoxyribonucleic acid.

senescence   the physiological processes or manifestations of ageing.

sequela (*pl.* **sequalae**)   any disorder or illness resulting from a preceding disease or accident.

soma   the entire body excluding germ cells.

structuralism   in social studies and the humanities, an approach to the study and interpretation of social formations which draws from the work of Marx and begins with an analysis of the principal interest groups or economic classes in a society and the manner in which social institutions confer differential advantages. Elements of structuralism have informed most recent social analysis, as in the notion of structured dependency (q.v.) without becoming a dominant paradigm (q.v.).

substrate   a structure on which others may be built or attached, for example, an enzyme substrate is the substance on which an enzyme (q.v.) acts, and DNA may be a substrate for mRNA construction.

syndrome   a complex of apparently unrelated symptoms which characterise a specified disease state.

thanatology   the study of death, its causes and phenomena.

third age   a term borrowed from the French rendering and gaining currency in

Europe especially to describe the phase of life following childhood (first age) and the period of maximum work (second age). Favoured instead of retirement (q.v.) because it does not connote the absence of a role and because it may be applied equally to men and women and to those who were not in paid employment. Hence, University of the Third Age.

Werner's syndrome a syndrome (q.v.) affecting individuals who appear normal during childhood but usually cease growth during early teenage years and who develop features of ageing during their twenties and thirties.

GUIDE TO FURTHER READING

Research papers, research monographs and textbooks in the field of gerontology are all multiplying rapidly at the present time. The following selected list of introductory and study volumes is intended as a guide to those who wish to pursue any of the themes raised in this volume, not least to those whose interests have previously been relatively confined to a small part of the subject's disciplinary spectrum. The selection has been guided by the recommendations of the authors of this book, other colleagues and recent book reviews.

ENCYCLOPAEDIA AND COMPENDIA

Binstock, R.H. and Shanas, E. (Eds) (1985). *Handbook of Aging and the Social Sciences*, 2nd edition. Van Nostrand Reinhold, New York.

Birren, J.E. and Clayton, V. (Eds) (1985). *Handbook of the Psychology of Aging*, 2nd edition. Van Nostrand Reinhold, New York.

Finch, C.E. and Schneider, E.L. (Eds) (1985). *Handbook of the Biology of Aging*, 2nd edition. Van Nostrand Reinhold, New York.

Maddox, G.L. (Ed.) (1987). *Encyclopedia of Aging.* Springer Publishing Co., New York.

BIOLOGY OF AGEING

Bittles, A.H. and Collins, K.J. (Eds) (1986). *The Biology of Human Ageing.* Cambridge University Press, Cambridge.

Comfort, A. (1982). *The Biology of Senescence*, 3rd edition. Churchill Livingstone, Edinburgh.

Strehler, B.L. (1977). *Time, Cells and Ageing*, 2nd edition. Academic Press, London.

Warner, H.R., Butler, R.N., Sprott, R.L. and Schneider, E.L. (1987). *Modern Biological Theories of Aging.* Raven, New York.

PSYCHOLOGY OF AGEING AND ELDERLY PEOPLE

Bromley, D.B. (1988). *Human Ageing.* Penguin, London.

Coleman, P.G. (1986). *Ageing and Reminiscence Processes: Social and Clinical implications.* John Wiley & Sons, Chichester.

Erikson, E.H., Erikson, J.M. and Kivnick, H.Q. (1987). *Vital Involvement in Old Age: The Experience of Old Age in Our Time.* W.W. Norton, London.

SOCIOLOGY OF AGEING AND ELDERLY PEOPLE

Fennell, G., Phillipson, C.R. and Evers, H. (1988). *The Sociology of Old Age.* Open University Press, Milton Keynes.

Hendricks, J. and Hendricks, C.D. (1986). *Aging in Mass Society: Myths and Realities*, 3rd edition. Little, Brown & Co., Boston, Massachusetts.

Phillipson, C.R. (1982). *Capitalism and the Construction of Old Age.* Macmillan, London.

Victor, C.R. (1987). *Old Age in Modern Society: A Textbook in Social Gerontology.* Croom Helm, London.

ECONOMICS OF AGEING POPULATIONS AND LATER LIFE

Clark, R.L. and Spengler, J.J. (1980). *The Economics of Individual and Population Ageing.* Cambridge University Press, Cambridge.

Schulz, J.H. (1985). *The Economics of Aging*, 2nd edition. *Wadsworth, Belmont, California.*

GEOGRAPHICAL AND ENVIRONMENTAL ASPECTS OF THE OLDER POPULATION

Altman, I., Lawton, M.P. and Wohlwill, J.F. (Eds) (1984). *Elderly People and the Environment.* Plenum, New York.

Warnes, A.M. (Ed.) (1982). *Geographical Perspectives on the Elderly.* John Wiley & Sons, Chichester.

SOCIAL AND PUBLIC POLICY RELATED TO ELDERLY PEOPLE

Fogarty, M.P. (Ed.) (1982). *Retirement Policy: The Next Fifty Years.* Heinemann, London.

Markides, K.S. and Cooper, C.L. (Eds) (1987). *Retirement in Industrial Societies.* John Wiley & Sons, Chichester.

Means, R. and Smith, R. (1985). *The Development of Welfare Services for the Elderly.* Croom Helm, London.

Phillipson, C.R. and Walker, A. (Eds) (1986). *Ageing and Social Policy: A Critical Assessment.* Gower, Aldershot.

Tinker, A. (1984). *The Elderly in Modern Society*, 2nd edition. Longman, London.

MEDICINE, NURSING AND HEALTH IN OLD AGE

Andrews, K. and Brocklehurst, J.C. (1987). *British Geriatric Medicine in the 1980s.* King Edward VII's Hospital Fund for London, London.

Brocklehurst, J.C. (Ed.). (1985). *Textbook of Geriatric Medicine and Gerontology*, 3rd edition. Churchill Livingstone, Edinburgh.

Pathy, M.S.J. (Ed.) (1985). *Principles and Practice of Geriatric Medicine.* John Wiley & Sons, Chichester.

Redfern, S.J. (Ed.) (1986). *Nursing Elderly People.* Churchill Livingstone, Edinburgh.

SUBJECT INDEX

cells   7–12, 20–6
  cultures   12
  germ   3
  population doubling level   33
  somatic   3, 15
  transformed   26
centenarians   50
Centre for Policy on Ageing   197
children, help and support from   83–95, 109
  Child Poverty Action Group   79
  childlessness   103
  child–parent relationship   86–92, 109, 173
choice, consumer   115, 150
chromosomes   6, 23, 24
chronically ill   126
'clocks', biological   3, 31
cohort differences and effects   77, 86–92,
    163–77, 193
  independence and willingness to accept
      help   109
collaboration among agencies   114
collagen   7, 15, 19, 20
communicating with elderly people   146,
    153
community care   77, 110, 114, 122, 127, 129,
    141, 205
  community health care   119–34
confusion among elderly people   151
Conservative Governments and Party   78,
    204–5
continuing care   146
control, self-   150
cross-linking of molecules   20, 25
cytology   32
cytoplasm   8

data, evidence and findings   199–201
  elderly people's need for help   86–92, 108
  health status and profiles   121, 123–5, 137
  nursing practice   147, 151
  patient behaviour and attitudes   153, 156
  social exchange and support   86–92
  see also experiments, Family Expenditure
      Survey, General Household Survey,
      Office of Population Censuses and
      Surveys
day centres   126
deamidation   17, 23
deaths
  causes of   60–1, 193
  rates   49, 59–60, 125
Declaration of Human Rights   178
  and education   178
demand for services   108, 115
dementia sufferers   112, 114
  see also Alzheimer's disease
demography, demographic ageing   47–66,
    193
  projections   73
denaturation, protein   18–19, 211
Denmark
  folk high schools   187
  nursing home care in   149
deoxyribonucleic acid (DNA)   8–13, 23–5,
    31, 35
Department of Education and Science
  Unit for the Development of Adult and
      Continuing Education   189

Department of Health and Social
    Security   148
  The Reform of Social Security 1985   73
dependants, dependency
  induced dependency hypothesis   149–50
  of individual elderly people   92, 149
  ratios   73
  structured   69–72
diabetes   42, 45
  and diet   45
diarrhoea   42
disease   45
  prevention of   128
  versus normal ageing   137
disposable soma theory   *see* theories of
    ageing
Down's syndrome   6, 24
drugs   *see* medication
dyads   86

eaters, eating   147, 151
economics   41
  cost of supporting elderly people   73, 79,
      193–4, 205
education   178–91
  attainment and experience of elderly
      people   166, 170, 174–5
  continuing and lifelong   131, 180
  curriculum   182, 188
  educational rights   180
  formal sector   181–2, 184, 189
  geriatrics or gerontology   142–3, 178, 195–
      7
  health   45–6, 128–9, 198
  informal sector   182, 184, 189
  local education authorities   184
  needs   180
  of medical students   142
  of nurses   152, 155
  Open University students, elderly people
      among   183
  stereotypes of old age   143, 183, 188
  subjects of study   184, 188
  systems   181–2
elderly people
  attitudes of   83–95, 131, 163–77
  attitudes towards   79, 83–95, 112, 147,
      183, 189, 192–4
  behaviour of   151
  communicating with   146
  employment   69
  frail   108, 112, 148
  health of   121
  help for   101, 108
  independence of   77, 102, 148
  living arrangements and social
      support   96–106
  providers of care   131
  quality of life   157, 183
electro-convulsive therapy   153
electron transport chain   31
employment   69
energy supply, in metabolism   9, 12, 29, 34
entertainment   169–70
enzymes   4, 6, 10, 17, 19, 23, 25
equal opportunities   185, 188

intervention, operative and non-
    operative   138
intimacy   84
inverse care law   97
investigations   *see* data
in vitro experiments and evidence   6, 12,
    32–5
involvement   *see* participation

Japan, ageing of   56

kin   *see* relatives
King's College London   viii, 192

Labour Governments and Party   78–9, 163,
    166, 168
learning   *see* education
leisure   169–75
lens
    crystallins   8–9, 13, 15, 20, 23, 41–3, 45
    implantation   42
less developed countries, ageing in   52, 57–8,
    193
life
    course   83–95, 199
    expectancy   12, 48–50, 59–60, 199
    quality of   75, 150, 163–77
    span   10, 12, 51
        biology and   3, 10, 29, 48
lipids   10, 23, 31
lipofuscin   11, 15
liver   8, 11, 32
living arrangements   96–106
    living alone   98, 125
living standards   75
local government authorities   129
    education authorities   184
    Inner London Education Authority   184–5,
        188
    residential homes   148
local planning   119–24
London
    elderly population profiles in
        Camberwell   125
    Inner London Education Authority   184–5,
        188
    New Survey of London Life and Labour
        1931   167
    University of the Third Age   187
longitudinal studies   5, 93, 199–201
    see also Office of Population Censuses and
        Surveys
long-stay care   146
lymphocyte   32

macrophages   25
management
    in medicine   136
    nursing homes   149
    primary health care   119
marginalisation   70
marriage, marital status   59, 100
meals and mealtimes   151
    meals-on-wheels   109
medical practice, medicine   135–45
    academic departments   142
    acute   121, 138, 146
    excessive specialisation in   121, 136

medical profession   147
    preventive   128, 139–40
    primary   119–34
    rehabilitative   121, 147
medication   151, 153
    drug therapy   138–9
membranes   31
    mitochondrial   33
menopause   7
metabolism   12
    drug   138
miscoding drug   23
mitochondria   12–13, 22–3, 29–37
    membranes and   13, 33
mobility, physical   78, 108
molecules   7–13, 15
    macromolecular synthesis   8, 13, 29
mortality   48–52, 59–61, 103, 139, 198
    basal vulnerability   49–50
motivations, of carers   111
multi-disciplinary and multisectoral
    services and planning   128, 137–8
myopia   42, 45–6

National Conference on Old Age Pensions
    (UK)   78
National Federation of Old Age Pensions
    Associations (UK)   77
National Health Service (UK)   78, 129, 140,
    168, 205
    nursing homes   148, 149
National Institute on Aging (USA)   62, 83,
    195
National Old People's Welfare Committee
    (UK)   78
National Readership Survey (UK)   165–6
National Survey of Black Americans
    (USA)   86–92
National Three Generation Family Study
    (USA)   86–92
needs
    health care   119–20
    special educational   184, 185, 188
    support   107–18
neighbours and relationships with   84, 111
nerves, nerve system   5, 13, 15
nicotinamide adenine dinucleotide
    phosphate (NADPH)   35
norms of behaviour   84
Nottingham Health Profile   124–6, 202
nucleic acid synthesis   35
nurses   146
    career choices of   152
    interpersonal communication skills of   146
    nurse–patient communication through
        touch   146
    student nurses' attitudes towards elderly
        people   152
nursing   146–59
    district   108, 116, 127, 141
    geriatric   152
    models of   127, 149
    Nursing Development Unit at Burford
        Cottage Hospital   147
    nursing homes   148, 149
nutrients   31–3
nutrition   167

AUTHOR INDEX

Page numbers in *italic* indicate Reference entries.